Integrated Systematic Nephrology

Integrated Systematic Nephrology

Fourth Edition

Edited by Desmond Yap, Tak Mao Chan, and Man Kam Chan

HKU
PRESS
香港大學出版社

Hong Kong University Press
The University of Hong Kong
Pokfulam Road
Hong Kong
https://hkupress.hku.hk

ISBN 978-988-8528-70-7 (*Paperback*)

British Library Cataloguing-in-Publication Data
A catalogue record for this book is available from the British Library.

10 9 8 7 6 5 4 3 2 1

Printed and bound by Sunshine (Caimei) Printing Co., Ltd. in Hong Kong, China

Contents

Preface to the Fourth Edition

Nephrology is often perceived as a complex specialty. The clinical practice of nephrology is intricately related to many medical disciplines, as the kidneys are often important targets of injury in various conditions. In addition, renal insufficiency not only causes complications in various organ systems, but also impacts the choice and dosing of treatments for diseases affecting other organs. The causes and mechanisms of kidney diseases are often complex and multifactorial. These attributes have rendered nephrology a challenging subject for medical undergraduates and young clinicians alike. The first and second editions of this book, written by Professor M. K. Chan, then Chief of Nephrology at the Department of Medicine of the University of Hong Kong, was an immediate success when published in 1986 and 1989 respectively as the work provided a much-welcomed comprehensive, yet succinct and systematic coverage of topics in nephrology relevant to the level required of medical students and physician trainees. The popularity of this book continued with its extensively revised and updated third edition (2006), edited by Chief of Nephrology Professor T. M. Chan with contributions from the nephrology community in Hong Kong.

The field of nephrology has witnessed many advances in knowledge and therapeutics in the fifteen years since the last edition of this book. There are new nomenclature and classification systems for acute kidney injury, chronic kidney disease, and renal parenchymal diseases. Progress in basic science and translational research has increased understanding of the molecular and mechanistic pathways of kidney diseases and expedited the clinical application of new knowledge, resulting in the advent of new treatments. The incidence and prevalence rates of various kidney diseases have also changed because of evolving demographics and socio-economic developments. In response to these changes, the current fourth edition, with Associate Professor Dr Desmond Yap as the lead editor, has been extensively revised based on the latest knowledge and evidence. New chapters or sections such as critical care nephrology, new modalities of haemodialysis, advances in kidney transplantation across immunological barriers, geriatric nephrology, palliative or supportive care, and renal rehabilitation have been added.

As in previous editions, this book aims to bridge the gap between two types of textbooks on the subject of nephrology—at one end, the sizeable multi-author textbooks with exhaustive bibliographies, and at the other, handbooks or point-form notes on selected topics. Our book is positioned as one that is manageable in depth and breadth, encompassing the entire scope of nephrology. Clinical pertinence and significance is the overarching emphasis throughout, and a practical approach has been adopted in all chapters so that the contents will prove useful to a frontline clinician. It is at a level appropriate to the clinical practice of a junior renal physician and can serve as a quick nephrology reference for a general practitioner. It is also intended for students, physician trainees, and clinicians with a keen interest in renal medicine.

This book is a concerted effort of all contributors and our publisher. The authors include not only nephrologists in various hospitals, but also specialists in different disciplines such as urology, radiology, pathology, histocompatibility, paediatrics, palliative care, obstetrics, critical care medicine, emergency medicine, haematology, clinical pharmacology, basic science, and renal nursing. We would like to thank all the authors for their support and important contributions.

Desmond Yap and Tak Mao Chan
May 2021

Preface to the Third Edition

The subspecialty of nephrology is closely associated with other medical disciplines. Acute or chronic renal failure can be a consequence of various systemic diseases, mostly immunological or metabolic, and renal impairment results in pathophysiological changes pertaining to diverse bodily functions, such as endocrine, haematological, or cardiovascular abnormalities. Worldwide, the prevalence of chronic renal failure is increasing by more than 5% annually, and the cost of renal replacement therapy has an increasing impact on health economics in both developed and developing countries. In this context, the past few decades have witnessed significant progress in the management of kidney diseases and the prevention of the dire consequence of end-stage renal failure.

Fifteen years have passed since the second edition of this book was published. The present edition is the contribution of many authors. Apart from contributing some chapters, the editors have ensured consistency in the level and the format of individual chapters. The contributors comprise most, if not all, of the leading local nephrologists, everyone writing from his or her own extensive clinical experience. The chapters have been completely re-written so as to take into account advances in this field in the past fifteen years. The emphasis is on practical clinical nephrology. While the contents are evidence-based, some of the clinical approaches and emphases are guided by experience and personal opinion.

This book, like its two previous editions, aims to bridge the gap between two types of publications on the subject of nephrology—at one end, the huge multi-author reference books with exhaustive bibliographies; and at the other, handbooks or lecture notes which are too brief or too concise. The editors' aim is to develop a textbook that is manageable in size and comprehensive in content, covering the entire field of nephrology at a level appropriate to the clinical practice of an average renal physician, but not exhaustive on the detailed pathogenetic mechanisms of individual conditions. It is intended for students, trainees preparing for membership examination, and general physicians with an interest in renal medicine.

Daniel T. M. Chan and M. K. Chan
2006

Preface to the Second Edition

The satisfaction that the first edition of this book has been well received by medical students, renal nurses and junior doctors has more than offset the pressure to keep the book up-to-date with recent advances in the field of nephrology, dialysis and renal transplantation. In this revised edition, I have maintained the concept of having a compact book which contains all the essential and clinically relevant information. Again I have written entirely from personal experience and biases are unavoidable. I have tried my best to keep the size of the book manageable. The language is precise and at times the student may, on first reading, find it difficult to comprehend the clinical significance of a particular section. I am sure a bit of patience and clinical exposure should render the meaning obvious. The original layout has been preserved. Many illustrations have been added. Most of the important recent advances have been included, albeit occasionally with only a few sentences. In particular, to render the book more useful for renal nurses and junior doctors, the sections on dialysis and renal transplantation have been considerably expanded.

The continued encouragement of my wife, Ying Wa, and of my dear friend Mr W. T. Lee, has been a prime mover behind this second edition. Dr K. W. Chan has kindly provided Figures 40, 41, 42, 44, 45, and 46. The cost of the book has also been kept within reach of most medical students by The Medical Faculty Grant for Medical Publications and the Development of Medical Training awarded by the Faculty of Medicine, University of Hong Kong, which I gratefully acknowledge. The efforts of Mr S. P. Hung at Hong Kong University Press have made it possible to produce this revised edition within 6 months of completion of the revised manuscript which is a remarkable achievement!

M. K. Chan
1989

Preface to the First Edition

The thought of writing a textbook on nephrology first came to me when I was working at the Royal Free Hospital in London. I remember being asked by senior house officers as to which textbook on nephrology I would recommend.

It suddenly dawned on me that there was no suitable textbook for beginners. The multi-authored American textbooks are too taxing to read, and the serial lecture notes are too simple and cannot even satisfy the inquisitive medical students. There were one or two medium-sized texts which, however, were either grossly out of date or ill-balanced in their approach.

On joining the University of Hong Kong, I soon started working on a textbook that was intended to bridge the gap between the serial lecture notes and the multi-authored reference books. The three-part text emphasizes equally on applied renal physiology, bread-and-butter conventional nephrology and renal replacement therapy. I wrote entirely from personal experience in clinical practice, and so every now and then personal biases would surface in the text.

This book is intended for use by inquisitive medical students, post-graduate doctors preparing for the Member of Royal College of Physicians (MRCP) examination, and junior doctors at the beginning of their training in nephrology. It is intended to be as self-contained as possible, and hence some rare entities which I have seen are also included. The content is abound with diagrams to help students to grasp, at a glance, the complicated pathogenesis of various clinical syndromes, for students remember a disease better if they understand its pathogenesis. A systematic approach is adopted in the layout of the chapters to integrate the text in such a way that little distinction is made between nephrology and urology where the disease demands a combined approach by the two related disciplines.

I sincerely hope that my book will stimulate students' interests in nephrology and serve to lead them into the specialty. I am deeply indebted to my friend, W. T. Lee, who has generously donated a grant towards the publication of this book. I gratefully acknowledge the skill of the Medical Illustration Unit in making the diagrams, the hard work of R. Fan in typing out the manuscript, and the help of my colleague I. K. P. Cheng, in proofreading. K. W. Chan kindly provided Figs. 26, 27, 28, and 30. The excellent cooperation of the staff at Hong Kong University Press, especially editor Amy Y. Ma, is deeply appreciated.

M. K. Chan
1986

Contributors

Editors

Desmond YAP, Clinical Associate Professor, Honorary Consultant, Department of Medicine, Queen Mary Hospital, the University of Hong Kong

Tak Mao CHAN, Chair Professor and Chief of Nephrology, Yu Chiu Kwong Professor in Medicine, Honorary Consultant, Department of Medicine, Queen Mary Hospital, the University of Hong Kong

Man Kam CHAN, author and editor of the first edition

Chapter Authors

(In alphabetic order)

Eugene CHAN, Associate Consultant, Department of Paediatrics and Adolescent Medicine, Hong Kong Children's Hospital

Gary CHAN, Associate Consultant, Department of Medicine, Queen Mary Hospital, the University of Hong Kong

Gavin CHAN, Consultant and Division Head (Anatomical Pathology), Department of Pathology, Queen Mary Hospital, the University of Hong Kong

Kwok Wah CHAN, Clinical Associate Professor, Department of Pathology, Queen Mary Hospital, the University of Hong Kong

Kwok Ying CHAN, Consultant and Chief of Service, Palliative Medicine Unit, Grantham Hospital, Hong Kong

Zi CHAN, Associate Consultant, Department of Medicine and Geriatrics, United Christian Hospital, Hong Kong

Yuk Lun CHENG, Consultant and Chief of Nephrology, Department of Medicine and Intensive Care Unit, Alice Ho Miu Ling Nethersole Hospital, Hong Kong

Bernard CHEUNG, Clinical Professor, Department of Medicine, Queen Mary Hospital, the University of Hong Kong

Simon C. Y. CHEUNG, Consultant, Department of Medicine, Queen Elizabeth Hospital, Hong Kong

Siu Fai CHEUNG, Consultant and Chief of Service (Medicine), Department of Medicine and Geriatrics, Yan Chai Hospital, Hong Kong

Stella CHIM, Consultant, Department of Paediatrics and Adolescent Medicine, Queen Mary Hospital, the University of Hong Kong

Kelvin CHOI, Associate Consultant, Department of Radiology, Queen Mary Hospital, the University of Hong Kong

Chik Cheung CHOW, Associate Consultant, Department of Medicine, Pamela Youde Nethersole Eastern Hospital, Hong Kong

Kai Ming CHOW, Consultant and Chief of Service (Medicine), Department of Medicine and Therapeutics, Prince of Wales Hospital, the Chinese University of Hong Kong

Cindy CHOY, Consultant, Department of Medicine, Queen Mary Hospital, the University of Hong Kong

Ferdinand CHU, Consultant, Department of Radiology, Queen Mary Hospital, the University of Hong Kong

Wai Ling CHU, Renal Nurse Specialist, Department of Medicine, Tung Wah Hospital, Hong Kong

Samuel Ka Shun FUNG, Consultant and Division Chief (Nephrology), Department of Medicine and Geriatrics, Princess Margaret Hospital, Hong Kong

Harry GILL, Clinical Assistant Professor, Department of Medicine, Queen Mary Hospital, the University of Hong Kong

Lorraine KWAN, Associate Consultant, Department of Medicine, Queen Mary Hospital, the University of Hong Kong

Janette KWOK, Consultant and Division Head (Transplantation and Immunogenetics), Department of Pathology, Queen Mary Hospital, the University of Hong Kong

Kar Neng LAI, Honorary Professor, Department of Medicine, Queen Mary Hospital, the University of Hong Kong

Wai Ming LAI, Consultant, Department of Paediatrics and Adolescent Medicine, Hong Kong Children's Hospital

May Ki LAM, Nursing Consultant, Department of Medicine, Queen Mary Hospital, the University of Hong Kong

Kit Ming LEE, Resident, Department of Medicine, Queen Mary Hospital, the University of Hong Kong

Victor LEE, Associate Consultant, Department of Radiology, Queen Mary Hospital, the University of Hong Kong

Chi Bon LEUNG, Consultant, Department of Medicine and Therapeutics, Prince of Wales Hospital, the Chinese University of Hong Kong

Patrick Siu Chung LEUNG, Clinical Assistant Professor of Emergency Medicine Practice, Emergency Medicine Unit, Li Ka Shing Faculty of Medicine, the University of Hong Kong

Chao LI, Attending Physician, Division of Nephrology, Peking Union Medical College Hospital, Chinese Academy of Medical Sciences and Peking Union Medical College

Philip Kam Tao LI, Consultant and Honorary Professor, Department of Medicine and Therapeutics, Prince of Wales Hospital, the Chinese University of Hong Kong

Xue-mei LI, Professor, Division of Nephrology, Peking Union Medical College Hospital, Chinese Academy of Medical Sciences and Peking Union Medical College

Xue-wang LI, Professor, Division of Nephrology, Peking Union Medical College Hospital, Chinese Academy of Medical Sciences and Peking Union Medical College

Davina LIE, Resident Specialist, Department of Medicine, Queen Mary Hospital, the University of Hong Kong

Wai Kei LO, Honorary Professor, Department of Medicine, Queen Mary Hospital, the University of Hong Kong

Sing Leung LUI, Consultant and Chief of Service (Medicine), Honorary Professor, Department of Medicine, Tung Wah Hospital, Hong Kong

Alison MA, Consultant and Service Head (Nephrology), Department of Paediatrics and Adolescent Medicine, Hong Kong Children's Hospital

Becky MA, Resident Specialist, Department of Medicine, Queen Mary Hospital, the University of Hong Kong

Maggie MA, Consultant and Co-director of Combined Renal Replacement Services, Department of Medicine, Queen Mary Hospital, the University of Hong Kong

Siu Ka MAK, Head of Nephrology, Department of Medicine and Geriatrics, Kwong Wah Hospital, Hong Kong

Maggie Ming Yee MOK, Associate Consultant, Department of Medicine, Tung Wah Hospital, Hong Kong

Pearl PAI, Consultant and Chief of Service (Medicine), Honorary Professor, Department of Medicine, HKU-Shenzhen Hospital, Shenzhen, China

Yat Fung SHEA, Associate Consultant, Department of Medicine, Queen Mary Hospital, the University of Hong Kong

Noel SHEK, Consultant and Chief of Obstetrics, Department of Obstetrics and Gynaecology, Queen Mary Hospital, the University of Hong Kong

Hoi Ping SHUM, Consultant and Chief of Service (Adult Intensive Care Unit), Adult Intensive Care Unit, Pamela Youde Nethersole Eastern Hospital, Hong Kong

Benjamin SO, Resident, Department of Medicine, Queen Mary Hospital, the University of Hong Kong

Cheuk Chun SZETO, Professor and Chief of Nephrology, Honorary Consultant, Department of Medicine and Therapeutics, Prince of Wales Hospital, the Chinese University of Hong Kong

Alex TANG, Clinical Assistant Professor and Honorary Associate Consultant, Department of Pathology, Queen Mary Hospital, the University of Hong Kong

Hon Lok TANG, Consultant, Department of Medicine and Geriatrics, Princess Margaret Hospital, Hong Kong

Sydney TANG, Chair Professor, Yu Professor in Nephrology, Honorary Consultant, Department of Medicine, Queen Mary Hospital, the University of Hong Kong

James TSU, Consultant and Chief of Urology, Director of Combined Renal Replacement Services, Department of Surgery, Queen Mary Hospital, the University of Hong Kong

Sik Hon TSUI, Chief of Service and Honorary Clinical Associate Professor, Department of Accident and Emergency, Queen Mary Hospital, the University of Hong Kong

Chiu Cheuk WONG, Consultant, Department of Surgery, Queen Mary Hospital, the University of Hong Kong

Ping Nam WONG, Consultant, Department of Medicine and Geriatrics, Kwong Wah Hospital, Hong Kong

Sunny WONG, Consultant, Department of Medicine and Geriatrics, United Christian Hospital, Hong Kong

Wing Wa YAN, Consultant, Adult Intensive Care Unit, Pamela Youde Nethersole Eastern Hospital, Hong Kong

Shing YEUNG, Consultant, Department of Medicine, Tseung Kwan O Hospital, Hong Kong

Terence YIP, Consultant, Honorary Clinical Associate Professor, Department of Medicine, Tung Wah Hospital, Hong Kong

Susan YUNG, Associate Professor, Department of Medicine, the University of Hong Kong

Normal Structure and Function of the Kidneys

Benjamin So, Desmond Yap, and Sing Leung Lui

Introduction

The kidneys are vital organs responsible for body homeostasis. Key functions of the kidneys include the excretion of waste products, control of blood pressure and fluid status, regulation of electrolyte and acid–base balance, and production of hormones. This chapter provides an overview of the structure and functions of the kidneys, which is a prerequisite to understanding the pathophysiology and treatments of renal disorders.

The Nephron

Each kidney contains about a million nephrons, which serve as the functional units of the kidney. Fluid is filtered from the blood via the glomerular capillary tuft, into the surrounding Bowman's capsule, and subsequently flows through the proximal convoluted tubule, the loop of Henle, and the distal convoluted tubule, before emptying into the collecting duct. Collecting ducts from different nephrons eventually drain into the duct of Bellini, which opens into a renal calyx.

Tubular cells are differentiated to facilitate their functions of reabsorption and secretion. Epithelial cells of the proximal tubule are cuboidal in appearance, with a brush border and numerous mitochondria, as necessitated by their high metabolic activity. Distal renal tubular cells are relatively more flattened than their proximal counterparts.

The juxtaglomerular apparatus is situated between the afferent arteriole and the distal segment of the ascending loop of Henle and is made up of juxtaglomerular cells (also known as granular cells), the macula densa, and pericytes (Lacis cells) (Figure 1.1). It is an important component of tubuloglomerular feedback (see below).

There are two types of nephrons, namely the cortical and juxtamedullary nephrons. The latter have longer loops of Henle that penetrate deep into the medulla, which have important roles in the osmoregulation of the medullary interstitium.

Renal Blood Supply

The kidneys receive 20% of the total cardiac output. The renal artery progressively branches to form the interlobar arteries, the arcuate arteries, and the interlobular arteries. The interlobular arteries give rise to the afferent arterioles as they course through the cortex, branching into tufts of glomerular capillaries to form the glomeruli. The glomerular capillaries then coalesce to form the efferent arteriole. The blood supply to the renal tubules is then derived from post-glomerular efferent arterioles. Corticomedullary efferent arterioles give rise to vasa recta, which penetrate deep into the renal medulla adjacent to the loops of Henle.

Glomerular Filtration

The glomerular capillary membrane is much more permeable to water and solutes than capillary membranes elsewhere, while remaining largely impermeable to proteins. A small driving pressure is thus sufficient to effect ultrafiltration. This filtration pressure is a function of the hydrostatic and colloid osmotic pressures across the glomerular membrane. The single nephron glomerular filtration rate is given as a product of the filtration pressure (P_{uf}), the

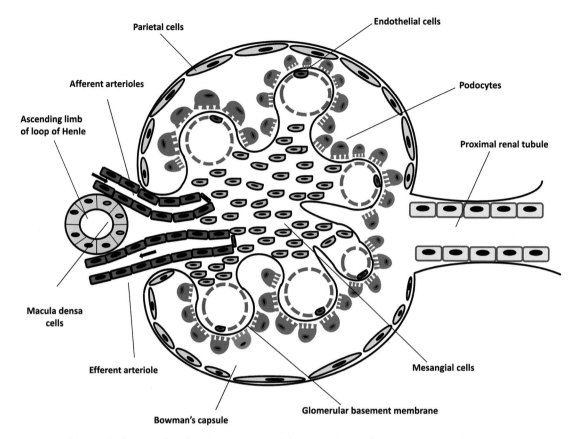

Figure 1.1: Schematic diagram showing the structures of the juxtaglomerular apparatus and the glomerulus

surface area of the glomerular capillaries (*S*), and the hydraulic permeability coefficient of the glomerular capillaries (*k*). Disease states that affect any of these factors can thus alter the glomerular filtration rate (GFR).

Autoregulation of Renal Blood Supply and GFR

Renal blood flow is maintained at a relatively constant level within a wide range of perfusion pressures, via autoregulatory mechanisms. A myogenic mechanism has been proposed: blood vessels respond to increased wall tension by contraction of vascular smooth muscle, thus preventing excessive stretch of the vessel. In addition, the juxtaglomerular apparatus senses volume delivery to the distal tubule and mediates a neurohormonal response to regulate renal blood flow.

Stimulation of the sympathetic nervous system, such as by endogenous catecholamine release from

the adrenal medulla, causes vasoconstriction and reduces renal blood flow. At low doses, dopamine preferentially stimulates dopaminergic receptors leading to renal vasodilation. Angiotensin II is synthesized in the systemic circulation as well as in the kidney; in the kidney, it preferentially leads to vasoconstriction of the efferent arteriole. Autacoids may also alter renal blood flow: locally secreted endothelin is a renal vasoconstrictor whereas nitric oxide, prostaglandins, and bradykinin tend to dilate renal vessels and increase renal blood flow. Drugs that affect these neurohormonal pathways (e.g. inhibitors of prostaglandin synthesis such as non-steroidal anti-inflammatory drugs) can therefore affect renal haemodynamics and cause renal vasoconstriction.

GFR is further regulated by a system of tubuloglomerular feedback, orchestrated by the juxtaglomerular apparatus. A decrease in the delivery of sodium chloride to the macula densa cells leads firstly to afferent arteriolar vasodilation, thereby increasing GFR; and secondly to renin release from juxtaglomerular cells. Increased angiotensin

II metabolized from this pathway constricts the efferent arterioles to maintain GFR.

Unless the drop in blood pressure is too precipitous or prolonged, GFR is maintained at a relatively constant level. However, GFR autoregulation is often impaired in kidney disease, causing significant fluctuations in GFR when the blood pressure changes. Thus, patients with chronic kidney disease are more susceptible to acute haemodynamic changes.

Structure and Permselectivity of the Glomerular Capillaries

Glomerular capillary haemodynamics enable filtration of large volumes of plasma while effectively retaining proteins and cellular elements within the circulation. The filtration barrier comprises 3 layers—an inner fenestrated capillary endothelium, the glomerular basement membrane (GBM), and an outer layer of podocytes with interdigitating foot processes separated by slit diaphragms. The movement of larger molecules across the filtration barrier is determined by their size, shape, and charge.

The GBM consists of an inner dense zone known as the lamina densa, and inner and outer lucent zones known respectively as the laminae rara interna and externa. It is an amorphous structure of 300–350 nm thickness, composed of both collagenous and non-collagen glycoproteins including type IV collagen, laminin, entactin, fibronectin, and heparan sulphate. Type IV collagen is assembled into a lattice-like network, forming a scaffold to which other matrix components adhere, and providing tensile strength and support to the GBM. Laminin is another major component of the GBM, and is believed to play an important role in cell differentiation and adhesion as well as providing structural integrity. It logically follows that antibodies directed against these GBM components are usually nephritogenic. For example, antibodies directed against the non-collagenous NC1 domain of the a3 chain of type IV collagen cause anti-GBM disease resulting in rapidly progressive glomerulonephritis.

Two important heparan sulphate proteoglycans, perlecan and agrin, have been identified in the GBM. Glycosaminoglycan chains are covalently attached to the core protein structure of these proteoglycans, conferring a net negative electrochemical charge. Damage to these structures is associated with effacement of the podocyte foot processes, resulting in loss of glomerular permselectivity and thus proteinuria.

Renal Tubular Functions and Mechanisms of Regulation

The formation of urine by ultrafiltration of plasma is highly efficient for the elimination of waste products. However, the renal tubules are essential for determining the final composition of urine through coordinated reabsorption and secretion of water and solutes (Figure 1.2). This is important for maintaining fluid balance, as well as electrolyte and acid–base homeostasis. Disorders of the proximal tubules can give rise to wasting of potassium (K^+), bicarbonate (HCO_3^-), phosphate (PO_4^{3-}), urate, glucose, and amino acids; whereas dysfunction of the distal tubules is often associated with abnormalities in reabsorption/excretion of K^+ and failure to acidify urine. The loop of Henle and the collecting ducts are key sites for regulating urinary dilution and concentration.

The following sections will highlight specific renal tubular functions responsible for handling several key electrolytes, which are often regulated by a cross-talk between glomerular and tubular functions (i.e. glomerulo-tubular balance).

Renal Handling of Sodium

Sodium (Na^+) is the most abundant cation in the extracellular fluid. It is extensively reabsorbed by renal tubules after it is filtered by the glomerulus, such that less than 1% of the filtered load is actually excreted in the urine. The bulk of Na^+ reabsorption occurs in the proximal tubules by indirect active transport. A concentration gradient is created as Na^+ is actively transported out of proximal tubular cells into the surrounding intercellular space by the Na^+-K^+-ATPase in the basolateral membranes. Na^+ therefore passes down the concentration gradient from the tubular lumen into the proximal tubular cells, accelerated by cotransport with glucose and amino acids. Some Na^+ also enters proximal tubular cells with chloride (Cl^-), in exchange for hydrogen ion (H^+). Water reabsorption follows Na^+ in the proximal tubules; due to the development of an osmotic gradient created with increased Na^+ reabsorption, water is transported across the basolateral cell membrane and tight junctions into the interstitium, and eventually into peritubular capillaries, mediated by Starling forces. Due to the active transport of Na^+ from the lumen,

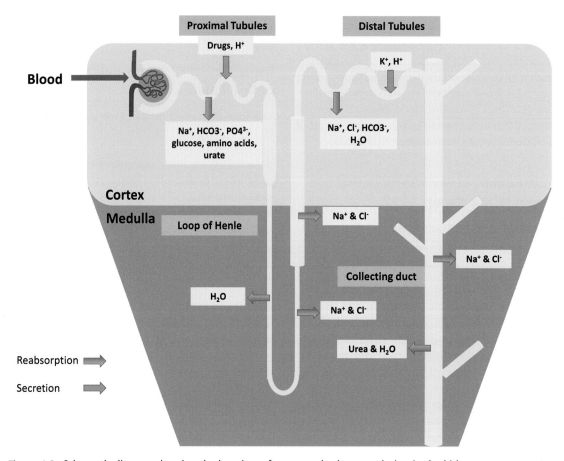

Figure 1.2: Schematic diagram showing the key sites of water and solute regulation in the kidney

the transepithelial membrane potential gradient is negative in the proximal tubules.

In the thick ascending limb of the loop of Henle, Na^+ reabsorption follows the active Cl^- transport out of the tubular lumen via the $Na^+/K^+/Cl^-$ cotransporter 2 (NKCC2). The transepithelial potential difference in this segment of the nephron is positive in the lumen.

In the distal convoluted tubules and the collecting tubules, Na^+ reabsorption is by active transport. The epithelium in this segment of the nephron, unlike in the proximal tubule, is only poorly permeable to Na^+. Na^+ reabsorption here is stimulated by aldosterone, and is coupled with the tubular secretion of K^+ and H^+ ions. The net transepithelial potential difference is normally orientated negatively in the lumen. Although the Na^+ reabsorption capacity of the distal convoluted tubule and collecting duct is low (about 10% of the filtered load), final adjustments in the Na^+ concentration in the urine are made in this part of the nephron.

Physical and hormonal factors affecting sodium handling

Physical forces determine the extent of Na^+ and water reabsorption especially at the level of the proximal tubules. This is mainly a function of the hydrostatic and colloid osmotic forces in the peritubular capillaries and the renal interstitium. In the case of dehydration, the hydrostatic pressure in the peritubular capillaries is relatively low while the colloid osmotic pressure in the capillaries is high due to haemoconcentration, favouring reabsorption of water and Na^+ from the renal interstitium.

The reabsorption of Na^+ is highly influenced by severe important hormones:

1. Aldosterone stimulates the Na^+-K^+-ATPase pump on the basolateral membrane of the principal cells of the cortical collecting tubule to increase Na^+ reabsorption while increasing K^+ secretion.

Increased K^+ concentrations and angiotensin II levels stimulate aldosterone secretion.

2. Angiotensin II increases in cases of low effective circulating volume, such as hypotension or dehydration. It retains Na^+ through stimulation of aldosterone activity, and also directly promotes Na reabsorption in the proximal tubules, the loop of Henle, the distal tubules and the collecting tubules. In addition, it leads to constriction of the efferent arterioles, thereby reducing peritubular capillary hydrostatic pressure, and favouring reabsorption of Na^+ and water.

3. Atrial natriuretic peptide (ANP) is released into the circulation in volume-expanded states to regulate blood volume. In the kidney, the ANP prohormone is further modified by the addition of four amino acids to form urodilatin. ANP reduces Na^+ and water reabsorption in the renal tubules especially in the collecting ducts, and also inhibits the renin-angiotensin-aldosterone system. The family of natriuretic peptides is gaining recognition for their impacts on the cardiovascular system as well.

Dilution and Concentration of Urine

The spatial configuration of the hairpin loop of Henle and the vasa recta creates a counter-current multiplier mechanism useful for the dilution and concentration of urine (Figure 1.3). The descending loop of Henle (A) is highly permeable to water with high concentrations of aquaporin-1 channels but less permeable to Na^+ and Cl^-. As such, the tubular fluid at the descending loop of Henle progressively becomes more concentrated due to water moving into the interstitium by osmosis. To reduce the buildup of hydrostatic pressure in the interstitium (B), the vasa recta transport accumulated fluid away to maintain the concentration of solutes in the medullary interstitium. The thin and thick ascending limbs of the loop of Henle are virtually impermeable to water but allow reabsorption of Na^+ and Cl^-. In the thick ascending limb of the loop of Henle (C), Na^+, Cl^- and other ions move into the interstitium by active transport and also through paracellular pathways. These mechanisms facilitate the generation of high osmolarity in the interstitium but very dilute tubular fluid within the loop of Henle.

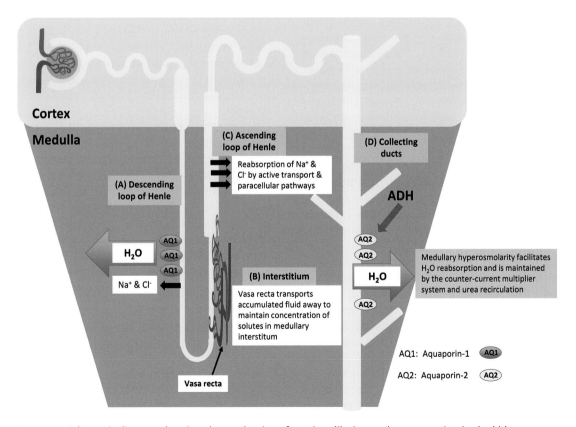

Figure 1.3: Schematic diagram showing the mechanisms for urine dilution and concentration in the kidney

Urinary concentration is achieved by the actions of antidiuretic hormone (ADH), also known as vasopressin, at the collecting duct (D). The collecting duct is usually impermeable to water. ADH is released from the posterior pituitary in response to various osmotic and non-osmotic stimuli, and binds to V2 vasopressin receptors at the basolateral membrane, leading to water reabsorption via apical aquaporin-2 channels. As the collecting duct passes through the hypertonic medullary interstitium, water can be reabsorbed efficiently. Thus, the urine concentration and the amount of free water loss are modified by ADH action based on blood osmolality as well as other variables. Deficiency of ADH or resistance to the actions of ADH results in diabetes insipidus, with the production of excessively dilute urine; conversely, excessive ADH, such as in syndrome of inappropriate antidiuretic hormone, results in impaired free water excretion.

The maintenance of a hyperosmotic renal medullary interstitium is of paramount importance in facilitating water reabsorption in the collecting ducts and urine concentration. There are two key mechanisms for maintaining a hyperosmotic renal medullary interstitium.

The first mechanism is known as the countercurrent multiplier. Ions are actively pumped into the medullary interstitium in the thick ascending limb of the loop of Henle. As the descending limb of the loop of Henle remains permeable to water, the osmolarities in the descending limb and medullary interstitium equilibrate through osmosis of water. However, this results in concentrated tubular fluid then reaching the ascending limb of the loop of Henle, where solutes are pumped into the interstitium. Na^+ and Cl^- continue to flow into the loop of Henle from the proximal tubule, thus perpetuating this process. The net effect is that the osmolarity in the medullary interstitium is significantly higher at 1,200–1,400 mOsm/L compared to the surrounding tubules.

The second mechanism is urea recirculation. Along the renal tubules, urea becomes progressively more concentrated as it is not as permeable as water and is thus reabsorbed to a lesser degree. Some urea is also passively secreted into the tubular fluid in the thin loop of Henle from the medullary interstitium. The thick ascending limb of the loop of Henle, distal tubules, and cortical collecting tubules are relatively impermeable to urea. Especially in the presence of high ADH levels, water is reabsorbed rapidly in the collecting duct, resulting in a very high urea concentration in the tubules. The urea then diffuses into the medullary interstitium down a concentration gradient facilitated by specific urea receptors, contributing to about 40–50% of the osmolarity of the medullary interstitium. Some of this sequestrated urea eventually diffuses back into the tubular fluid at the thin loop of Henle as described above, recirculating through the latter parts of the tubular system before excretion. The importance of urea in urinary concentration is underscored by the fact that subjects that take high-protein diets can concentrate their urine better, due to the higher concentration of nitrogenous waste products they produce. Conversely, urine concentration is impaired in malnourished individuals.

Renal Handling of Potassium

K^+ is a predominantly intracellular cation, with only 2% of the body's K^+ store being in the extracellular space. As even small changes in the blood K^+ level can affect cellular function and may precipitate cardiac arrhythmias, homeostasis and regulation of K^+ must be efficient and responsive to changes in the blood K^+ level.

Filtration of K^+ at the glomerulus is relatively constant. 65% of the filtered load of K^+ is reabsorbed in the proximal tubules and another 30% in the loop of Henle via the NKCC2 (coupled with Na^+ and Cl^- as described above) as well as paracellular pathways. Fine-tuning of K^+ excretion is primarily mediated by secretion at the level of the distal and cortical collecting tubules.

Na^+-K^+-ATPase pumps in the basolateral membranes of principal cells in the late distal and cortical collecting tubules are stimulated by high extracellular concentrations of K^+, leading to the transfer of K^+ from the interstitium into the intracellular space in exchange for Na^+. K^+ then diffuses rapidly into the renal tubules down an electrochemical gradient. Under conditions of K^+ depletion, however, K^+ is reabsorbed via H^+/K^+-ATPase transporters located on the apical side of intercalated cells in the collecting duct.

Factors affecting potassium secretion and reabsorption in distal and collecting tubules

1. Increased mineralocorticoid activity, mostly by secretion of aldosterone from the adrenal cortex in response to hyperkalaemia, stimulates K^+ secretion through direct action on the Na^+/

K^+-ATPase pump, and also stimulates activity and expression of H^+/K^+-ATPases.

2. Increased distal tubular flow rate due to volume expansion, diuretic treatment, or a high Na^+ diet can stimulate K^+ secretion as the secreted potassium is rapidly flushed away. Thus a steep electrochemical gradient is maintained, promoting K^+ secretion.

3. Acid–base disturbances affect the movement of K^+ in different cell types and also K^+ secretion in the kidneys. In acute acidosis, increased H^+ ion concentration inhibits the Na^+/K^+ ATPase pump in the basolateral membrane of tubular cells throughout the nephron, reducing K^+ secretion in the kidneys. In chronic acidosis, proximal tubular NaCl and water reabsorption is inhibited, which increases Na^+ delivery to the distal tubules and overrides the initial effect of acidosis on K^+ secretion.

4. During pregnancy, high circulating levels of progesterone favour the reabsorption of K^+ via H^+/K^+-ATPase transporters to meet the increased K^+ requirements of pregnancy.

Renal Handling of Calcium

Most of the body's calcium (Ca^{2+}) is stored in the bone. However, serum Ca^{2+} levels affect myocardial and neuromuscular functions and a fine balance between gastrointestinal absorption and renal excretion is typically maintained. Just under half of serum Ca^{2+} is not filtered, as it is protein-bound; thus total ultrafiltratable Ca^{2+} equals the sum of ionized Ca^{2+} and complexed Ca^{2+} (i.e. Ca^{2+} bound to phosphate or citrate). Up to 98–99% of the filtered Ca^{2+} load is eventually reabsorbed.

Around 55–60% of Ca^{2+} is reabsorbed at the proximal tubules, 20–25% in the loop of Henle, and the remaining at the distal tubules. Much of the reabsorption of Ca^{2+} in the proximal tubules is via paracellular pathways and parallels reabsorption of Na^+ and water, with a smaller percentage attributable to active transport. In the thick ascending loop of Henle, a lumen-positive transepithelial potential difference drives paracellular reabsorption of Ca^{2+}, a process that is regulated by the calcium-sensing receptor (CaSR) in response to changes in blood Ca^{2+} levels; active transport also occurs in this segment. While only around 10–15% of Ca^{2+} reabsorption takes place at the terminal nephron, it is here that fine-tuning of the final Ca^{2+} content of urine takes place. Active transport mediated by a receptor called transient receptor potential cation channel subfamily V member 5 (TRPV5) in distal tubular cells is required for Ca^{2+} reabsorption as this takes place against the electrochemical gradient (which is lumen-negative in this segment).

Factors affecting calcium reabsorption and excretion

1. Parathyroid hormone (PTH) is the most important hormone governing Ca^{2+} reabsorption. Except in subjects who have an autonomously functioning parathyroid adenoma, the parathyroid gland detects Ca^{2+} levels via CaSR and adjusts PTH secretion accordingly. In the renal tubules, PTH promotes Ca^{2+} reabsorption through effects on TRPV5 activity as well as intracellular Ca^{2+} transporter proteins.

2. Volume status affects Na^+ delivery to the renal tubules and by extension, the extent of Na^+ reabsorption. As passive Ca^{2+} reabsorption mirrors that of Na^+ and water, an expansion of extracellular volume reduces Ca^{2+} reabsorption.

3. Blood Ca^{2+} levels directly affect renal Ca^{2+} excretion. Increases in serum Ca^{2+} level increases the filtered load, though such increase in filtered load is partially offset by hypercalcaemia-induced renal vasoconstriction and reduced GFR. Furthermore, hypercalcaemia also reduces Ca^{2+} reabsorption by suppressing PTH actions and also via PTH-independent effects such as activation of CaSR in the loop of Henle.

4. Acidosis increases renal Ca^{2+} excretion. This occurs by increasing the filtered load of Ca^{2+} as acidosis increases the ionized fraction of Ca^{2+}, and also mobilizes additional Ca^{2+} from the bone as H^+ ion is buffered in the bone. Additionally, acidosis also directly inhibits Ca^{2+} reabsorption by reducing the channel conductance of TRPV5 in the renal tubules.

5. Calcitriol (1, 25-$(OH)_2$-vitamin D) increases renal Ca^{2+} excretion through several mechanisms: (a) through increasing Ca^{2+} levels and thus the filtered Ca^{2+} load; (b) through suppression of PTH activity; and (c) through direct effects on the distal tubules. The vitamin D receptor is expressed in multiple sites of distal tubular cells, and affects Ca^{2+} transport through the apical and basolateral membranes as well as intracellular transport.

6. Calcitonin does not appear to have direct effects on renal reabsorption of Ca^{2+}, but instead inhibit calcitriol synthesis and promote calcitriol degradation in the proximal renal tubular cells.

7. Diuretics affect renal Ca^{2+} excretion in different ways. Loop diuretics bind to the NKCC2 transporter in the loop of Henle, which decreases Na^+ reabsorption, and hence inhibits Ca^{2+} reabsorption and promotes calciuresis. Conversely, thiazide diuretics bind to the thiazide-sensitive Na^+/Cl^- cotransporter, thereby reducing intracellular Na^+ concentrations in distal tubular cells. This triggers increased expression of the basolateral Na^+/Ca^{2+}-exchanger to replete intracellular Na^+ stores, which results in hypocalciuria.

Renal Handling of Phosphate

Most of the body's stores of phosphorus are in the bones, with less than 1% present as serum phosphate (PO_4^{3-}). However, maintenance of PO_4^{3-} within a relatively normal range is important for various cellular processes and is a result of the interplay of gastrointestinal absorption, exchange with bone, and renal excretion.

In the nephron, about 85% of the filtered PO_4^{3-} load is reabsorbed at the proximal tubules. Three Na^+-PO_4^{3-} cotransporters have been identified in the apical brush border of the proximal tubules. The remaining 15% of reabsorption appears to take place in the distal tubules, but the exact transporters remain unknown. Hormonal or dietary factors that affect PO_4^{3-} reabsorption appear to do so primarily by changing the quantity of transporters expressed. For example, a high PO_4^{3-} diet reduces the transporters available, thereby reducing renal PO_4^{3-} reabsorption, and vice versa for a low PO_4^{3-} diet.

Factors affecting phosphate reabsorption

1. Like with Ca^+, PTH is the most important hormonal influence on PO_4^{3-} handling. In subjects with normal renal function, it promotes phosphaturia by reducing the number of Na^+/PO_4^{3-} cotransporters available for reabsorption.
2. Fibroblast growth factor 23 (FGF23) is gaining recognition as an important hormone in bone turnover and PO_4^{3-} metabolism. It is synthesized by osteoblasts in response to serum PO_4^{3-} levels. FGF23 functions at the proximal tubules in the presence of a locally produced cofactor known as Klotho to reduce the expression of PO_4^{3-} transporters and promote phosphaturia. FGF23 also inhibits PTH synthesis. In addition, FGF23 also downregulates 1α-hydroxylase and thus reduces calcitriol synthesis, while upregulating

24-hydroxylase to break down calcitriol. As PO_4^{3-} levels increase in chronic kidney disease, FGF23 levels increase dramatically but often fail to compensate for the excessive retention of PO_4^{3-}. In patients with normal renal function, autonomous secretion of FGF23 in oncogenic osteomalacia results in phosphate wasting.
3. Calcitriol exhibits complex effects on renal PO_4^{3-} handling: on the one hand, it enhances PO_4^{3-} reabsorption at the proximal tubules, while on the other hand, it also increases blood Ca^{2+} levels and suppresses PTH actions.
4. Metabolic acidosis inhibits PO_4^{3-} transporter activity in the proximal tubules to increase the PO_4^{3-} available to buffer against acidaemia.
5. Insulin promotes PO_4^{3-} reabsorption at the proximal tubule in phosphate-depleted states through a stimulatory effect on transporters.
6. Very high glucose levels with glycosuria inhibit PO_4^{3-} reabsorption due to the codependence of both systems on the generation of an electrochemical Na^+ gradient.
7. Other neurohormonal pathways can also have an impact on renal PO_4^{3-} handling. For example, glucocorticoids, oestrogen and dopamine all induce phosphaturia by reducing the number of Na^+-PO_4^{3-} cotransporters available at the proximal tubule. The role of oestrogen is underscored by the finding that healthy post-menopausal women, who have lower levels of oestrogen, show lower urinary PO_4^{3-} clearance compared to pre-menopausal women. Conversely, older men have higher levels of oestrogen compared to younger men and may have increased urinary PO_4^{3-} clearance.
8. Thyroid hormone can increase urinary PO_4^{3-} reabsorption by upregulating transcription and expression of PO_4^{3-} transporters.

Acidification of Urine

The maintenance of body pH within the physiological range is vital for cellular functions and therefore is tightly regulated. Alterations in body pH are corrected acutely by the body's buffer systems, namely, the bicarbonate (HCO_3^-) and PO_4^{3-} buffer systems, then later by respiratory and renal compensations. The kidney's response is relatively slow (occurs within several days) but is by far the most powerful mechanism to regulate acid–base balance. Excretion of acid generated during the body's metabolism is also effected through the kidney.

The kidney reclaims the filtered HCO_3^- and generates new HCO_3^- to compensate for the loss of HCO_3^- consumed in the titration of H^+ ions. Throughout the tubular system, H^+ ions are buffered by other systems, including the PO_4^{3-} and ammonia (NH_3) buffers, as well as less important systems such as urate and citrate.

Very little HCO_3^- is directly reabsorbed. Instead, H^+ is secreted by active transport via the Na^+/H^+ exchanger in the proximal tubules. In the tubular lumen, H^+ reacts with HCO_3^- to form H_2CO_3 (carbonic acid), which dissociates to form carbon dioxide (CO_2) and water (H_2O). The CO_2 passes into the tubular cell where it reconstitutes with water to generate H_2CO_3 again, a process catalysed by carbonic anhydrase. The H_2CO_3 in the tubular cell dissociates to form HCO_3^- and H^+ again. The HCO_3^- is reabsorbed through the basolateral membrane in tandem with Na^+. 85% of filtered HCO_3^- is reclaimed in this way. The process of active secretion of H^+ into the tubular lumen to control acid–base homeostasis is known as renal acidification.

In the late distal and collecting tubules, intracellular CO_2 dissolves in water under the effects of carbonic anhydrase to form H_2CO_3, which in turn generates HCO_3^- and H^+ (Figure 1.4). The hydrogen ion so formed is secreted into the tubular lumen by active transport while the HCO_3^- is reabsorbed. The secretion of H^+ in the distal and collecting tubules is important in forming maximally acidic urine and is upregulated in the face of systemic acidosis.

H^+ ion also combines with PO_4^{3-} and NH_3 buffer systems to generate HCO_3^- to replenish extracellular stores. H^+ reacts with $NaHPO_4^-$ in the tubular lumen to form NaH_2PO_4, which is then excreted in the urine (Figure 1.4). The HCO_3^- that is formed during the synthesis of H^+ in the tubular cell is absorbed into the interstitium and then into the peritubular capillaries, generating a new HCO_3^- ion.

Furthermore, glutamine release from skeletal muscles and the liver is upregulated during acidosis, which is then delivered to tubular cells in the proximal tubules, the thick ascending limb of the loop of Henle, and distal tubular cells for renal ammoniagenesis (Figure 1.5). The process generates new HCO_3^- to buffer against H^+ in the blood. NH_4^+ (ammonium ion) formed is secreted into the tubular lumen in exchange for Na^+, where it binds with Cl^- ion and is excreted. In the collecting duct, NH_3 and H^+ are both secreted into the tubular lumen by dedicated transporters, where they combine to form NH_4^+, which is then passed into the urine (Figure 1.6). HCO_3^- is also generated in this process.

Net acid excretion is calculated as NH_4^+ excretion + urinary titratable acid − HCO_3^- excretion. While NH_4^+ and HCO_3^- can be quantified, urinary titratable acid is derived by measuring the amount of strong base that has to be added to the urine to achieve a pH of 7.4. It should be remembered that net acid excretion is not the same as net renal secretion of H^+ ion. In acute metabolic alkalosis, the amount of filtered bicarbonate exceeds the capacity of the

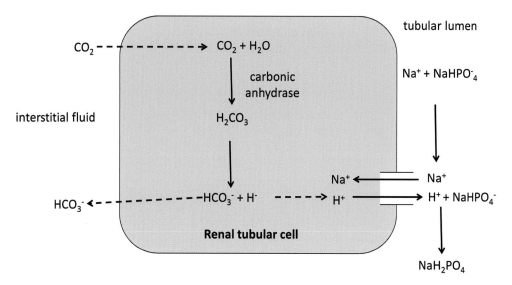

Figure 1.4: Schematic diagram showing the processes for hydrogen ion excretion in the kidney

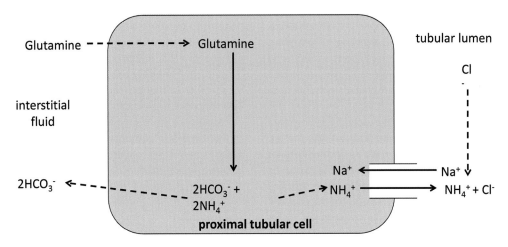

Figure 1.5: Schematic diagram showing the process of ammoniagenesis and secretion of ammonium ion in proximal renal tubular cells

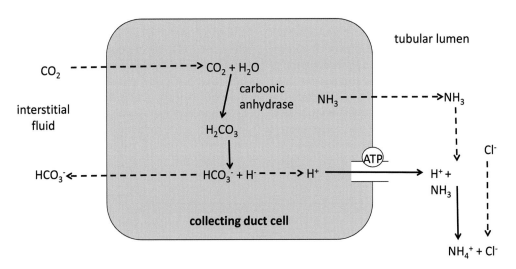

Figure 1.6: Schematic diagram showing the process for ammonium excretion in the collecting ducts

proximal tubular reabsorption and titration by distal tubular secretion of H^+, resulting in bicarbonaturia and a high urine pH. Net renal secretion of H^+ ion is positive to titrate against the large HCO_3^- load, but net acid excretion is negative.

Factors affecting hydrogen ion secretion in the proximal tubules

1. Carbonic anhydrase activity: inhibition of carbonic anhydrase activity limits the conversion of CO_2 and H_2O to H_2CO_3, a critical step in H^+ secretion and HCO_3^- reabsorption; thus carbonic anhydrase inhibitors such as acetazolamide may cause metabolic acidosis.
2. K^+ store: chronic K^+ depletion leads to intracellular acidosis, which increases H^+ secretion.
3. Glutamine metabolism: acute acidosis alters the intra-renal metabolism of glutamine, such that renal ammoniagenesis is increased several-fold to cope with the acute load of acid.
4. pCO_2 in peritubular blood: elevated pCO_2, including that due to respiratory acidosis, increases the availability of intracellular CO_2 that can be converted to H_2CO_3, which then forms HCO_3^- and H^+ to be secreted into the tubular lumen.
5. Extracellular fluid volume: as Na^+ is exchanged for H^+ in the proximal tubules, enhanced Na^+ reabsorption in face of a low effective circulating volume is associated with increased H^+ secretion and HCO_3^- reabsorption, and thus metabolic alkalosis.
6. Hormonal influences: adrenergic agonists and angiotensin II can stimulate HCO_3^- reabsorption/ H^+ secretion in acute acidosis, while PTH inhibits HCO_3^- reabsorption/H^+ secretion. In chronic acidosis, endothelin-1 is upregulated leading to enhanced Na^+/H^+ exchange and thus increased H^+ secretion; and glucocorticoids may also play a role in promoting HCO_3^- reabsorption.

Factors affecting hydrogen ion secretion in the distal nephron

1. Intracellular or extracellular acidosis: the mechanisms affecting H^+ ion secretion is similar to that in proximal renal tubules.
2. Transepithelial potential difference: the apical H^+-ATPase responsible for H^+ secretion is very sensitive to electrochemical gradients. Thus, increased lumen-negative voltage, such as that caused by increased sodium reabsorption or the presence of non-resorbable anions, will promote H^+ secretion.
3. Hormonal influences: mineralocorticoids such as aldosterone stimulate H^+ secretion in the distal nephron. The role of angiotensin II and endothelin-1 in distal renal tubular H^+ secretion has also been reported.

2

Symptoms and Signs of Kidney Diseases and Investigative Procedures

Kit Ming Lee, Desmond Yap, and Pearl Pai

Introduction

Although different types of renal diseases may have their own distinctive clinical features, some of them bear common symptoms and signs, especially in connection with chronic renal impairment. This chapter provides an overview of the common clinical manifestations in kidney diseases and the relevant investigative procedures.

Clinical Manifestations in Renal Diseases

Many symptoms and signs of renal disease are related to changes in urinary habits or characteristics of urine.

Urinary symptoms

1. Polyuria: The term refers to increased frequency and volume of urine. It can be a symptom of diabetes mellitus, diabetes insipidus, compulsive water drinking, the effect of diuretics, and the early stages of chronic kidney disease (CKD).
2. Oliguria: This is marked by a reduction of urine volume to less than 0.5 ml per kilogram body weight per hour, which is the lowest amount of water excretion required to remove metabolic waste by the kidneys. It is often seen in patients with acute kidney injury or those with advanced CKD.
3. Nocturia: The term means frequent urination during night time, which can be an early manifestation of impaired urinary concentrating ability. Nocturia can also be due to bladder neck abnormalities such as prostatism.

4. Urinary retention: This can be acute or chronic and is often related to prostatic obstruction in men. Acute retention of urine is usually painful, while chronic retention of urine is usually asymptomatic. Longstanding urinary retention can lead to obstructive uropathy.
5. Lower urinary tract symptoms (LUTS): These include storage symptoms (urinary urgency, frequency, nocturia) and voiding symptoms (weak stream, terminal dribbling, incomplete voiding/urinary retention). These symptoms can be related to prostatism in men, which are commonly caused by benign prostatic hyperplasia. In women, the presence of LUTS is suggestive of urinary tract infections (UTIs).
6. Haematuria: The term signifies the presence of blood in urine. It can be classified as gross or macroscopic haematuria (visible to the naked eye), or microscopic haematuria. Microscopic haematuria can be detected in various glomerulonephritis and is a common presentation of IgA nephropathy. Gross haematuria may or may not be accompanied by pain during micturition. Painful gross haematuria can be a symptom of cystitis or renal stone disease, while painless gross haematuria can be seen in IgA nephropathy or urinary tract neoplasms.
7. Proteinuria: This term refers to the presence of protein in urine. Asymptomatic proteinuria is common in patients with renal disorders and should be taken seriously with further work-up. Frothy urine (i.e. bubbles in urine) may be present in patients with a higher quantity of proteinuria.
8. Incontinence: There are different types of urinary incontinence. Overflow incontinence may occur in the background of a distended bladder.

Stress incontinence occurs typically in women when they laugh or cough, and is often due to a weakened pelvic floor following previous labour and childbirth. Urge incontinence is related to bladder detrusor overactivity with urinary frequency. Functional incontinence can be related to environmental, psychosocial, or neurological disabilities that affect accessibility to toilets.

9. Renal colic: The term describes a colicky pain radiating from the loin down to the external genitalia. It is often manifested as an excruciating pain during the passage of a stone or blood clot down the ureter.

10. Loin mass/pain: Early renal cell carcinoma, renal angiomyolipoma, and polycystic kidneys are often asymptomatic. However, they may also present with ballotable loin masses with or without tenderness. Acute onset of loin pain may signify acute bleeding or acute pyelonephritis.

11. Turbidity and discolouration of urine: Turbid urine can be the result of pus in the urine (pyuria) secondary to UTIs or excessive phosphate in the urine. Milky appearance of urine may indicate the presence of chyle in urine (chyluria), which is often the result of lymphatic obstruction. Certain antimicrobials (e.g. rifampicin and pyridium) can cause orange discolouration of urine, whereas methylene blue can cause a tinge of blue discolouration of the urine. The ingestion of beetroot can give rise to reddish urine mimicking gross haematuria. Rhabdomyolysis may cause myoglobulinuria, leading to red urine discolouration.

Other systemic symptoms

1. Oedema: Pitting oedema over dependent regions (e.g. ankle oedema or sacral oedema) is a common manifestation of renal diseases, and can be the result of fluid retention or hypoalbuminemia secondary to proteinuria. Oliguric/anuric patients may experience shortness of breath due to pulmonary oedema secondary to fluid overload.

2. Hypertension: While hypertension may cause kidney damage, it can also be a manifestation of CKD, glomerulonephritis, or renovascular disease.

3. Symptoms associated with connective tissue diseases: Patients with renal involvement secondary to autoimmune diseases (e.g. systemic lupus erythematosus or ANCA vasculitis) may show systemic manifestations of these collagen vascular disorders. The presence of these systemic symptoms (e.g. skin rash, arthralgia, hair loss, oral ulcers, and peripheral numbness) may be a clue to the underlying diagnosis.

4. Symptoms associated with electrolyte disturbances: Disturbances in blood sodium concentration (hypernatraemia and hyponatraemia) can lead to altered mental state and, in severe cases, may even induce seizures or coma. Patients with significant hyponatraemia, hypokalaemia, or hyperkalaemia may experience muscle weakness and paralysis. Fatal cardiac arrhythmias can be precipitated by serious electrolyte abnormalities (e.g. hypokalaemia, hyperkalaemia, hypocalcaemia, and hypomagnesaemia). Profound hypocalcaemia causes tetany with demonstrable classical Chvostek or Trousseau signs. Clinical manifestations of hypercalcaemia include neuropsychiatric symptoms, renal calculi, abdominal pain (peptic ulcer or constipation), and bone pain. Patients with severe metabolic acidosis show a deep and laboured breathing pattern known as Kussmaul breathing.

5. Symptoms associated with hereditary renal diseases: Patients with renal angiomyolipoma due to tuberous sclerosis may show cutaneous lesions such as adenoma sebaceum, Shagreen patches, and ashleaf macules. Sensorineural deafness can occur in patients with Alport's syndrome. Patients with nail-patella syndrome show typical nail dystrophy and absence of patella. Patients with Lowe Syndrome (a condition associated with proximal renal tubular acidosis and hypercalciuria) may show low-set ears.

6. Symptoms associated with uraemia: Patients with advanced CKD may experience malaise, loss of appetite, nausea, and generalized itchiness. Patients with later stages of CKD often appear to have a dark skin complexion accompanied by pallor, described as 'cafe au lait' complexion. Patients with terminal uraemia (without dialysis) may develop drowsiness, seizure, or even coma.

Investigations for Renal Diseases

Urine tests

Urinalysis

Urine dipstick is a simple screening test for renal diseases. The presence of white blood cells, nitrite, or leukocyte esterase is suggestive of a UTI, while the presence of red blood cells or protein may be an early sign of glomerular disease. Abnormalities in the urinalysis can often provide clues to the underlying causes of renal disease (Table 2.1).

Table 2.1: Findings in urinalysis and their clinical correlations

Urinalysis findings	Remarks
Red blood cells	• Can be a result of microscopic (e.g. GN) or macroscopic haematuria (e.g. renal stones, or neoplasms of kidneys, bladder or ureters)
White blood cells	• Indicative of UTI, especially in the presence of nitrite and leukocyte esterase
Protein	• Indicates the presence of albumin in urine • Positivity may suggest glomerular proteinuria or post-renal proteinuria related to UTI
Specific gravity	• Reflects urine concentration; normal SG is 1.002–1.030 • High SG can be related to dehydration, UTI, glycosuria, RAS, hepatorenal syndrome, and SIADH • Low SG can be related to DI, excessive fluid intake, AIN, ATN, and renal failure
Cellular casts	
Red blood cell cast	• Red blood cells embedded in Tamm–Horsfall mucoprotein • The presence of red blood cell cast is highly indicative of GN; occasionally seen in severe tubular injury • A high proportion of dysmorphic red blood cells is indicative of a glomerular cause for the haematuria
White blood cell cast	• Indicate possible kidney infection (pyelonephritis) or inflammation of tubular cells, for example AIN
Renal tubular epithelial cell cast	• Indicative of ATN when coexisting with muddy brown casts
Oval fat bodies	• Represent degenerated tubular cells filled with fat globules • Frequently seen in nephrotic syndrome with lipiduria • Characteristic 'maltese cross' appearance under polarized light
Acellular casts	
Hyaline cast	• Consists of Tamm–Horsfall protein, which is synthesized by thick ascending limb of loop of Henle • Can be present in a wide range of conditions
Granular cast	• Degenerated tubular cells • Mostly non-specific (except for muddy brown casts, which are characteristic of ATN)
Telescope sediment	• Comprises of all varieties of cellular and acellular casts, and occur in active glomerular inflammation (e.g. LN or ANCA-associated GN)
Crystals	
Uric Acid crystal	• Rhomboid-shaped crystals; usually found in acidic urine
Calcium oxalate crystal	• Bi-hydrated crystals show 'envelope' shape while mono-hydrated crystals show 'dumbbell' shape
Calcium phosphate crystal	• Pleomorphic appearances; usually precipitate in alkaline urine
Triple phosphate crystal	• Usually comprises magnesium ammonium phosphate; 'coffin lid' appearance and precipitate only in alkaline urine
Cystine crystal	• Hexagonal in shape and often stack on each other; only found in acidic urine

AIN, acute interstitial nephritis; ANCA, anti-neutrophil cytoplasmic antibodies; ATN, acute tubular necrosis; DI, diabetes insipidus; GN, glomerulonephritis; LN, lupus nephritis; RAS, renal artery stenosis; SG, specific gravity; SIADH, syndrome of inappropriate anti-diuretic hormone secretion; UTI, urinary tract infection

Urinary protein measurement

There are different types of proteinuria, including transient proteinuria, glomerular proteinuria, tubular proteinuria, overflow proteinuria, and post-renal proteinuria. Transient proteinuria can occur in patients with fever or after strenuous exercise. Glomerular proteinuria is detectable by urinary dipstick test due to the presence of urinary albumin. Tubular proteinuria refers to low molecular weight proteins such as β2 microglobulins and retinol-binding protein. Overflow proteinuria occurs when there is overproduction of low molecular weight proteins (e.g. Bence Jones proteins and excessive light chain production in plasma cell dyscrasias), that overwhelm the renal handling mechanisms of these proteins. Post-renal proteinuria is often associated with UTI.

The physiological limit for urinary protein excretion is below 150 mg per day. Excessive urinary protein excretion above the physiological limit usually warrants further investigations. The conventional method for quantifying proteinuria is a 24-hour urine collection. However, this method is cumbersome and under-collection is not uncommon. The urine volume, and sodium and creatinine level of a collected sample can sometimes inform the adequacy of collection. Spot urine protein to creatinine ratio (UPCR) is an alternative quantitative test. UPCR tends to be less accurate in patients with low or very high levels of proteinuria, and is affected by the diurnal variation of urinary protein excretion and rate of creatinine excretion. For instance, UPCR may underestimate the severity of proteinuria in subjects with greater muscle mass (higher rate of creatinine production and excretion).

Renal function tests and estimation of glomerular filtration rate

Renal clearance is an indicator of kidney function and is determined by the glomerular filtration rate (GFR) (defined as the volume of fluid filtered from the renal glomerular capillaries into the Bowman's capsule per unit time).

For a given substance S, the renal clearance of S, $C_S = (U_S \times V) \div P_S$

in which, P_S is the plasma concentration of S, U_S is urine concentration of S, and V is the volume of urine.

When the daily production rate of S is constant, the GFR is equal to the clearance of S when S is freely filtered through the glomerulus and without any renal tubular reabsorption or secretion. In this context, the gold standard for GFR measurement is by inulin, or by radioactive tracers such as chromium-51 or technetium-99m. In daily clinical practice, creatinine (Cr) or creatinine clearance (CrCl) is commonly used as a surrogate marker for kidney function because Cr is freely filtered through the glomeruli and with little renal tubular secretion. Renal function test is an important and commonly used investigation in both in- and out-patient settings. The serum levels of urea, Cr, sodium (Na), potassium (K), and chloride (Cl) are generally included in a renal function test. Elevated levels of serum urea and Cr are highly indicative of impaired renal function, and yet relying solely on increased serum Cr level to detect renal impairment can sometimes be misleading, especially in patients with small muscles or severe wasting. Other surrogate markers for GFR include cystatin C, which is a 13-kDa protein produced by all cells at a constant rate and is filtered by glomerulus without any renal tubular absorption or secretion. The clearance of cystatin C may be used to estimate GFR, but its measurement is not routinely available in many clinical laboratories. The CrCl can be measured by 24-hour urine collection, but this method is troublesome and under-collection of urine remains a problem. To overcome these issues, various equations have been developed to estimate GFR (Table 2.2), each of which has its distinct merits and shortcomings.

Renal tubular function tests

Following glomerular ultrafiltration, and tubular reabsorption and secretion, the tubular fluid contains a certain amount of glucose, amino acids, bicarbonate, acids, and other electrolytes. Water reabsorption primarily occurs in the collecting ducts under the influence of antidiuretic hormone (ADH). Virtually all glucose (given normal blood glucose level), amino acids, and bicarbonate are reabsorbed by proximal tubules and therefore proximal tubular dysfunction would result in glycosuria, aminoaciduria, and bicarbonaturia, as well as electrolyte and acid–base disturbances (e.g. hypokalaemia and normal anion gap metabolic acidosis). Similarly, distal tubular and collecting duct dysfunctions can also cause distinct patterns of electrolyte disturbance and changes in urinary concentration.

To evaluate renal tubular function, tubular secretion or reabsorption of a substance can be measured by dividing the amount of substance reabsorbed or secreted by the amount of substance filtered (i.e. GFR).

Assuming the GFR is equal to CrCl, the fractional excretion of Na can be calculated as follows (see p. 18):

Table 2.2: Different formulas for the estimation of glomerular filtration rate

	Formula	Remarks
Cockcroft–Gault	eCrCl = (140−Age) × 0.85(female) × BW(kg)/ (72 × Scr)	– A simple equation for estimation of CrCl – Depends on Cr and BW, and is therefore less accurate for patients who are markedly obese, have fluid overload, or are cachexic – Can also be confounded by drugs that interfere with tubular reabsorption and secretion of Cr
Ix equation	eCrCl = (Ecr/1440)/(0.01 × Scr) Ecr = 880−6.2 × Age + 12.5 × BW(kg) + 35(black)−380(female)	– Validated using a larger group of subjects than the CG equation – The race variable is included compared with the CG equation – Not very accurate for patients who are markedly obese, have fluid overload or are cachexic
MDRD equation	eGFR/1.73m² = 175 × (Scr)$^{-1.154}$ × (Age$^{-0.203}$ × (0.742 if female) × (1.210 if black)	– The MDRD equation is initially developed from a cohort of Caucasians without diabetes; a modified equation validated in Chinese is now available – Normalized GFR to body surface area and hence does not include a BW variable – Most accurate in patients with moderate CKD, but less accurate at extremes of GFR
CKD-EPI-Creatinine	eGFR/1.73m² = 141 × min(SCr/κ,1)^α × max(SCr/κ,1)^−1.209 × 0.993^Age × 1.018 [female] × 1.159[Black]	– Validated using a larger group of subjects compared with MDRD equation – Better accuracy for eGFR >60 ml/min compared with MDRD equation
CKD-EPI-Cystatin C	eGFR/1.73m² = 133 × min(Scys/0.8,1)^(−0.499) × max(Scys/0.8,1)^1.328 × 0.996^Age × 0.932[female]	– More accurate than MDRD and CKD-EPI-Creatinine equations – Measurement of cystatin C is not routinely available in clinical laboratories
CKD-EPI-Creatinine-Cystatin C	eGFR/1.73m² = 135 × min(SCr/κ,1)^α × max(SCr/κ,1)^(−0.601) × min(Scys/0.8,1)^−0.375 × max(Scys/0.8,1)^−0.711 × 0.995^Age × 0.969[female] × 1.08[black]	– More accurate than CKD-EPI-Cystatin equation, especially in younger subjects – Measurement of cystatin C is not routinely available in clinical laboratories

BW, body weight; CKD, chronic kidney disease; CKD-EPI, Chronic Kidney Disease-Epidemiology Collaboration; Cr, creatinine; CrCl, creatinine clearance; Ecr, 24-hour urine excretion rate in mg/day; GFR, glomerular filtration rate; κ = 0.7 (females) or 0.9 (males); α = −0.329 (females) or −0.41 (males); MDRD, Modification of Diet in Renal Disease; max(SCr/κ,1), maximum of SCr/κ or 1; max(Scys/0.8,1), maximum of Scys/0.8 or 1; min(SCr/κ,1), minimum of SCr/κ or 1; min(Scys/0.8,1), minimum of Scys/0.8 or 1; Scr, serum creatinine measured in mg/dL; Scys, standardized serum cystatin C in mg/l;

$FeNa$ = Amount of Na^+ excreted / Amount of Na^+ filtered

$= U_{Na} / (CrCl \times P_{Na})$ or $(U_{Na} \times Pcr) / (Ucr \times P_{Na})$

Similarly, the reabsorption of PO_4^{3-} can be calculated as follows:

TR_{PO4} = Amount of PO_4^{3-} reabsorbed / Amount of PO_4^{3-} filtered

= (Amount of PO_4^{3-} filtered − Amount of PO_4^{3-} excreted) / Amount of PO_4^{3-} filtered

= 1 − Amount of PO_4^{3-} excreted / Amount of PO_4^{3-} filtered

= 1 − $U_{PO4} / (CrCl \times P_{PO4})$ or 1 − $(U_{PO4} \times Pcr) / (Ucr \times P_{PO4})$

A water deprivation test is used to determine whether a patient with polyuria has underlying diabetes insipidus (DI) or other causes of polyuria. The test is designed to test the concentration ability of the collecting ducts. The patient is subject to water deprivation and their body weight, plasma, and urine osmolality are repeatedly measured. Those who fail to show an appropriate rise of urine osmolality following >3% weight loss during the test may have a concentration defect. If the urine osmolality rises after vasopressin, then the concentration ability of the collecting ducts is likely to be normal and implies a lack of ADH centrally. Patients who show no significant rise in urine osmolarity after vasopressin indicates a defective renal response to ADH (i.e. nephrogenic DI).

Tests for urinary acidification

The kidneys are responsible for removing excess acids to maintain normal acid–base balance in the body. Acidification of the urine is achieved by reabsorption of bicarbonate (HCO_3^-) in the proximal tubules and excretion of hydrogen ions in the distal tubules. Various investigations can help to establish the diagnosis and determine the type of renal tubular acidosis (RTA). Urine anion gap (UAG) is a convenient way to estimate the amount of ammonium (NH_4^+) ions in urine, and is often used as a screening test in patients with suspected RTA. The UAG is calculated by subtracting urinary Cl^- from urinary Na^+ and K^+. In patients with metabolic acidosis, the UAG is usually negative because Cl^- is excreted together with NH_4^+. Therefore, in patients with normal anion gap acidosis, a positive UAG indicates distal acidification dysfunction. Proximal and distal RTA can be further confirmed by the $NaHCO_3$ infusion or NH_4 salt loading tests respectively. In patients with proximal RTA, the infusion of $NaHCO_3$ will increase the serum

HCO_3^- concentration, urine pH and fractional excretion of HCO_3^- (> 15–20%). However, it is not usually necessary to proceed with this test if bicarbonaturia is present in spite of a low blood HCO_3^- level. Distal acidification ability is assessed by urinary pH after being challenged by an acidifying agent. The NH_4 salt loading test is used to assess distal acidification defect, but should be performed with caution in patients with severe metabolic acidosis. After administration of NH_4Cl, normal functioning distal tubules should be able to excrete excessive NH_4^+ ions, leading to a decrease in urinary pH. Unchanged urinary pH after NH_4Cl administration confirms a distal acidification defect.

Blood tests

Haematological tests

Low haemoglobin levels are often seen in CKD patients. Renal anaemia is the result of multiple factors including lack of erythropoietin, iron deficiency due to poor gut absorption, uncontrolled hyperparathyroidism, aluminium toxicity (ingestion of aluminium-containing medications), and anaemia of chronic illness secondary to chronic inflammation. The iron profile should be monitored in CKD patients, especially before and during treatment with erythropoietin-stimulating agents. Other haematological abnormalities, such as the presence of pancytopenia, eosinophilia, and fragmented red cells with thrombocytopenia, may provide a clue to the underlying causes of renal impairment.

Immunological tests

The measurement of immunological parameters can help to pinpoint the diagnosis of immune-mediated glomerular diseases (Table 2.3). Some of these immunological markers can also be used to monitor disease activity and treatment response in immune-mediated glomerulonephritis.

Blood tests for bone mineral diseases

Patients with CKD can develop a spectrum of mineral bone diseases including renal osteodystrophy as a result of secondary/tertiary hyperparathyroidism, adynamic bone disease, and osteomalacia. In this context, the bone profile (i.e. calcium, phosphate, and alkaline phosphate levels), and parathyroid hormones should be regularly monitored in CKD patients.

Table 2.3: Common immunological tests and their clinical use in renal diseases

Immunological test	Clinical utility and remarks
ANA	• Show high sensitivity for the diagnosis of SLE • May be positive in other connective tissue diseases (e.g. Sjögren syndrome or ANCA vasculitis)
Anti-dsDNA	• Shows high specificity for the diagnosis of SLE • Shows association with clinical disease activity in SLE and LN
C3 and C4	• Decreased complements raises suspicion of some forms of GN (e.g. LN, MPGN, C3 glomerulopathy, post-infectious GN) • Both C3 and C4 are depressed in active SLE patients • Low C3 with normal C4 signifies activation of alternative pathway (e.g. post-infectious GN, MPGN, C3 glomerulopathy, HUS, aHUS)
ANCA	• Associated with pauci-immune crescentic glomerulonephritis • MPO-ANCA: suggestive of microscopic polyangiitis, also present in 50% of eosinophilic granulomatosis with polyangiitis • PR3-ANCA: suggestive of granulomatosis with polyangiitis • Antibody titre correlates with disease activity, renal prognosis and risk of recurrence
Anti-GBM	• Associated with Goodpasture disease • Antibody titre correlates with disease activity, renal prognosis, and risk of recurrence
C reactive protein (CRP)	• May reflect clinical disease activity in ANCA vasculitis
Ig pattern and serum immunoelectrophoresis (SIEP)	• Serum IgA is only elevated in 50% of patients with IgAN • Monoclonal bands can be detected in multiple myeloma, monoclonal gammopathy of renal significance, and amyloidosis
Cryoglobulins	• Can be seen in MPGN associated with viral hepatitis infection or haematological disorders (e.g. B-cell lymphoproliferative disease)

aHUS, atypical haemolytic uremic syndrome; ANA, antinuclear antibodies; ANCA, antineutrophil cytoplasmic antibodies; anti-dsDNA, anti-double stranded DNA antibody; GBM, glomerular basement membrane; GN, glomerulonephritis; HUS, haemolytic uremic syndrome; IgAN, IgA nephropathy; LN, lupus nephritis; MPGN, membranoproliferative glomerulonephritis; MPO, myeloperoxidase; PR3, proteinase 3; SLE, systemic lupus erythematosus

Blood tests to screen for infections

The virology status of hepatitis B virus (HBV), hepatitis C virus (HCV), and human immunodeficiency virus (HIV) should be established in patients with suspected renal diseases. HBV, HCV, and HIV infections are associated with various forms of glomerulonephritis. HBV and HCV may reactivate and cause fulminant hepatitis in glomerulonephritic or transplant patients undergoing immunosuppressive therapy. The HBV and HCV status is also important for the allocation of kidney allografts and dialysis machines in patients requiring haemodialysis. The liver function may be abnormal in certain renal disorders (e.g. leptospirosis, hantavirus infection, or hepatorenal syndrome).

Imaging for renal diseases

Ultrasonography

Ultrasonography (US) is a simple and non-invasive imaging modality of the urinary system. US of the urinary system provides important information on the kidney size, echotexture, and the presence of renal mass and obstruction. Congenital anomalies such as solitary kidney, atrophic kidney, or horseshoe kidney can be detected by US assessment. Doppler US of renal arteries and veins can be used to detect abnormalities in the renal vasculatures (e.g. renal artery stenosis or renal vein thrombosis). The detailed applications of US assessment of the kidneys will be discussed in Chapter 21.

Computed tomography and magnetic resonance imaging scans

Non-contrast computed tomography (CT) is the gold standard for the evaluation of renal stone disease, and for assessing the level and nature of the ureteric obstruction. Either contrast CT or magnetic resonance imaging (MRI) scans can be used to evaluate and stage renal tumours. CT or MR angiography and venography are the gold standards for diagnosis of renal artery stenosis and renal vein thrombosis respectively. CT and MRI can also be used to assess the total kidney volume in patients with adult polycystic kidney disease. The applications of CT and MRI in renal diseases will be further discussed in Chapter 21.

Skeletal survey

Skeletal survey may be used to assess renal osteodystrophy in patients on dialysis. It involves X-rays of the skull, limbs, spine, pelvis, and chest.

Bone density scan

Dual-energy X-ray absorptiometry scan can be used to screen and monitor the development of steroid-induced osteoporosis in kidney transplant recipients including the treatment response to bisphosphonates. Its use in dialysis patients is limited and is not recommended.

Radionuclide renal scans

Different radio-isotopes are used in functional scan assessment of the kidneys. They are preferable to CT scans in the case of paediatric patients because of less radiation. These tests are especially useful for evaluating perfusion or drainage abnormalities of native or allograft kidneys. The most commonly used isotopes include diethyl-triamino-penta-acetic acid (DTPA), mercaptoacetyltriglycine (MAG3) and dimercaptosuccinic acid (DMSA). DTPA is exclusively filtered by the glomeruli and is used to obtain dynamic images of the kidneys. It can be used to assess perfusion, excretion, and drainage of the kidneys into the bladder. A 'perfusion index' is obtained by dividing the counts over the kidney by the counts over the iliac artery in the first 15 seconds. The differential uptakes of isotope by the two kidneys provide a basis for comparison of differential renal functions. During the drainage phase, the level of obstruction can be evaluated by the pooling of isotope. MAG3 is predominantly excreted by tubules and is not used to assess GFR. MAG3 showed a higher renal extraction ratio and better image quality than DTPA. It is the preferred tool for the assessment of renal excretory function and drainage. MAG3 scan can also be used to evaluate the effective renal plasma flow. DMSA scan is a static scan. DMSA binds to the renal tubules and is often used to evaluate focal renal scarring.

Parathyroid imaging

US and sestamibi parathyroid (MIBI) scans can help to localize parathyroid glands for renal patients that are scheduled for parathyroidectomy. Tc99m-sestamibi is selectively taken up by active parathyroid cells. It is used as a tracer in parathyroid isotope scan and is superior to US scan in identifying ectopic parathyroid tissue.

Positron emission tomography scan

Various forms of renal diseases are associated with solid organ or haematological malignancies. Positron emission tomography (PET) scan (often combined with CT scan) may be used to work up suspected cases of tumour-associated glomerulonephritis, especially in elderly patients. It may also be used to evaluate occult infections or neoplasms in dialysis or kidney transplant recipients.

Renal biopsy

Renal biopsy is necessary for the definitive diagnosis of renal parenchymal disease. Besides providing clinicians with a histological diagnosis, it also provides important information on severity, activity, chronicity, and reversibility of the disease. Percutaneous renal biopsy is commonly performed under US guidance and local anaesthesia. A CT-guided or open renal biopsy may be considered in very difficult cases. The patient should lie prone during a native kidney biopsy and in a supine position in the case of an allograft biopsy. In general, one or more cores of the renal cortex are obtained using a renal biopsy needle. Renal biopsy should be avoided in patients with bleeding tendency or uncontrolled hypertension (Table 2.4). Patients on antiplatelet agents or anticoagulation are required to discontinue these medications for a sufficient period of time before the procedure. Inability to lie flat (e.g. pulmonary oedema), large body habitus, thin renal cortex, or the presence of renal cysts are relative contraindications to kidney biopsy. A solitary kidney is not an absolute contraindication to renal biopsy, but this should only be attempted if there is a strong indication for histological diagnosis. The most common complication of renal biopsy is post-procedure bleeding, which can vary from transient haematuria to perinephric or retroperitoneal haematoma to uncontrolled haemorrhage. The patient should remain in bedrest for 24 hours after kidney biopsy to reduce the risk of bleeding. Heavy manual duties should be avoided in the subsequent four weeks. Mild haematuria post-biopsy usually resolves spontaneously. In case of uncontrolled haemorrhage, urgent imaging with embolization or even nephrectomy may be required (see Chapter 21).

The standard histological examinations of renal tissue include light microscopy (LM), immunofluorescence (IF) and electron microscopy (EM) (Table 2.5). The kidney tissues are examined under LM using different stains that reveal distinct histological features. IF studies are performed on fresh samples to detect the patterns of immunoglobulins and complements deposition on different kidney structures. EM can provide information on the presence and location of any electron-dense deposits, the structure of the basement membrane, and podocyte foot processes effacement. Special staining for C4d, SV40, PLA2R, and other virus antigen may be undertaken to aid specific diagnoses.

Table 2.4: Absolute and relative contraindications for renal biopsy

Absolute contraindications

1. Bleeding diathesis
2. Uncooperative patients
3. Uncontrolled hypertension
4. On antiplatelets or anticoagulants

Relative contraindications

1. Morbid obesity
2. Solitary kidney
3. Hydronephrosis
4. Acute pyelonephritis
5. Small kidneys
6. Large cysts or tumor

Table 2.5: The common staining methods and examinations of kidney biopsy

	Remarks
Light microscopy staining	
H&E	• A standard staining for the evaluation of general structures, cellular characteristics, and types of inflammation
PAS	• For better delineation of glomeruli, including composition of matrix and changes of basement membrane • Also useful for evaluation of arterial hyalinosis and fibrinoid necrosis
Methamine-silver	• Most useful for assessment of basement membrane (e.g. spikes)
Congo red	• Used for demonstration of renal amyloidosis
Immunofluorescence staining	• Common staining includes IgG, IgA, IgM, C1q, and C3 • Each disease entity is associated with a distinct IF staining pattern • Lambda and kappa light chains for suspected plasma cell dyscrasia
Electronic microscopy	• EM is useful to assess: (1) the presence and location of electron-dense deposits; (2) basement membrane structure and thickness; and (3) podocyte foot process effacement
Other special staining	• C4d staining for antibody-mediated rejection in kidney allografts • SV40 staining for BK virus infection in kidney allografts • Glomerular PLA2R staining for membranous nephropathy

C4d, Complement 4 degradation products; EM, electron microscopy; H&E, haematoxylin and eosin; IF, immunofluorescence; PAS, periodic acid-Schiff; PLA2R, phospholipase A2 receptor

3

Water Metabolism, Hyponatraemia, and Hypernatraemia

Gary Chan

Introduction

Water is essential for life. In a normal adult, the minimal loss of water from the body includes losses through the mucosal surfaces of respiratory and gastrointestinal tracts, perspiration from the skin, and obligatory urinary loss to excrete nitrogenous wastes. Typically, these insensible losses are often exceeded by water intake, which must be excreted to maintain water and sodium (Na^+) balance.

Water Balance

Under normal circumstances, the kidneys maintain water balance by adjusting the degree of water excretion. This is mediated by antidiuretic hormone (ADH) in the presence of an intact counter-current exchange mechanism. ADH is synthesized in the hypothalamus, stored in the posterior hypophysis, and released in response to alterations in plasma volume and osmolality. The mechanism of action and effect of ADH has been discussed in Chapter 1. Suffice to say that hypovolaemia induced non-osmotic release of ADH takes precedence over the need to maintain plasma osmolality.

Volume receptors are situated in the cardiopulmonary circulation, carotid sinuses, aortic arch, and the afferent glomerular arterioles. A low effective circulatory volume is sensed as a reduced degree of 'stretch' and promotes ADH release. In situations where the volume status of an individual is normal, ADH release becomes dictated by plasma osmolality, which is sensed by osmoreceptors located in the anterior hypothalamus. The normal plasma osmolality is held within 275–290 mOsmol/kg and values exceeding this range trigger the increased release of ADH, the amount of which is proportional to the level of hyperosmolality. Regulation of plasma volume and osmolality therefore represent two separate but inter-related homeostatic mechanisms to influence water balance.

Water Distribution

The total body water (TBW) accounts for approximately 50% and 60% of the total body weight in females and males respectively. It is distributed in two main compartments and exists as intracellular fluid (ICF) or extracellular fluid (ECF). ICF accounts for two-thirds of the TBW and the remaining is distributed extracellularly in the interstitial space, the vascular compartment, and a small transcellular compartment (i.e. cerebrospinal, synovial, pleural, pericardial, and gut fluid inside the gut). The ICF and ECF are separated by the cell membrane, which is freely permeable to water but not electrolytes. Hence, electrolytes impart an osmotic gradient across the cell membrane to affect water movement and distribution.

Na^+ salts account for the major proportion of the ECF electrolyte composition and are therefore the main determinants of ECF osmolality. Abnormalities in Na^+ concentrations are common and, as will be highlighted in this chapter, usually represent a disorder in water regulation. Where hyponatraemia is the consequence of free water accumulation, hypernatraemia represents an excess loss of water, relative to Na^+.

Hyponatraemia

Under normal circumstances, the plasma Na+ concentration is maintained between 136 and 145 mEq/L by the aforementioned regulatory mechanisms. Hyponatraemia is defined by a plasma Na+ concentration of less than 135 mEq/L and severe hyponatraemia by a value of less than 120 mEq/L. It is the most common electrolyte abnormality in hospitalized patients and correlates with patient mortality.

Clinical manifestations

The symptoms of hyponatraemia are a direct consequence of cerebral oedema. There is reduced plasma osmolality in true hyponatraemia, which produces an osmotic shift of free water into the relatively hypertonic intracellular space. In acute hyponatraemia, this process occurs more rapidly than the ability of the brain to adapt. As a consequence, cerebral oedema develops to give rise to neurological manifestations.

The earliest findings include headache, nausea, and malaise, which may be observed with a plasma Na+ concentration of 125–130 mEq/L. Delirium, seizures, and eventually coma may occur with a further drop in plasma Na+ concentration below 120 mEq/L. In chronic hyponatraemia, the brain is able to compensate by reducing intracellular osmolality and patients are usually asymptomatic. However, subtle neurological symptoms such as fatigue, dizziness, and attention deficits can manifest in the vulnerable elderly population. Seizures and coma are rare and most likely represent an acute exacerbation of underlying chronic hyponatraemia.

Diagnostic evaluation

The approach to a patient with hyponatraemia should be systematic (Figure 3.1). The following construct illustrates a systematic approach to delineate the cause of hyponatraemia.

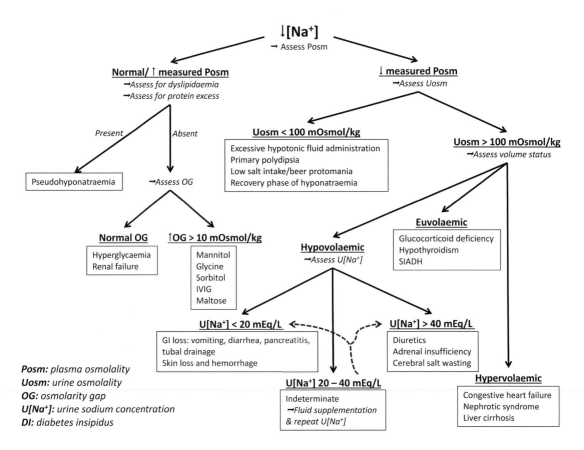

Figure 3.1: Major differential diagnoses of and approach to hyponatraemia

Step 1: Assessment of plasma osmolality

Plasma Na$^+$ concentration is the major determinant of plasma osmolality and the first step in the approach to hyponatraemia is to evaluate plasma osmolality. In patients where the plasma osmolality is normal or elevated, the cause of hyponatraemia can be logically deduced by following steps 2 and 3. One may proceed to steps 4 and 5 in cases of hypo-osmolar hyponatraemia.

Step 2: Exclusion of pseudohyponatraemia

In the clinical scenario where the measured plasma osmolality is normal, pseudohyponatraemia should first be excluded. Common causes of pseudohyponatraemia include hyperlipidaemia and hyperproteinaemia, where plasma water as a fraction of total plasma is proportionately reduced. Hence, the measured concentration of Na$^+$ in plasma water, corrected per volume of total plasma, is decreased and constitutes a laboratory artefact. This error can be avoided by measuring the plasma Na$^+$ concentration using specific Na$^+$-selective electrodes.

Step 3: Assessment for circulating osmoles

In the setting where pseudohyponatraemia has been dismissed, hyponatraemia associated with normal or elevated measured plasma osmolality points to the excess presence of an osmotically active solute within the extracellular space. These circulating osmoles draw out water from the intracellular space to dilute plasma Na$^+$ concentration while maintaining plasma osmolality. To differentiate the nature of this osmotically active solute, the osmolar gap can be evaluated.

The calculated plasma osmolality may be derived from the plasma Na$^+$, urea, and glucose concentrations by equation [A], which allows the determination of the underlying osmolar gap by equation [B]:

[A] Calculated Plasma Osmolality = (2 × Plasma [Na$^+$]) + [Urea] + [Glucose]

[B] Osmolar Gap = Measured Plasma Osmolality − Calculated Plasma Osmolality

A normal osmolar gap represents a calculated plasma osmolality that closely approximates the measured value. Both hyperglycaemia and the presence of excess urea in the extracellular space are causes of hyponatraemia without a raised osmolar gap. In hyperglycaemia, the plasma Na$^+$ concentration may be corrected by 1.6–2.4 mEq/L for each 5.5 mmol/L increase in glucose concentration, to

determine its contribution towards hyponatraemia. With raised urea concentrations in renal failure, however, the *in vitro* measurement of plasma osmolality is an inaccurate reflection of the true *in vivo* value. This is because urea is an ineffective osmole by virtue of its ability to freely equilibrate between intra- and extracellular spaces. Hyponatraemia in this setting is therefore associated with a normal *in vitro* plasma osmolality without a significant osmolar gap. However, the effective plasma osmolality, which determines intra- and extracellular water distribution, would be low and can be deduced by equation [C]:

[C] Effective Plasma Osmolality = (2 × Plasma [Na$^+$]) + [Glucose]

This concept is true of all solutes that can freely equilibrate across cellular membranes and must be accounted for to elucidate the underlying hypotonic hyponatraemia under *in vivo* conditions. Sometimes, hyponatraemia in the absence of hypo-osmolality is the result of an unmeasurable osmotically active solute. The administration of mannitol or intravenous immunoglobulin and the absorption of glycine or sorbitol used in urogynaecological procedures are potential examples. These invisible osmoles reveal themselves only via the presence of a sizeable osmolar gap on the background of a compatible history.

Step 4: Assessment of ADH activity

In hyponatraemic patients with a low measured plasma osmolality, the presence of ADH should be evaluated by measuring the urine osmolality. Under normal circumstances, individuals are able to produce dilute urine with osmolality less than 100 mOsm/kg in the absence of ADH. Therefore, in the context of hyponatraemia, the ability of the kidneys to dilute urine appropriately implicates excessive hypotonic fluid administration or primary polydipsia. Rarely, it can also be seen in extremely low dietary solute intake, such as in beer protomania. Conversely, a failure to dilute urine to less than 100 mOsm/kg suggests the elevated presence of circulating ADH. An assessment of the patient's volume status is then required, in order to delineate the primary driver of non-osmotic ADH secretion and hence hypotonic hyponatraemia (Step 5).

Step 5: Assessment of volume status

In patients with volume depletion, the necessity to maintain adequate perfusion pressure takes precedence over the regulation of plasma osmolality. In this circumstance, non-osmotic release of ADH occurs to preserve volume, resulting in hyponatraemia. There are multiple causes of hypovolaemic hyponatraemia and the assessment of urine Na^+ concentration provides a useful tool to categorize fluid loss from an extra-renal or a renal aetiology. Typically, a urine Na^+ concentration < 20 mEq/L is indicative of volume depletion from an extra-renal cause. This is on the premise that an intact renin-angiotensin system exists in the absence of advanced renal failure. However, urine Na^+ concentration > 20 mEq/L suggests volume depletion resulting from conditions rendering obligatory renal Na^+ and water loss, to cause hypovolaemic hyponatraemia. In hypervolaemic patients with low effective circulatory volumes, there is also avid water retention with hyponatraemia from non-osmotic ADH release. The most common cause of euvolaemic hyponatraemia is the syndrome of inappropriate ADH (SIADH), which results in inadequate urinary dilution. The urine Na^+ concentration is characteristically > 40 mEq/L. This syndrome is associated with a multitude of drugs, malignancies, pulmonary, and central nervous system diseases (Table 3.1). It must be remembered that SIADH is a diagnosis of exclusion since glucocorticoid deficiency and hypothyroidism may present similarly.

Table 3.1: Causes of syndrome of inappropriate antidiuretic hormone

---

Increased endogenous ADH production

   Central Nervous System disorders:
meningoencephalitis, abscess, stroke, primary or metastatic neoplasia, vasculitis, Guillain-Barré syndrome, post-transsphenoidal pituitary surgery, and head injury

   Pulmonary: pneumonia (especially those due to atypical organisms), tuberculosis, aspergillosis, abscess, pneumothorax

   Drugs: psychotropics, SSRIs, opiates, cytotoxics

   Post surgery

Ectopic ADH production

   Carcinoma: lung (small cell), duodenum, pancreas, prostate, thymus

Exogenous ADH administration

   Obstetrics: oxytocin

   Endocrine/Renal: desmopressin

   ICU: vasopressin

ADH, antidiuretic hormone; ICU, intensive care unit; SSRI, selective serotonin reuptake inhibitor

Management

Principles

The general management of hyponatraemia centres upon two important principles. Firstly, therapy should only be directed towards hyponatraemia with low plasma osmolality. Implicitly, pseudohyponatraemia must be identified in order to prevent unnecessary treatment. Secondly, correction of plasma Na^+ concentration must occur at a safe rate. Overzealous correction of hyponatraemia can result in rapid osmotic movement of water into the relatively hypertonic extracellular space. In the brain, this results in osmotic demyelination giving rise to severe and potentially irreversible neurological sequelae (e.g. central pontine myelinolysis). Henceforth, the maximum rate of plasma Na^+ correction should not exceed 8 mEq/L in a 24-hour period. In order to avoid overcorrection, a more conservative elevation of 4 to 6 mEq/L in a 24-hour period is generally recommended. For cases of acute symptomatic hyponatraemia, this 24-hour goal can be achieved earlier with hypertonic saline to abate neurological symptoms in an intensive care setting. Thereafter the plasma Na^+ level should be held at a constant level for the remainder of the 24-hour period to prevent overcorrection.

Specific management

In addition to treating the inciting aetiology, several measures can be used to treat chronic hyponatraemia, which is defined by the presence of low plasma Na^+ concentration for more than 48 hours. These specific measures are dictated by the patient's volume status. In hypovolaemic hyponatraemia, therapy is directed at correcting the volume deficit with intravenous administration of isotonic saline, which is relatively hypertonic. Moreover, it removes the non-osmotic stimulus for ADH release to facilitate renal excretion of free water.

In SIADH, the mainstay of therapy is to restrict fluid intake to counteract against impaired urinary dilution. A common mistake is to administer isotonic saline, which leads to a paradoxical lowering of plasma Na^+ concentration. If fluid must be given, the fluid osmolality must be higher than that of urine, such that obligatory water excretion is required for solute clearance. It therefore follows that NaCl supplementation can be employed to augment renal excretion of free water in SIADH. In some situations, loop diuretics can be beneficial by interfering with the renal counter-current mechanism to induce functional ADH resistance. Vasopressin receptor antagonists are an option in select cases and interferes with the effect of ADH. However, significant safety concerns arise from the side effect profile of vasopressin receptor antagonists and, more importantly, their use is associated with a risk of plasma Na^+ overcorrection.

In hypervolaemic scenarios, water removal is the principal aim of management. Salt and water restrictions in combination with diuretics are the mainstays of treatment, while vasopressin receptor antagonists may also have a role.

Hypernatraemia

Hypernatraemia is defined by a plasma Na^+ concentration greater than 145 mEq/L and severe hypernatraemia is defined by a plasma Na+ concentration greater than 160 mEq/L. It is frequently the result of excessive free water loss rather than Na^+ retention. In this situation, thirst is stimulated and ADH secretion is increased to restore water balance. Therefore, it is difficult for hypernatraemia to develop in patients with a normal mental state and an intact thirst mechanism unless access to water is prohibited or that there is a defect in urinary concentration.

Clinical manifestations

Hypernatraemia represents a hyperosmolar state, which imparts an osmotic gradient to shift water from the intracellular space to the extracellular compartment. Depending on the acuteness and severity, cellular dehydration is associated with a spectrum of neurological symptoms in the brain. The earliest symptoms include irritability, lethargy and weakness, and can progress to seizures, coma and death. Similar to chronic hyponatraemia, chronic hypernatraemia is usually asymptomatic due to brain adaptation. However, it carries an attendant risk of cerebral oedema when corrected rapidly.

Diagnostic evaluation

The approach to hypernatraemia should also be systematic. ADH release is stimulated by plasma hyperosmolality to enhance water reabsorption, which can produce a maximum urine osmolality of 800–1400 mOsmol/kg. Therefore, the cause of hypernatraemia can be categorized according to urine osmolality (Figure 3.2).

Urine osmolality greater than 800 mOsmol/kg

This indicates an adequate renal concentrating ability to suggest appropriate endogenous ADH secretion and effect. In this context, hypovolaemic hypernatraemia is the result of water loss from an extra-renal cause or, in rare cases, primary hypodipsia. This is supported by a low estimated fractional excretion of Na^+ (urine Na^+ concentration may be elevated by urinary concentration). Conversely, in hypervolaemic hypernatraemic patients, a raised urine Na^+ concentration is suggestive of excessive Na^+ administration.

Urine osmolality less than 300 mOsmol/kg

A failure to concentrate urine in the presence of hypernatraemia is indicative of diabetes insipidus (DI). Central and nephrogenic DI can be differentiated by the administration of exogenous ADH during a water deprivation test. Following administration, the urine osmolality rises concurrently with a reduction in urine volume in central DI, but not in nephrogenic DI. It is possible for polyuric individuals with cranial or nephrogenic DI to compensate by increasing water intake, such that plasma Na^+ concentration remains in the normal range.

Urine osmolality between 300 and 800 mOsmol/kg

In this scenario, urinary concentration is present but suboptimal. Osmotic diuresis can induce hypernatraemia associated with an intermediate range of urine osmolality. The cause of osmotic diuresis is most commonly due to glycosuria from hyperglycaemia or increased urea excretion in the recovery phase of acute kidney injury, and is usually evident from the clinical history. Where doubt exists, the total urinary excretion of solute can be calculated. If osmotic diuresis has been excluded, the patient should be evaluated for partial central or nephrogenic DI with exogenous ADH administration.

Reset osmostat

Endocrinopathies resulting in a state of mineralocorticoid excess, such as Cushing's syndrome and hyperaldosteronism, can manifest with mild and clinically insignificant hypernatraemia. A more typical presentation, however, is a plasma Na^+ concentration in the high–normal range with or without hypokalaemia. In these conditions, there is subclinical but persistent hypervolaemia, which resets the

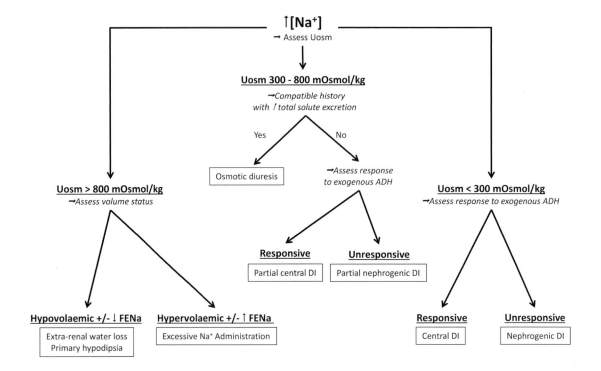

Uosm: urine osmolality
FENa: fractional excretion of sodium
DI: diabetes insipidus

Figure 3.2: Major differential diagnoses of and approach to hypernatraemia

osmostat to regulate thirst and ADH release at a higher threshold.

Management

Principles

The key consideration in the management of hypernatraemia lies in the rate of correction. Chronic hypernatraemia, defined by the presence of a raised plasma Na^+ concentration for 48 hours or more, must be reversed slowly. Rapid correction in this setting results in cerebral oedema, via a shift of water into the relatively hypertonic intracellular space, which can lead to seizures and death. It is generally recommended to lower the plasma Na^+ concentration by a rate of less than 12 mEq/L per day. Acute hypernatraemia is uncommon and occurs mainly in DI patients without access to water or from osmotic diuresis due to severe hyperglycaemia. Under these circumstances, the plasma Na^+ concentration can be lowered rapidly to achieve a near-normal level in less than 24 hours to prevent osmotic demyelination.

Specific management

Fluid administration is the mainstay of treatment for patients with hypovolaemic hypernatraemia. The water deficit to be replaced in order to lower the plasma Na^+ concentration at the target rate can be estimated by the following equation:

$$\text{Water Deficit} = TBW \times \{(\text{Current } [Na^+] - \text{Desired } [Na^+])/\text{Desired } [Na^+]\}$$

The TBW is approximately 50% and 60% of the lean body weight in women and men respectively. It is important to remember that this formula does not account for the isosmotic fluid deficit or the ongoing insensible losses, which must also be replaced. In reality, the calculated rate of replacement is only an approximation and serial measurements of plasma Na^+ concentration must be obtained to ensure the desired rate of correction is being achieved.

Central and nephrogenic DI can be acquired or congenital (Table 3.2). The underlying aetiology should be identified and reversed if possible. Where the aetiology is not rapidly correctable or the condition is irreversible, the specific treatment of DI hinges upon manipulation of the renal counter-current mechanism, as described in Chapter 1. Thiazide and potassium-sparing diuretics are commonly used, which act by inducing mild volume depletion to increase Na^+ reabsorption in the proximal tubules. This increases medullary interstitial osmolality to mediate water reabsorption at the loop of Henle, where the descending limb remains water-permeable. Importantly, loop diuretics potentiate the problem and must not be prescribed. This class of drugs would further impair the urine concentrating ability of the kidney by inhibiting the counter-current mechanism. The fixed urine osmolality of DI provides an adjunctive therapeutic option of using a low salt and protein diet. The reduction in urine output is directly proportional to the decrease in solute excretion. However, adherence to this therapeutic modality is usually suboptimal. These interventions are applicable to both central and nephrogenic DI. Additionally, exogenous ADH supplementation in the form of desmopressin can be used in central DI. However, it is prudent to remember that the resulting artificial ADH activity is no longer under physiological regulation by plasma osmolality. Therefore, the minimal dose of desmopressin required to control diuresis and permit adequate sleep is prescribed to prevent the risk of water retention and hyponatraemia.

In hypervolaemic hypernatraemic patients resulting from primary Na^+ overload, treatment involves removing excess Na^+ with the use of diuretics and preventing further Na^+ administration. Where there is inadequate renal function, Na^+ removal can only be achieved by dialysis.

Table 3.2: Causes of central and nephrogenic diabetes insipidus (DI)

Central DI	Nephrogenic DI
Hereditary	**Hereditary**
Idiopathic	**Drugs**: lithium, cidofovir, foscarnet, tolvaptan, amphotericin B, demeclocycline, ifosfamide, ofloxacin, orlistat
Malignancy: craniopharyngioma, pituitary and suprasellar tumours, secondary (lung, leukaemia, and lymphoma)	
	Electrolytes: hypercalcaemia, hypokalaemia
Infiltrative disease: histiocytosis X, sarcoidosis	**Kidney Diseases**: polycystic kidney disease, reversal of urinary obstruction, renal amyloidosis, Sjögren's syndrome
Trauma: hypoxic brain injury, head trauma, transphenoidal surgery	
Autoimmune: IgG4-related disease, granulomatosis with polyangiitis	
Other: meningo-encephalitis, post-supraventricular tachycardia, anorexia nervosa	

4

Electrolyte and Acid–Base Disorders

Lorraine Kwan, Yuk Lun Cheng, and Wai Kei Lo

Introduction

Electrolytes and acid–base disorders are important and commonly encountered clinical problems. This chapter illustrates the regulatory mechanisms of acid–base and some important electrolytes, and also highlights the pathophysiology and clinical management of their disturbances.

Regulation of Potassium by the Kidney

Potassium (K^+) is the most abundant intracellular cation. About 2% of total body K^+ is extracellular, while 98% is intracellular. The concentration difference of intracellular and extracellular K^+ is maintained by Na^+-K^+-ATPase pump in the cell membrane, and is the major determinant of the resting membrane potential and stability of excitable membranes such as cardiac and nerve tissues. The kidney is primarily responsible for K^+ homeostasis, in which 90% of the K^+ load is excreted in urine while faecal K^+ loss accounts for the remaining 10%. Around 90% of the filtered K^+ is reabsorbed in the proximal convoluted tubule and loop of Henle. K^+ secretion begins in the early distal convoluted tubule and progressively increases along the distal nephron into the cortical collecting duct. Increasing the permeability of the luminal membrane for K^+ will increase the rate of urinary K^+ secretion. This is determined by:

1. Mineralocorticoid activity: Aldosterone increases intracellular K^+ concentration by stimulating Na^+-K^+-ATPase activity in the basolateral membrane. It also promotes Na^+ reabsorption across the luminal membrane, which increases the electronegativity of the lumen, thereby augmenting the

electrical gradient favouring K^+ secretion. Lastly, aldosterone has a direct effect on the luminal membrane to enhance K^+ permeability.
2. Rate of distal delivery of Na^+ and water: Increased distal delivery of Na^+ stimulates distal Na^+ absorption, which renders the luminal potential more negative and thus enhances K^+ secretion. Increased flow rates also trigger intracellular signals to open up the maxi-K channels, thereby promoting K^+ secretion.

Renal K^+ excretion occurs over several hours; therefore, changes in extracellular K^+ concentration are initially buffered by the movement of K^+ into or out of the skeletal muscle. The influx or efflux of K^+ are influenced by: (1) insulin; (2) β-adrenergic activity; and (3) acid–base status. In this context, β2-adrenergic activity and insulin both promote K^+ uptake by stimulating Na^+-K^+-ATPase activity primarily in skeletal muscles. In metabolic acidosis, more than one-half of the excess H^+ is buffered in the cells and electroneutrality is maintained in part by efflux of intracellular K^+ into the extracellular fluid.

Hyperkalaemia

Causes of hyperkalaemia include:

1. Disorder in the internal balance of K^+ (i.e. a shift of K^+ from intracellular to extracellular compartments)
   a. Metabolic acidosis
   b. Extensive tissue breakdown (e.g. rhabdomyolysis, intravascular haemolysis, tumour lysis syndrome)
   c. Insulin deficiency

d. Hyperkalaemic periodic paralysis—an autosomal dominant disorder in which episodes of weakness or paralysis are usually precipitated by cold exposure, rest after exercise, fasting, or the ingestion of small amounts of K^+. During the episode of muscle weakness or paralysis, the release of K^+ from the muscles will cause an acute rise in the blood K^+ concentration.

2. Disorder in external balance
   a. Reduced urinary excretion
      i. Reduced aldosterone secretion (e.g. Addison's disease and hyporeninaemic hypoaldosteronism) or aldosterone hyporesponsiveness
      ii. Reduced distal Na^+ and water delivery as a result of effective blood volume depletion
      iii. Advanced renal impairment (e.g. GFR < 30 ml/min)
      iv. Drugs: K^+-sparing diuretics, angiotensin-converting enzyme inhibitors (ACEI), angiotensin-receptor blockers (ARB), non-steroidal anti-inflammatory agents, calcineurin inhibitors
   b. Excessive K^+ intake in the context of limited excretory capacity e.g. in renal failure

Clinical manifestations

The manifestations of hyperkalaemia usually occur when blood K^+ level ≥ 7 mmol/L in chronic hyperkalaemia. However, they may occur earlier if there is an acute rise in serum K^+ level. Patients may present with muscle weakness or paralysis, and cardiac arrhythmias. Early electrocardiogram (ECG) changes may show tall peaked T waves with a shortened QT interval. These are followed by the prolongation of PR interval and QRS duration, then the disappearance of P wave, and ultimately the widening of QRS complex to a sinusoidal pattern and cardiac arrest.

Evaluation of patients with hyperkalaemia

It is important to exclude pseudohyperkalaemia related to a haemolysed blood sample. A detailed dietary, drug, and family history should be elicited in patients with true hyperkalaemia. However, increase dietary K^+ alone cannot account for hyperkalaemia if there are no underlying abnormalities of aldosterone secretion or responsiveness, or renal impairment. The acid–base status should also be determined in patients with hyperkalaemia. Transtubular potassium gradient (TTKG), calculated as $\{[K^+]_{Urine} \times blood\ osmolality\} \div \{urine\ osmolality \times [K^+]_{blood}\}$, can also help differentiate between renal and extra-renal causes of hyperkalaemia. It is also important to appreciate that the measurement of TTKG should be based on the assumptions that, firstly, urine osmolality is higher than blood osmolality reflecting the presence of vasopressin activity, which is required for potassium excretion, and, secondly, urine sodium is > 25 mmol/L, which signifies adequate sodium delivery to the cortical collecting duct.

Management of hyperkalaemia

Severe hyperkalaemia is a medical emergency. Emergency treatment includes administration of intravenous calcium chloride or gluconate which stabilizes the myocardial cell membrane and reduce the risk of arrhythmia. Treatment with intravenous glucose-insulin infusion rapidly but temporarily shifts the K^+ into the intracellular space. Correction of metabolic acidosis with sodium bicarbonate can also help lower blood K^+ levels by shifting K^+ intracellularly. Definitive treatment requires removal of K^+ which can be achieved by increasing K^+ loss via the gastrointestinal tract (e.g. potassium-binding resins like sodium or calcium resonium and sodium zirconium cyclosilicate) or kidneys (e.g. intravenous loop diuretics). Haemodialysis is most effective in correcting severe hyperkalaemia, particularly in patients with oliguria or severe renal impairment.

Chronic hyperkalaemia, which mostly occurs in patients with advance chronic kidney disease, should be managed by educating the patient about a low-potassium diet, dosage adjustment or cessation of ACEI or ARB, correction of chronic metabolic acidosis, and use of oral loop diuretics or thiazides.

Hypokalaemia

Causes of hypokalaemia include:

1. Inadequate oral intake
2. Increased intracellular shift
   a. Increased availability of insulin
   b. Elevated $\beta 2$-adrenergic activity (e.g. $\beta 2$-agonist)
   c. Hypokalaemic periodic paralysis (sometimes associated with thyrotoxicosis)
   d. Increase in blood cell production (e.g. lympho- or myelo-proliferative disorder)
   e. Hypomagnesaemia (as magnesium is a cofactor of Na^+-K^+-ATPase)
3. Increased intestinal loss
   a. Small bowel diarrhoea

b. Villous adenoma of the colon (due to high K^+ content in the mucous secretion)
c. Loss from drains
d. Laxative abuse
4. Increased urinary loss
   a. Use of diuretics (thiazide and loop diuretics)
   b. Mineralocorticoid excess
      i. endogenous sources: Conn's syndrome, Cushing's syndrome, ectopic Adrenocorticotropic hormone (ACTH), renal artery stenosis (RAS)
      ii. Exogenous sources: Liquorice abuse, steroid therapy
   c. Osmotic diuresis (e.g. non-reabsorbable anion)
   d. Renal tubular acidosis (RTA) type I and II
   e. Hypomagnesaemia
   f. Amphotericin B
   g. Salt-wasting nephropathies (e.g. Bartter or Gitelman syndrome)
   h. Diuretic phase of acute tubular necrosis
   i. Protracted vomiting—metabolic alkalosis as a result of gastric acid loss, results in bicarbonaturia and increase Na^+ delivery to the distal convoluted tubules, leading to increase urinary K^+ secretion.

Clinical manifestations

Muscle weakness and even rhabdomyolysis can occur in severe hypokalaemia. Characteristic ECG changes include depressed ST segments, inverted T wave and prominent U waves. Life-threatening arrhythmias such as atrioventricular block, and ventricular tachycardia or fibrillation may also occur.

Evaluation of patients with hypokalaemia

Like in hyperkalaemia, dietary, drug, and family history should be elicited for patients with hypokalaemia. Gastrointestinal loss (e.g. vomiting, diarrhoea) should be excluded. TTKG can also be used to help distinguish between renal and extra-renal causes of hypokalaemia. Other relevant investigations include blood magnesium (Mg^{2+}) levels, acid–base status and endocrine tests (e.g. thyroid function tests, plasma renin-aldosterone, and 24-hour urine cortisol). Doppler ultrasonography can also be performed in patients with suspected RAS. Type I or II RTA should be suspected in patients with hypokalaemia in the face of normal anion gap (AG) acidosis.

Management of hypokalaemia

The goal of treatment is to prevent potentially life-threatening cardiac arrhythmia or neuromuscular disorder, then correct the underlying cause. Oral K^+ replacement is preferred for patients with mild hypokalaemia. Intravenous K^+ replacement is used for severe hypokalaemia with serum $K^+ < 2.5$ mmol/L or when ECG abnormalities are present. The standard concentration of intravenous K^+ is 20–40 mmol in 1 L of normal saline, and correction typically should not exceed 20 mmol/hour. Higher concentrations of K^+ should only be infused via a central line.

Homeostasis of Calcium and Phosphate

Calcium ions (Ca^{2+}) plays essential roles in bone formation, cardiac and neuromuscular electrical activity and contractility, blood coagulation, and cellular signalling. The level of blood Ca^{2+} has to be maintained within a very tight physiological range to ensure proper functions of various biological processes. Most intestinal Ca^{2+} absorption takes place in the upper intestine, and more than 99% of our total body Ca^{2+} is stored in the skeleton as calcium phosphate complexes, primarily as hydroxyapatite. Serum Ca^{2+} comprises free ions (~51%), protein-bound complexes (~40%), and ionic complexes (~9%). The proportion of free ionic calcium is affected by the change of pH in blood, with more ionic calcium in acidemia and vice versa. Phosphate (PO_4^{3-}) is an essential component in the formation of cell membranes and nucleic acids. It is also involved in bone formation, generation of high-energy bonds (e.g. intracellular adenosine triphosphate or ATP), metabolic pathways, and regulation of cellular functions. Ca^{2+} and PO_4^{3-} homeostasis involves an interplay between bones, intestine, and kidneys. Calcium homeostasis is regulated by: (1) parathyroid hormone (PTH) and PTH-sensing receptor (PTHR); (2) 1,25-dihydroxyvitamin D [1,25(OH)$_2$D3] and vitamin D receptor (VDR); and (3) serum-ionized calcium and calcium-sensing receptors (CaSR). A decrease in serum Ca^{2+} inactivates the CaSR in the parathyroid glands to increase PTH secretion, which acts on the PTHR in the kidneys to increase tubular Ca^{2+} reabsorption, and in the bones to increase net bone resorption. The increased PTH also stimulates 1,25(OH)$_2$D3 production by the kidneys, which in turn activates the VDR in the gut to promote Ca^{2+} absorption, decrease PTH secretion in the parathyroid glands, and increase bone resorption. The decrease in serum Ca^{2+} also deactivates the CaSR in the kidney to increase Ca^{2+} reabsorption and potentiate the effect of PTH. This integrated hormonal response restores serum Ca^{2+} and closes the negative feedback loop, which serves to maintain total serum Ca^{2+} levels in healthy individuals within a relatively narrow physiologic range.

Vitamin D3 (cholecalciferol) is primarily obtained through synthesis in the skin in the presence of ultraviolet light or through diet. Cholecalciferol is hydroxylated in the liver to form 25-hydroxyvitamin D (calcidiol, 25(OH)D3), and with further metabolism in the kidneys to become the activated form 1, 25 dihydroxycholcaliferol (calcitriol 1,25(OH)$_2$D3). 1,25(OH)$_2$D3 promotes intestinal absorption of Ca^{2+}, and bone reabsorption and renal absorption of Ca^{2+} and PO_4^{3-}. Ca^{2+} can also directly influence renal Ca^{2+} handling via CaSR signalling.

Hypercalcaemia

Causes of hypercalcaemia include:

1. Increased intestinal Ca^{2+} absorption: 1,25(OH)$_2$D3-dependent active transport accounts for the majority of gut Ca^{2+} absorption. Increased active vitamin D can be seen in sarcoidosis and granulomatous disorders, vitamin D poisoning, or excessive intake of calcitriol or its analogues.
2. Increased bone resorption: Increased net bone resorption occurs in osteoclastic metastatic bone cancer, multiple myeloma, primary hyperparathyroidism, vitamin D or A poisoning, hyperthyroidism, or prolonged immobilization. In CKD patients with adynamic bone disease, hypercalcaemia develops as a result of impaired Ca^{2+} uptake by bones.
3. Reduced urinary Ca^{2+} excretion: Urinary Ca^{2+} excretion is mainly determined by tubular calcium reabsorption and filtered Ca^{2+} load. Increased tubular reabsorption is observed in primary hyperparathyroidism, Na^+ depletion, dehydration, use of thiazide, and inactivating mutations in the CaSR. Hypercalcemia can also occur in children and patients with CKD when the input of Ca^{2+} to the circulation exceeds its removal by the kidney's filtration rate.

Clinical manifestations

Mild hypercalcaemia is usually asymptomatic. Symptoms of hypercalcaemia can be non-specific which include constipation, fatigue, nausea, or vomiting. Severe hypercalcaemia or a rapid rise in Ca^{2+} level may cause polyuria, polydipsia, anorexia, ventricular arrhythmia, and change in sensorium. Peptic ulcer disease, pancreatitis, nephrolithiasis, and tubulointerstitial disease can occur in chronic hypercalcaemia. Metastatic calcification can also be seen, especially when the PO_4^{3-} level is also high. While patients with hyperparathyroidism usually present with chronic mild hypercalcaemia which is asymptomatic, malignancy-associated hypercalcemia usually gives rise to higher Ca^{2+} levels and more symptoms.

Evaluation of patients with hypercalcaemia

Blood Ca^{2+} level should be interpreted after correction for serum albumin levels. As Ca^{2+} is highly bound to albumin, the blood calcium level is affected by the serum albumin level without a change in the ionized Ca^{2+} level. To adjust for the influence of albumin level, the formula *adjusted [Ca](mmol/L) = total [Ca](mmol/L) + 0.02 (40 − [albumin] (g/L))* is commonly used. Direct measurement of ionized Ca^{2+} level is preferred in case of severe hyper- or hypoalbuminaemia, and in the presence of significant acidemia or alkalemia. Assessment of PTH level helps differentiate between PTH-mediated and non-PTH-mediated hypercalcaemia. An elevated PTH level points towards primary hyperparathyroidism due to a single adenoma (80%) or diffuse hyperplasia (15%). Primary hyperparathyroidism may occur as part of the multiple endocrine neoplasia (MEN) syndromes. Tertiary hyperparathyroidism in renal failure patients also presents with hypercalcaemia and a high PTH level. Patients with familial hypocalciuric hypercalcemia may show PTH levels at the upper limit of normal range. A low normal or low PTH level indicates a non-PTH-mediated hypercalcaemia (e.g. osteolytic metastasis and multiple myeloma). PTH-related protein (PTHrp) and vitamin D metabolites should also be measured to identify humoral hypercalcemia of malignancy (e.g. advanced squamous cell carcinomas, or renal, bladder, breast or ovarian carcinomas) and vitamin D intoxication.

Management of hypercalcaemia

Treatment of the underlying cause and adequate hydration may suffice for patients with asymptomatic hypercalcaemia (Ca^{2+} < 3 mmol/L). For patients with mild symptoms and Ca^{2+} level 3.0–3.5 mmol/L, intravenous normal saline and bisphosphonates can be used in addition to the treatment of the underlying cause. Loop diuretics can be used to augment urinary

Ca^{2+} excretion after the fluid status has been corrected. Patients with Ca^{2+} level > 3.5 mmol/L warrant more aggressive treatment, including calcitonin to rapidly suppress Ca^{2+} levels. For malignancy-associated hypercalcaemia, Ca^{2+} levels can be lowered by bisphosphonates or denosumab (in patients with contraindications to bisphosphonates) and treatment of underlying neoplasm. Specific treatment of underlying causes (e.g. parathyroidectomy or calcimimetics for hyperparathyroidism, corticosteroids for sarcoidosis) will also improve hypercalcaemia. Acute haemodialysis with low calicum dialyzate should be considered in refractory severe hypercalcaemia, especially when there is concomitant renal failure.

Hypocalcaemia

Causes of hypocalcaemia include:

1. Decreased intestinal absorption
   a. Reduced dietary intake
   b. Malabsorption (e.g. chronic pancreatitis or intestinal resection/small bowel disease)
   c. Decreased production of 25(OH)D3—in severe liver disease
   d. Increased loss of 25(OH)D3—in nephrotic syndrome
   e. Decreased production of $1,25(OH)_2D3$—in hyperphosphataemia, renal failure or hypophosphataemic rickets
   f. Increased metabolism of vitamin D (e.g. use of anticonvulsants)
   g. End-organ resistance to $1,25(OH)_2D3$—hereditary or acquired
2. Decreased mobilization from bone
   a. Hypoparathyroidism
   b. Pseudohypoparathyroidism
   c. Hypomagnesaemia (functional hypoparathyroidism)
3. Loss of Ca^{2+} from circulation
   a. Hungry bone syndrome after parathyroidectomy
   b. Acute pancreatitis
   c. Hyperphosphataemia (e.g. tumour lysis syndrome, acute rhabdomyolysis, or chronic renal failure)
   d. Acute respiratory alkalosis
4. Drugs
   a. Calcium chelators (e.g. citrate, lactate, foscarnet)
   b. Antiresorptive agents (e.g. bisphosphonates, denosumab)

   c. Calcimimetic drugs (e.g. cinacalcet)
   d. Chemotherapeutic agents (e.g. cisplatin)

Clinical manifestations

Symptoms in acute hypocalcaemia are due to neuromuscular irritability. Paraesthesia, muscle twitching, carpopedal spasm, Trousseau's sign, or Chvostek's sign may be present. Seizure, laryngospasm, and bronchospasm can occur in severe cases. Prolonged QT interval on ECG is characteristic of hypocalcaemia. In chronic hypocalcaemia, ectopic calcification of the basal ganglia, dry skin, abnormal dentition, or brittle hair may be seen. Children with vitamin D deficiency may have muscle weakness and hypotonia, motor retardation, and stunted growth.

Evaluation of patients with hypocalcaemia

As for hypercalcaemia, correction for albumin level or obtaining an ionized calcium level is important to ensure there is true hypocalcaemia. The family, drug and surgical history, physical findings, renal and liver function tests, alkaline phosphatase (ALP), PO_4^{3-} and Mg^{2+} levels, serum PTH and vitamin D levels, and urinary calcium may give hints to underlying aetiology. PTH and ALP are elevated in hypocalcaemia due to chronic kidney disease, vitamin D deficiency, and pseudohypoparathyroidism. A low or inappropriately normal PTH points towards hypoparathyroidism. PTH is also low or low normal in hypomagnesemia.

Management of hypocalcaemia

Oral calcium supplement can be used to correct hypocalcaemia, and vitamin D should also be added in patients with evidence of vitamin D deficiency. In case of symptomatic or severe hypocalcaemia, intravenous calcium (in the form of calcium gluconate or $CaCl_2$) should be administered. One should be careful in administering intravenous calcium as extravasation of calcium can result in severe tissue necrosis, especially when $CaCl_2$ is used for its higher calcium content. Hypomagnesemia, if present, should also be corrected. Calcium supplement and $1,25(OH)_2D3$ should be prescribed together in patients with hypoparathyroidism. In patients with CKD, $1,25(OH)_2D3$ should be given while in patients with liver disease the use of 25(OH)D3 may suffice.

Hypophosphataemia

Causes of hypophosphataemia include:

1. Redistribution of PO_4^{3-} from the extracellular fluid into cells
   a. Stimulation of glycolysis by the administration of glucose or insulin (e.g. refeeding syndrome, during treatment of diabetic ketoacidosis, administration of dextrose-containing intravenous fluid to hospitalized alcoholics)
   b. Hungry bone syndrome after parathyroidectomy
   c. Acute respiratory alkalosis
2. Decreased intestinal absorption of phosphate
   a. Prolonged parenteral nutrition (poor oral intake alone usually does not cause significant hypophosphataemia as PO_4^{3-} is abundant in most food)
   b. Use of aluminium or magnesium-based antacids or PO_4^{3-} binders
   c. Malabsorption, severe steatorrhoea or chronic diarrhoea
3. Increased urinary phosphate excretion
   a. Primary hyperparathyroidism
   b. Secondary hyperparathyroidism (e.g. in post-renal transplant patients when PTH act on the graft kidney)
   c. Vitamin D deficiency or resistance
   d. Primary renal PO_4^{3-} wasting e.g. X-linked hypophosphataemic rickets
   e. Proximal renal tubular defects (e.g. Fanconi's syndrome)
4. Excessive removal by intensive dialysis

Clinical manifestations

Symptoms usually occur when serum PO_4^{3-} level falls below 0.6 mmol/L. The symptoms are attributed to intracellular PO_4^{3-} depletion, leading to firstly, a fall in red cell 2,3-diphosphoglycerate levels, thereby increasing haemoglobin affinity for oxygen to cause tissue hypoxia. Secondly, the fall in ATP levels leads to impaired cellular functions that are dependent upon energy-rich PO_4^{3-} compounds. Neuromuscular manifestations include proximal myopathy, dysphagia, and ileus. Rhabdomyolysis can ensue in severe cases. Metabolic encephalopathy can manifest as irritability, paraesthesia, or even seizure. Hypercalciuria may be present as a result of an increase in Ca^{2+} load due to increased 1,25-$(OH)_2$D3 synthesis. Osteomalacia and pathological fracture are also complications of chronic hypophosphataemia.

Evaluation of patients with hypophosphataemia

As in other electrolyte disturbances, a careful dietary, drug, and family history should be obtained. A 24-hour urinary PO_4^{3-} excretion $\geq$ 3.2 mmol or a fractional excretion of phosphate (FE_{PO4}) $\geq$ 5% indicates renal PO_4^{3-} wasting. Other useful investigations include levels of Ca^{2+}, PTH, ALP, and vitamin D. In patients with hypokalaemia and normal AG acidosis, the urine glucose, amino acids, and PO_4^{3-} levels should be measured to identify possible proximal renal tubular disorders (Fanconi syndrome).

Management of hypophosphataemia

PO_4^{3-} level should be monitored and replacement given in situations when hypophosphataemia is anticipated. Concomitant vitamin D deficiency should also be treated. Mild hypophosphataemia can be managed by oral PO_4^{3-} supplementation, while severe symptomatic hypophosphataemia should be treated with intravenous KH_2PO4 solution until serum PO_4^{3-} level reaches $\geq$ 0.6 mmol/L.

Hyperphosphataemia

The serum PO_4^{3-} concentration is highly dependent on renal PO_4^{3-} excretion. The kidneys exhibit good capacity to excrete PO_4^{3-}, and thus hyperphosphataemia is usually seen in patients with severe renal impairment (e.g. eGFR < 15 ml/min).

Other causes of hyperphosphataemia include:

1. Increased release of intracellular PO_4^{3-} from cell breakdown (e.g. tumour lysis syndrome, rhabdomyolysis) and hypercatabolic state, especially when there is concomitant renal failure
2. An acute PO_4^{3-} load (e.g. laxatives containing PO_4^{3-}) that exceeds the renal excretory capacity
3. Hypoparathyroidism may give rise to mild hyperphosphataemia due to an increase in tubular PO_4^{3-} reabsorption

Management

Acute hyperphosphataemia may lead to metastatic calcification, especially when the Ca^{2+} level is also high. However, the main risk with hyperphosphataemia is severe hypocalcaemia as a response to the acute rise in PO_4^{3-} level, and therefore treatment should aim to correct hypocalcaemia. Saline infusion helps to increase PO_4^{3-} excretion. In patients with normal renal function, the PO_4^{3-} level will normalize within 6–12 hours. The management of chronic hyperphosphataemia in patients with CKD and ESRD will be discussed in Chapter 15.

Acid–Base Homeostasis

Acid–base homeostasis and pH regulation are critical for both normal physiology and cell metabolism and function. Normally, systemic acid–base balance is well regulated with arterial pH between 7.36 and 7.44, and the intracellular pH is usually approximately 7.2. An acid is a substance that releases hydrogen ions (H^+) on dissociation in solution (e.g. HCl, H_2CO_3, $NH4^+$ and $H_2PO_4^-$) whereas a base is a substance that in solution accepts H^+ ions (e.g. Cl^-, HCO_3^-, NH_3 and HPO_4^{2-}). Food and cellular metabolism result in net acid production. Acid–base balance is maintained by: (1) chemical buffering; (2) respiratory response; and (3) kidney response.

1. Buffer system

A buffer is made up of a weak acid and its conjugate base. Intracellular and extracellular buffers provide an immediate response to acid–base disturbances, minimizing changes in pH. Important buffer systems include H_2CO_3/HCO_3^-, H_2PO/HPO_4^{2-} and $H/Protein^-$ systems. The relationship between the pH of a buffer system and the concentration of its components is described by the Henderson–Hasselbalch equation:

$$pH = PKa + log\left(\frac{[anion]}{[weak\ acid]}\right)$$

where pKa is the dissociation constant of the weak acid.

The most important buffer system is the HCO_3^-/CO_2 buffer system catalysed by carbonic anhydrase.

$$H^+ + HCO_3^- \Leftrightarrow H_2CO_3 \Leftrightarrow CO_2 + H_2O \text{ (Equation 1)}$$

The Henderson–Hasselbalch equation for this process is:

$$pH = pKa + log[HCO_3^-]/0.03 \times pCO_2,$$

where pKa = 6.1, HCO_3 is in mmol/L, and pCO_2 is in mmHg

CO_2 concentrations can be regulated by pulmonary ventilation, and H^+ and HCO_3^- concentrations can be finely regulated by renal excretion.

2. Respiratory response

The respiratory system contributes to the balance of acids and bases in the body by regulating the blood levels of carbonic acid. Cellular metabolism produces CO_2. This stimulates the respiratory chemoreceptors to increase alveolar ventilation by increasing the depth of breathing and respiratory rate, thus removing CO_2 and driving equation 1 to the right. The respiratory centre is also stimulated by hypercapnoea, acidaemia, and hypoxia.

3. Renal response

The renal system controls serum pH via two mechanisms (see also Chapter 1):

a. Reabsorption of filtered HCO_3^- (up to 4,000–5,000 mmol/day)
b. Excretion of fixed acids (70–100 mmol/day)

The proximal convoluted tubule is responsible for reabsorbing HCO_3^- which is freely filtered at the glomerulus, and the production of ammonium (NH_4^+). Approximately 85–90% of the filtered HCO_3^- is reabsorbed by the proximal tubule. Filtered HCO_3^- combines with secreted H^+ to generate H_2CO_3. Carbonic anhydrase located at the brush border of the proximal tubular cells dissociates H_2CO_3 to produce CO_2 and H_2O. The CO_2, being lipid-soluble, crosses into the cytoplasm of the proximal tubular cell where it combines with OH^- to produce HCO_3^- and H^+. H^+ is excreted via the Na^+/H^+ antitransporter, while the HCO_3^- crosses the basolateral membrane via a Na^+/HCO_3^- symporter to enter the peritubular capillary blood. Reabsorption of HCO_3^- is affected by the luminal flow rate and concentration of HCO_3^-, arterial pCO_2 and angiotensin II via a decrease in cyclic AMP.

The excretion of H^+ as ammonium (NH_4^+) constitutes the major renal adaptive response to an acid load. The rate of NH_4^+ production and excretion can be regulated in response to physiological needs. NH_4^+ is produced from glutamine, which enters the cell from the peritubular capillaries (80%) and the filtrate (20%). Metabolism of glutamine via glutaminase generates two NH_4^+ and two HCO_3^-. Most of the NH_4^+ produced is removed from the tubular fluid into the medullary interstitium, and the NH_4^+ level in the distal convoluted tubular fluid is low. At the collecting tubules, the lipid-soluble ammonia (NH_3) passively diffuses from the medulla into the lumen and combines with secreted H^+ to form NH_4^+. NH_4^+ is lipid insoluble and is excreted in the urine.

Table 4.1: Changes in metabolic parameters in different acid–base disorders

	Respiratory		Metabolic	
	Acidosis	Alkalosis	Acidosis	Alkalosis
pCO_2	↑↑ (primary)	↓↓ (primary)	↓ (compensatory)	↑ (compensatory)
Blood HCO_3^-	↑ (compensatory)	↓ (compensatory)	↓↓ (primary)	↑↑ (primary)
pH	±↓	±↑	±↓	±↑
Urinary electrolytes	Sodium retention	Natriuresis	↑ in titratable acid + NH_4^+	Kaliuresis

Some weak acids (titratable acids) filtered at the glomeruli act as buffers to facilitate H^+ excretion in the distal tubules. Dibasic phosphate (HPO_4^{2-}) is the main buffer, followed by creatinine and urate. Their contribution to buffering 10–40 mmol H^+/day remains small. Disturbance in acid–base balance can be in the form of acidosis or alkalosis, the aetiology being respiratory or metabolic. The systemic pH can usually be maintained within a normal range at the initiation of acidosis or alkalosis because of compensatory mechanisms. However, if these conditions are left unopposed, the pH will deviate from the normal range, resulting in acidaemia (pH < 7.35) or alkalaemia (pH >7.45). The key changes in metabolic parameters are summarized in Table 4.1.

Respiratory Acidosis

Respiratory acidosis occurs when the rate of CO_2 production is greater than its removal by alveolar ventilation. A primary increase in pCO_2 above 6 kPa results in respiratory acidosis. This can be caused by an increase in CO_2 production or, more frequently, a decrease in CO_2 removal.

Metabolism of fat and carbohydrates lead to the production of a large amount of CO_2. Systemic pH decreases when CO_2 accumulates. The initial response to acute respiratory acidosis is buffered by plasma protein (cellular buffering), which occurs over minutes to hours. Cellular buffering leads to a mild rise in plasma HCO_3^-, around 1 mmol/L for each 1.3 kPa rise in pCO_2. In chronic respiratory acidosis, renal compensation sets in, and occurs over 2–3 days. Urinary excretion of H^+, in the form of $NH_4^{+,}$ is increased, and so is the reabsorption of HCO_3^-.

In acute respiratory acidosis, pCO_2 is high, with accompanying acidemia (pH < 7.35). In chronic respiratory acidosis, pCO_2 is high, but serum pH is near-normal due to renal compensation, and there is an elevated serum HCO_3^- (Table 4.1). Common causes of primary respiratory acidosis are listed in Table 4.2.

Table 4.2: Causes of primary respiratory acidosis

Increase in CO_2 production
- High carbohydrate diet with constant mechanical ventilation
- CO_2 insufflation during endoscopic procedures

Decrease in CO_2 removal
- Pulmonary disease
  - Asthma
  - Chronic obstructive airway disease
  - Pulmonary fibrosis
- Mechanical ventilation defect
  - Pneumothorax
  - Haemothorax/hydrothorax
  - Adult respiratory disease syndrome
  - Muscular or neuromuscular disease (e.g. Guillain–Barre syndrome)
- Defect in respiratory drive
  - Brainstem infarct
  - Sleep apnoea
  - Drugs (opiates and sedatives)
- Others
  - Cardiac arrest
  - Shock
  - Severe pulmonary oedema
  - Massive pulmonary embolism

Respiratory Alkalosis

Respiratory alkalosis occurs when alveolar ventilation removes CO_2 faster than its production from tissue metabolism. As in respiratory acidosis, the initial compensatory response is by cellular buffering. Blood HCO_3^- concentration decreases by 2 mmol/L for every 1.3 kPa fall in pCO_2. Renal compensation takes place in the chronic phase, and is completed within 48 hours. It is characterized by bicarbonaturia, natriuresis, and decreased NH_4^+ and titratable net acid excretion. Blood HCO_3^- concentration is decreased 4 mmol/L below 24 mmol/L for every 1.3 kPa decrease below 5 kPa in pCO_2. Common causes of primary respiratory alkalosis are listed in Table 4.3.

Metabolic Alkalosis

Metabolic alkalosis results from a primary rise in serum HCO_3^-, leading to a rise in arterial pH. Two factors need to be present simultaneously for metabolic alkalosis to be persistent:

1. A process that increases plasma HCO_3^- concentration
2. A process that prevents the excretion of excess HCO_3^- in the urine

A rise in plasma HCO_3^- concentration can be caused by an intracellular shift of H^+, gastrointestinal H^+ loss, excessive H^+ loss from the kidney, administration and retention of HCO_3^- or volume contraction in the face of a constant amount of extracellular HCO_3^-. Gastrointestinal and renal loss of H^+ is usually accompanied by Cl^- and K^+ loss, hence hypochloraemia and hypokalaemia are common features. Metabolic alkalosis results in bicarbonaturia, excreting the excess HCO_3^- in urine. The alkalosis can only persist if the ability to excrete excess HCO_3^- is impaired. The most common cause of impaired urinary HCO_3^- excretion is reduced effective arterial blood volume (Table 4.4).

Other causes include Cl^- depletion and hypokalaemia, both leading to increased renal reabsorption of HCO_3^- and reduced glomerular filtration rate or hyperaldosteronism. Extra-renal loss of acid can be caused by vomiting or high output from nasogastric tubes. Loop and thiazide diuretics increase distal Na^+ and water delivery, and also stimulate the release of renin, which, as a result, increase angiotensin and

Table 4.3: Causes of primary respiratory alkalosis

Increased central nervous system respiratory drive
- Anxiety
- Brain injury/trauma
- Sepsis, fever
- Drugs (salicylate, nicotine, doxapram)
- Tissue hypoxia
- Severe anaemia
- High altitude
- Cyanotic heart disease
- Pneumonia

Iatrogenic
- Mechanical ventilation

Table 4.4: Causes of metabolic alkalosis and their relationship with fluid status and urine [Cl^-]

Low spot urine [Cl^-] (< 20 mmol/L)
*Usually hypotensive or normal blood pressure
*Generally chloride (saline) responsive

- Gastrointestinal hydrogen loss
- Vomiting or nasogastric suction
- Congenital chloride diarrhoea (congenital chloridorrhea)

- Severe hypokalaemia causing both intracellular hydrogen shift and renal hydrogen excretion
- Villous adenoma (may manifest metabolic alkalosis, metabolic acidosis, or both)
- Laxative abuse (may manifest metabolic alkalosis, metabolic acidosis, or both)
- Cystic fibrosis

- Renal hydrogen ion loss
- Status post chronic hypercarbia
- Loop or thiazide diuretics—remote treatment (effect has dissipated)

- Alkali administration with reduced renal function
- Calcium–alkali syndrome (related to ingestion of excessive Ca^{2+} in conjunction with absorbable alkali)
- Bicarbonate ingestion/infusion with impaired renal function

High spot urine [Cl^-] (>20 mmol/L)
*Generally chloride (saline) unresponsive

Hypertensive	*Hypotensive or Normotensive*
• Primary mineralocorticoid excess (primary hyperaldosteronism, Cushing syndrome [usually associated with ectopic ACTH] exogenous mineralocorticoids) • Mineralocorticoid excess-like states • Liquorice ingestion • Liddle syndrome	• Bartter or Gitelman syndrome leading to excess renal hydrogen loss • Loop or thiazide diuretics—recent treatment (effect persists)

aldosterone levels. Urinary H^+ and K^+ secretion are enhanced, resulting in metabolic alkalosis. A patient's volume status and urinary Cl^- level are useful in differentiating different causes of metabolic alkalosis. A high spot urine K^+ level also points towards a renal cause.

Metabolic Acidosis

Metabolic acidosis occurs when there is a primary increase in the concentration of H^+ with reduced HCO_3^- concentration in the body. The pH of the patient may be low, high, or normal, depending on the coexistence of other acid–base disorders. It can be a result of increased H^+ input from dietary sources or from anaerobic tissue metabolism, loss of HCO_3^- or reduced renal acid excretion. In metabolic acidosis, respiratory compensation via increased alveolar ventilation decreases plasma pCO_2. This takes place within 30 minutes and completes in 12 to 24 hours. The kidney responds by increasing its H^+ secretory capacity. Increased reabsorption of HCO_3^- at the proximal tubules facilitates the H^+ secreted by distal tubules to be titrated against other buffers such as NH_3 and PO_4^{3-}. There may be increased K^+ excretion. That said, hyperkalaemia is frequent in metabolic acidosis due to the shift of intracellular K^+ to extracellular space. With acute acidosis due to mineral acids, for each decrease in pH of 0.1 pH units, plasma K^+ is expected to increase by 0.6 mmol/L. However, this does not occur with organic acid-induced acidosis. Metabolic acidosis can be classified into high AG metabolic acidosis and normal AG metabolic acidosis.

Anion gap

Anion gap is the difference between measured cations (Na^+) and anions (Cl^-, HCO_3^-) in serum, plasma, or urine.

Serum AG = $[Na^+]-[Cl^-]-[HCO_3^-]$

where [Na] = serum Na^+ concentration; $[Cl^-]$ = serum Cl concentration and $[HCO_3^-]$ = serum HCO_3^- concentration

The normal AG is 12±2 mmol/L. The AG reflects the difference between the concentration of 'unmeasured' cations and anions. Unmeasured cations include gammaglobulins, Ca^{2+}, Mg^{2+}, and K^+. The unmeasured anions include albumin, PO_4^{3-}, SO_4^{3-}, lactates, and other organic anions. Albumin normally constitutes most of the AG, and for every 10g /L decrease in serum albumin, the AG is reduced by 2.5 mmol/L. An increase in AG indicates the presence of unidentified anions.

High AG metabolic acidosis

High AG metabolic acidosis is caused by increased acid production or ingestion of acids (Table 4.5).

Table 4.5: Causes of high anion gap metabolic acidosis

Lactic acidosis

Type A
- Increase oxygen demand
  - Seizure
  - Vigorous exercise
- Decrease tissue oxygenation
  - Severe hypoxaemia/shock
  - Sepsis
  - Low cardiac output
  - Carbon monoxide poisoning
  - Cyanide intoxication

Type B
- Malignancy
- Diabetes Mellitus
- Liver failure
- Renal failure
- Hereditary/enzyme defect in glucose metabolism

Ketoacidosis
- Diabetes Mellitus (especially type 1)
- Starvation
- Alcohol

Toxin ingestion
- Methanol
- Ethylene glycol
- Toluene
- Salicylate
- Paraldehyde
- Acetaminophen

Uraemia
- Retention of acid load from protein metabolism (e.g. PO_4^{3-}, SO_4^{2-}, and urate)

Lactic acidosis

Lactic acidosis is usually caused by accumulation of L-Lactic acid which is derived from glucose metabolism via the glycolytic pathway. It is then oxidized to CO_2 and water, and is also used to generate glucose. Utilization primarily occurs in the liver, but also takes place in the kidneys, heart, and other tissue. Increased production or diminished utilization leads to lactic acidosis. Causes of L-lactic acidosis are classified as type A, which is due to reduced tissue oxygenation, and type B, which is due to toxin-induced impairment of cellular metabolism and regional ischemia. L-lactate is usually generated as a result of hypoxia. D-lactate acidosis can occur in patients with short bowel syndrome when the altered bowel flora metabolize starch and glucose to D-lactate.

Ketoacidosis

The most dominant acid in patients with ketoacidosis is beta-hydroxybutyric acid. Uncontrolled diabetes mellitus is the most common cause of ketoacidosis. Insulin deficiency stimulates increased lipolysis, and the free fatty acids are metabolized into ketoacids. Alcoholic ketoacidosis usually occur in malnourished patients with chronic alcoholism and a history of recent binge drinking. Hepatic generation of ketone bodies from fatty acid oxidation occurs in the setting of low insulin and high glucagon (i.e. during fasting or low carbohydrates intake). Ethanol withdrawal in alcoholics increases the level of catecholamine and cortisol, and amplifies the hormonal response to fasting, leading to enhanced lipolysis.

Salicylate overdose

Aspirin, acetylsalicylic acid, is converted to salicylic acid in the body. Excess of salicylic acid interferes with cellular metabolism (e.g. Kreb cycle), leading to accumulation of organic acids and hence high AG metabolic acidosis. Of note, salicylic acid also stimulates the respiratory centre at the medulla, resulting in hyperventilation and respiratory alkalosis.

Normal AG metabolic acidosis

Normal AG metabolic acidosis is frequently caused by processes leading to HCO_3^- loss or reduction in renal H^+ excretion (Table 4.6). With the loss of HCO_3^-, Cl^- is retained to maintain the electric neutrality, resulting in hyperchloraemia.

Gastrointestinal bicarbonate loss

In gastrointestinal HCO_3^- loss, there is a compensatory increase in renal NaCl reabsorption to maintain intravascular volume, thus resulting in normal AG acidosis.

Renal tubular acidosis

RTA is a group of disorder characterized by the development of normal AG metabolic acidosis despite a

Table 4.6: Causes of normal anion gap metabolic acidosis

Bicarbonate loss
- Gastrointestinal: diarrhoea, ileostomy, ureterosigmoidostomy, and pancreatic or biliary drainage
- Renal: Proximal (Type 2) RTA, post-chronic hypocapnia

Impaired renal acid excretion
- With hypokalaemia—Distal (Type 1) RTA
- With hyperkalaemia—Hypoaldosteronism (Type 4) RTA
- Impaired renal perfusion

Administration of chloride-containing acids
- NH_4Cl, HCl, Total parenteral nutrition

Administration of chloride-containing salts (oral administration)
- $CaCl_2$, $MgCl_2$, chloride containing anion exchange resins (cholestyramine)

Medications
- Acetazolamide (increase renal HCO_3^- loss)
- Amiloride (decrease renal acid excretion)

RTA, renal tubular acidosis

relatively preserved glomerular filtration rate. This is due to a net retention of H^+, or a net loss of Na^+ and HCO_3^-. There are different types of RTA, each with distinct clinical associations and electrolyte abnormalities (Table 4.7).

1. **Type 1—Distal RTA**
   There is impaired H^+ excretion in the collecting duct. The defect may be due to decreased activity of proton pumps in the distal nephrons or increased H^+ permeability of the luminal membrane. In distal RTA, patients cannot acidify their urine to a pH of below 5.3. Hypokalaemia is commonly present. Patients are also hypercalciuric and often develop renal stones (calcium phosphate stones). Type 1 RTA can be familial or idiopathic, but secondary causes have to be excluded (Table 4.7).

2. **Type 2—Proximal RTA**
   In proximal RTA, there is a reduced proximal HCO_3^- resorptive capacity, leading to HCO_3^- wasting until the serum HCO_3^- concentration has fallen to a level low enough to allow all filtered HCO_3^- to be reabsorbed. Fanconi syndrome describes the condition when there is a concomitant reduction in reabsorption of PO_4^{3-}, glucose, uric acid, and amino acids. Urine pH is variable in proximal RTA. In untreated proximal RTA, when serum HCO_3^- level falls below the capacity for the tubules to reabsorb HCO_3^-, urine can be acidified and pH

Table 4.7: Common clinical conditions that are associated with different types of renal tubular acidosis

Type 1 RTA	Type 2 RTA	Type 3 RTA	Type 4 RTA
• Autoimmune disorders: Sjogren's syndrome, RA, SLE	• Familial: e.g. cystinosis and Wilson disease	• Marble bone disease (congenital carbonic anhydrase deficiency)	• Hyporeninaemic hypoaldosteronism (Diabetic nephropathy, NSAIDs, CNI)
• Hypercalciuria: hyperparathyroidism, vitamin D intoxication, sarcoidosis	• Amyloidosis, multiple myeloma	• Topiramate misuse	• Hyper-reninaemic hypoaldosteronism (RAS blockers)
• Medications: Ifosfamide, amphotericin B, lithium, ibuprofen	• Drugs: ifosfamide, tenofovir, carbonic anhydrase inhibitor, aminoglycosides, cisplatin		• Primary adrenal insufficiency
• Toxin: Toluene (glue sniffing)	• Heavy metal: lead, cadmium, mercury, copper		• Aldosterone resistance Potassium sparing diuretics, and antibiotics like trimethoprim and pentamadine
• Others: Medullary sponge kidney, obstructive uropathy, Wilson disease, renal transplant rejection	• Others: vitamin D deficiency, PNH or Sjogren syndrome (less common)		

CNI, calcineurin inhibitor; NSAIDs, non-steroidal anti-inflammatory drugs; PNH, paroxysmal nocturnal haemoglobinuria; RA, rheumatoid arthritis; RAS, renin-angiotensin system; RTA, renal tubular acidosis; SLE, systemic lupus erythematosus

will then be < 5. However, with alkali loading, the tubules cannot reabsorb HCO_3^-, and urine pH will be inappropriately elevated.

To distinguish Type 1 (distal) and type 2 (proximal) RTA, a $NaHCO_3$ infusion test is done to raise the serum HCO_3^- concentration to 18–20 mmol/L. Urine pH and fractional excretion of HCO_3^- ($FEHCO_3^-$) are calculated.

	Urine pH after $NaHCO_3$ infusion	$FEHCO_3^-$
Type 1 RTA	No change	< 3%
Type 2 RTA	> 7.5	> 15–20%

RTA, renal tubular acidosis

3. **Type 3—Combined proximal and distal RTA**
   Type 3 is a rare clinical entity that shares features of proximal and distal RTA.
4. **Type 4—Hypoaldosteronism RTA**
   Type 4 RTA occurs when there is a low aldosterone level, or when the distal renal tubules do not respond to aldosterone. Typically, patients present with hyperkalaemia associated with mild metabolic acidosis which is a result of decreased urinary NH_4^+ excretion.

Evaluation of Patient with Acid–Base Disorder

Step 1

Careful *history taking* is important. Drug history, and gastrointestinal symptoms must be clarified. Assessment of fluid status is a must in a physical examination. Volume contraction is a potent stimulus for the maintenance of metabolic alkalosis. Cyanosis, a bounding pulse, and warm extremities are features of respiratory acidosis. Tetany is frequent in respiratory alkalosis; whereas deep, laboured breathing (Kussmaul breathing) is typical of severe metabolic acidosis.

Step 2

Arterial blood gas and electrolytes panels aid diagnosis of the nature and causes of acid–base disorders. A blood and urine toxicology screen is often helpful in patients with severe acid–base disturbances, especially in patients with metabolic acidosis. Acidaemia with high partial pressure of CO_2 ($PaCO_2$) indicates respiratory acidosis. In acute respiratory acidosis, serum HCO_3^- rises about 1 mmol/L per 1.3 kPa rise of $PaCO_2$. When chronic respiratory acidosis develops after a few days, with the kidney generates more HCO_3^-, serum HCO_3^- increases about 3 mmol/L per 1.3 kPa rise in $PaCO_2$. A low pH with low $PaCO_2$ points towards metabolic acidosis. In pure metabolic acidosis, $PaCO_2$ decreases by 0.13 kPa with every 1 mmol/L drop in serum HCO_3^-.

Alkalaemia accompanied by a low $PaCO_2$ suggests respiratory alkalosis. There will be a fall in HCO_3^- of 2 mmol/L per 1.3 kPa fall in $PaCO_2$. In the chronic phase, there will be a 4 mmol/L drop in serum bicarbonate for each 1.3 kPa decrease in $PaCO_2$. In metabolic alkalosis, each mmol/L increase in HCO_3^- leads to a 0.1 kPa rise in $PaCO_2$.

Step 3

After identifying the primary abnormality, one should *compare the observed compensatory response with the anticipated response* and determine if there are mixed acid–base abnormalities. For every 1.3 kPa change in $PaCO_2$, pH changes by 0.08 (in the opposite direction of the change in $PaCO_2$) if the process is acute, and by 0.03 if the process is chronic.

Plasma HCO_3^- rarely falls below 15 mmol/L as a result of compensation for respiratory alkalosis and rarely exceeds 45 mmol/L as a result of compensation for respiratory acidosis.

Respiratory acidosis

➤ Compensatory increase in HCO_3^- per 1.3 kPa rise in $PaCO_2$
  • < 1 mmol/L → additional metabolic acidosis
  • > 5 mmol/L → additional metabolic alkalosis

Metabolic acidosis

➤ Expected $PaCO_2$ (in kPa) = (1.5 × [HCO_3^- (in mmol/L)]+8) × 0.133 ± 0.3 (Winters' formula)
  • If higher → additional respiratory acidosis
  • If lower → additional respiratory alkalosis

Respiratory alkalosis

➤ Compensatory decrease in HCO_3^- per 1.3 kPa fall in $PaCO_2$
  • > 5 mmol/L → additional metabolic acidosis
  • < 2 mmol/L → additional metabolic alkalosis

Metabolic alkalosis

➤ Expected $PaCO_2$ (in kPa) = [0.7 × ([HCO_3^-] - 24) + 40] × 0.133 ± 0.3
  • If higher → additional respiratory acidosis
  • If lower → additional respiratory alkalosis

Step 4

Calculation of serum *AG* helps to identify the presence of primary metabolic acidosis. Normal AG is 12±2 mmol/L; an increase reflects an excessive accumulation of unmeasured acid anions such as acetoacetate and lactate. AG of > 20 signifies that AG metabolic acidosis must be present and this is always a primary abnormality. When the AG increases in magnitude as a result of metabolic acidosis, that increase should be compared with the magnitude of the fall in HCO_3. A fall in HCO_3^- smaller than expected suggests mixed metabolic acidosis and alkalosis.

Urine pH, urine anion gap (UAG), and urine osmolal gap (UOG) are also very helpful in delineating the causes of acid–base abnormalities. The usual renal response to metabolic acidosis is a reduction of urinary pH. However, in distal RTA, and metabolic acidosis due to chronic diarrhoea, urinary pH is persistently above 5.5. Their key difference is the high urine ammonium (NH_4^+) level with diarrhoea, but a low level with distal RTA. Measurement of urine UAG and UOG provides an estimate of urinary ammonium (NH_4^+) excretion. UAG is calculated from Urine (Na + K – Cl); whereas UOG is represented by the formula *Measured urine osmolality – [2 × (Urine Na+ Urine K) + Urine urea)]*. A positive UAG or UOG < 150 mmol/kg is indicative of low or normal NH_4^+ excretion, pointing towards distal RTA; whereas a negative UAG or UOG > 400 mmol/kg represents increased NH_4^+ excretion, as seen in metabolic acidosis related to chronic diarrhoea.

Step 5

Serum chloride level is also helpful. In the presence of hyperchloraemic metabolic acidosis, when the increase in plasma Cl^- is out of proportion with the decrease in serum HCO_3^-, there is coexisting metabolic alkalosis. In primary metabolic alkalosis, if the decrease in plasma Cl^- is much greater than the increase in serum HCO_3^-, concomitant metabolic acidosis present.

Common scenarios of mixed acid–base disorder

1. Respiratory and metabolic acidosis
   • Patients with acute cardiopulmonary emergencies. Acute hypercapnia from respiratory failure and lactic acidosis from cardiac arrest result in extreme acidaemia.

2. Respiratory alkalosis and metabolic alkalosis
   - Patients with chronic liver disease given diuretics for ascites often have this combination. There are shallow and rapid respirations that produce hypocapnia, while excessive diuresis causes hypokalaemic alkalosis. Severe alkalaemia is the consequence.
3. Metabolic acidosis and respiratory alkalosis
   - This picture is typical in salicylate poisoning. Salicylic acid gives rise to metabolic acidosis, and stimulation of the respiratory centre leads to hyperventilation, and hence respiratory alkalosis.
4. Respiratory acidosis and metabolic alkalosis
   - These often occur when patients with *cor pulmonale* are given overly vigorous diuresis. Chronic respiratory acidosis is common in chronic obstructive airway disease due to CO_2 retention. With vigorous diuresis, volume contraction and hypokalaemic alkalosis set in. The compensatory response is hypoventilation, which will further raise the pCO_2.
5. Metabolic acidosis and metabolic alkalosis
   - These commonly occur in severely uraemic patients who have repeated vomiting. Vomiting gives rise to metabolic alkalosis, which may mask the degree of metabolic acidosis in uraemia.

Management of Acid–Base Disturbances

In patients with metabolic acidosis, the underlying causes should be identified and managed. $NaHCO_3$ is used to correct metabolic acidosis. Oral $NaHCO_3$ can be used for milder cases, while intravenous $NaHCO_3$ should be used for severe metabolic acidosis. Coexisting respiratory acidosis should also be excluded prior to administration of $NaHCO_3$. One should appreciate that intravenous $NaHCO_3$ is unable to correct acidosis if the clinical conditions associated with rapid acid production (e.g. lactic acidosis or ketoacidosis) are not abrogated. Excessive $NaHCO_3$ infusion may cause overshoot alkalosis and, rarely, paradoxical cerebral acidosis. Specific antidotes may be considered in patients with metabolic acidosis related to toxin ingestion. Patients with type 1 or 2 RTA may require high doses of $NaHCO_3$ and potassium supplements (or potassium citrate). Type 4 RTA can be managed with discontinuation of culprit agents, low potassium diets, loop diuretics, and, in resistant cases, fludrocortisone.

For patients with metabolic alkalosis, the causes leading to an increase in plasma HCO_3^- level and the factors impairing HCO_3^- excretion have to be addressed. The underlying aetiology of alkalosis has to be treated (e.g. discontinuation of offending drugs and management of gastrointestinal disorders). To increase renal HCO_3^- excretion, volume repletion, and the correction of Cl^- and K^+ deficits are all important. Cl^--sensitive alkalosis is responsive to treatment with normal saline with KCl supplementation.

5

Acute Kidney Injury

Gary Chan and Sydney Tang

Introduction

Acute kidney injury (AKI) is a disease process characterized by an abrupt loss of glomerular filtration rate (GFR). This results in the accumulation of urea, creatinine, and other metabolic wastes that are normally cleared by the kidneys. The incidence of AKI is likely underestimated but has been reported to occur in up to 20% of hospitalized patients and 60% of patients admitted to intensive care units. The development of AKI is associated with potentially life-threatening complications requiring in-hospital care and specialist input.

Definition and Staging

Until recently, a consensus definition for AKI has been lacking. In 2004, the RIFLE criteria (Risk, Injury, Failure, Loss, and End-stage kidney disease) was introduced by the Acute Dialysis Quality Initiative working group to provide uniform standards of AKI definition and classification. Subsequent modifications of the RIFLE criteria led to a classification published by the Acute Kidney Injury Network. The most recent and preferred classification is the Kidney Disease: Improving Global Outcomes (KDIGO) definition and staging system (Table 5.1). Such classifications, however, are unable to distinguish between various aetiologies that may lead to AKI. Another limitation inherent to these constructs lies in their use of serum creatinine to define and stage AKI. Serum creatinine remains a crude measure of renal function and its use to detect early AKI is particularly flawed. Much effort has therefore been directed at developing biomarkers of renal injury with greater sensitivity and specificity. Such biomarkers will likely be incorporated into, if

not totally replace, future definition and staging classifications of AKI.

Evaluation of Patients with Acute Kidney Injury

It is of paramount importance to promptly identify the underlying aetiology of AKI. In many cases, addressing the underlying cause may reverse AKI and prevent excess morbidity and mortality. The diagnostic approach to AKI should be systematic and aetiology is best divided into pre-renal, intrinsic renal, and post-renal entities.

Pre-renal disease

Pre-renal disease is a common cause of AKI and is characterized by decreased renal perfusion. Often, this results from conditions in which true volume depletion or reduced effective circulating volume occurs. Both sympathetic and renin-angiotensin systems become activated to cause afferent and efferent arteriolar vasoconstriction in the kidney, effectuating a drop in GFR. In addition, certain drugs can lead to pre-renal failure by disrupting the autoregulation of glomerular haemodynamics. For example, non-steroidal anti-inflammatory drugs and angiotensin-converting enzyme inhibitors can decrease afferent arteriolar dilatation and efferent arteriolar constriction respectively, to lower intraglomerular pressure and thus GFR.

In pre-renal disease, the diminution of GFR is entirely due to the compromise in renal perfusion. The histological structure of the kidney is therefore intact, and AKI is reversible upon ameliorating the

Table 5.1: RIFLE, AKIN, KDIGO criteria for acute kidney injury

	RIFLE	AKIN	KDIGO	RIFLE/AKIN/KDIGO
	Serum creatinine	Serum creatinine	Serum creatinine	Urine output
		Diagnostic Criteria		
		↑ ≥ 0.3 mg/dL within 48 hrs or ≥ 50% within 48 hrs	↑ ≥ 0.3 mg/dL within 48 hrs or ≥ 50% within 7 days	< 0.5 mL/kg/hr for > 6 hrs
		Staging Criteria		
Risk (RIFLE) Stage 1 (AKIN/KDIGO)	↑ 1.5 times baseline	↑ ≥ 0.3 mg/dL or ↑ 1.5 times baseline	↑ ≥ 0.3 mg/dL or ↑ 1.5 times baseline	< 0.5 mL/kg/hr for 6–12 hrs
Injury (RIFLE) Stage 2 (AKIN/KDIGO)	↑ 2.0 times baseline	↑ 2.0 times baseline	↑ 2.0 times baseline	< 0.5 mL/kg/hr for 12–24 hrs
Failure (RIFLE) Stage 3 (AKIN/KDIGO)	↑ by ≥ 0.5 mg/dL to ≥ 0.4 mg/dL or ↑ ≥ 3.0 times baseline or start KRT	↑ by ≥ 0.5 mg/dL to ≥ 0.4 mg/dL or ↑ ≥ 3.0 times baseline or start KRT	↑ by ≥ 0.3 mg/dL to ≥ 0.4 mg/dL or ↑ ≥ 3.0 times baseline or start KRT	< 0.3 mL/kg/hr for ≥ 24 hrs or anuria ≥ 12 hrs
Loss (RIFLE)	Require KRT > 4 weeks			
End stage (RIFLE)	Require KRT > 3 months			

AKIN, Acute Kidney Injury Network; KDIGO, Kidney Disease: Improving Global Outcomes; RIFLE, Risk, Injury, Loss of Kidney Function and End-Stage Kidney Disease; KRT, Kidney Replacement Therapy
Serum creatinine: 1 mg/dL = 88.4 μmol/L

haemodynamic imbalance. However, pre-renal disease, if severe or prolonged, can lead to acute tubular necrosis (ATN).

Intrinsic renal disease

Intrinsic renal aetiologies resulting in AKI may be subclassified into four categories (Table 5.2). The following section focuses on renal tubular pathologies, while diseases affecting the glomeruli, kidney interstitium, and renal vasculature will be further elaborated in Chapters 7, 8, 9, and 10.

ATN accounts for the majority of in-hospital AKIs. Conceptually, there are four sequential phases of ATN. The initiation phase is characterized by renal tubular epithelial cell injury from an inciting event. Subsequently, there is an extension phase of injury propagated by an inflammatory response. The initiation and extension phases result in a disruption of cellular function and membrane transport, ultimately leading to apoptosis. The epithelial slough and tubular casts obstruct the renal tubular lumen to reduce urine output and GFR, which is further compounded by a back-leaking of filtrate into the interstitium. Histologically, there is effacement and loss of renal tubular brush border, which

is accompanied by proximal tubule dilatation and the presence of necrotic cells within the lumen (Figure 5.1). However, the decline in renal function may be out of proportion to the severity of damage observed histologically. One reason for this is the increased sodium delivery to the macula densa due to impaired proximal reabsorption, which activates tubuloglomerular feedback to mediate afferent arteriolar vasoconstriction and a further reduction of GFR. Following the extension phase, there is a prolonged maintenance phase typified by low or non-existent GFR, which manifests as a continued rise in urea and creatinine. The recovery phase is heralded by tubular epithelial cell repair and regeneration. Clearance of urea, creatinine, and other metabolic waste begins to resume and may be associated with brisk diuresis until epithelial cells fully dedifferentiate with recovery of membrane function. It is therefore prudent to be aware of the potential volume depletion and electrolyte disturbances, which may occur during the recovery phase of ATN. The maintenance and recovery phases are in fact highly variable. The presence of existing renal disease, duration and severity of the injurious event are synergistic factors, which modify the reversibility of ATN and renal outcome.

Table 5.2: Common intra-renal causes of acute kidney injury

	Cause of Intra-renal Acute Kidney Injury
Tubular	ATN
	Ischaemic
	Sepsis
	Nephrotoxins
	Tubular obstruction
	Cast nephropathy
	Haeme pigment-induced AKI
	Uric acid nephropathy
	Crystal-induced nephropathy
Glomerulus	Rapidly progressive GN
	Anti-GBM GN
	Immune complex-mediated GN
	Pauci-immune GN
	Idiopathic
	Microangiopathy
	HUS/TTP
	PE/HELLP
Interstitium	Tubulo-interstitial nephritis
	Drugs
	Infections
	Autoimmune
	Idiopathic
Vascular	Renal artery
	Thrombosis/emboli
	Dissection
	Vasculitis
	Renal vein
	Thrombosis
	Other
	Malignant hypertension
	Scleroderma renal crisis

AKI, acute kidney injury; ATN, acute tubular necrosis; GBM, glomerular basement membrane; GN, glomerulonephritis; HELLP, haemolysis, elevated liver enzymes, and low platelet count; HUS, haemolytic uraemic syndrome; PE, pre-eclampsia; TTP, thrombotic thrombocytopenic purpura

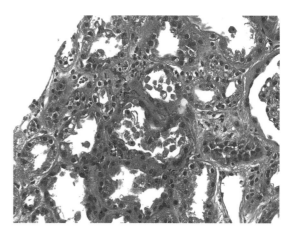

Figure 5.1: Acute tubular necrosis. Intra-tubular necrotic cells are present (PAS, ×400, Dr A. H. N. Tang).

The major causes of ATN include ischaemia, nephrotoxins, and sepsis. Of these, ischemic ATN is the most common and represents a severe continuum of pre-renal disease. A variety of nephrotoxins can also damage the renal tubules to cause ATN. Commonly used antibiotics such as aminoglycosides and cis-platin-containing chemotherapeutic regimens can directly induce cellular injury. Radioiodine contrast is tubulo-toxic per se but can also induce intra-renal vasoconstriction to give rise to contrast-induced AKI.

In some circumstances, epithelial cell damage occurs secondary to intra-tubular obstruction. Classical examples include tubular precipitation of uric acid and heme pigments in tumour lysis syndrome and rhabdomyolysis respectively. Sepsis-related AKI is often associated with systemic hypotension and renal hypoperfusion, which induces renal arteriolar vasoconstriction. However, the mechanism is likely to be more complex, involving neurohormonal and inflammatory mediators.

It can often be difficult to clinically differentiate pre-renal failure from ischemic ATN. A history of fluid loss or comorbidities resulting in reduced effective circulating volume is often present in both clinical scenarios. Therefore, the fractional excretion of sodium (FE_{Na}), which estimates the percentage of filtered sodium that is excreted in urine, is often used as a discriminatory tool:

$$FE_{Na} = (\text{Urine } [Na^+] \times \text{Serum } [\text{Creatinine}])/(\text{Serum } [Na^+] \times \text{Urine } [\text{Creatinine}]) \times 100$$

In pre-renal disease, tubular architecture and function remain intact and there is avid sodium reabsorption to give a FE_{Na} value of less than 1%, while a FE_{Na} value greater than 2% is indicative of ATN in the context of AKI. However, it must be noted that diuretic therapy or the presence of metabolic alkalosis, which would result in obligatory urinary sodium loss, precludes the use of FE_{Na}.

Post-renal disease

The post-renal causes of AKI can be subdivided into intra-luminal, luminal, and extra-luminal obstructive

Table 5.3: Common post-renal causes of acute kidney injury

| | Urinary Tract | |
	Upper	Lower
Intra-luminal	Nephrolithiasis Papillary necrosis Blood clot	Bladder stone Blood clot
Luminal	Transitional cell carcinoma	Transitional cell carcinoma Urethral stricture/valve
Extra-luminal	Intra-abdominal mass/malignancy Retroperitoneal fibrosis	Pelvic mass/malignancy
Functional		Neurogenic bladder

aetiology (Table 5.3). The majority of cases will exhibit hydronephrosis on ultrasonography or cross-sectional imaging. Depending on the level of obstruction, evidence of hydroureter may be present. It should be borne in mind that very early cases of obstruction or retroperitoneal fibrosis may yield negative imaging findings.

Management

AKI is prevalent and imposes a heavy burden of illness. Therefore, early risk stratification and prevention, via optimization of hydration status, is of critical importance. Observational studies have elucidated various risk factors for AKI (Table 5.4), from which predictive models of risk have been developed to

Table 5.4: Common risk factors for acute kidney injury

Risk Factors	
Exposures	Susceptibilities
• Critical illness	• Old age
• Sepsis	• Volume depletion
• Shock	• Female sex
• Trauma	• Black race
• Burns	• Chronic kidney disease
• Cardiac surgery and cardiopulmonary bypass	• Other chronic diseases, e.g. cirrhosis, heart failure
• Major non-cardiac surgery	• Diabetes mellitus
• Nephrotoxic drugs	• Cancer
• Iodinated contrast	• Anaemia
• Poisonous plants and animals	

facilitate individualization of monitoring and timely recognition.

The goals of AKI management are to treat and potentially reverse the underlying aetiology while providing supportive care to prevent and manage a plethora of associated complications. The general management of AKI and its principles are detailed below, but the specific treatment paradigms for individual diseases will be described in Chapter 7, 8, 9 and 10 respectively.

Drug administration and dosing

Patients with AKI require special attention to drug administration and dosing. In the first instance, nephrotoxic agents must be identified and discontinued to prevent further renal injury. The need for iodinated-contrast imaging studies should be carefully reviewed and alternative imaging modalities should be considered. Where the use of iodinated-contrast is unavoidable, the lowest possible dose of iso-osmolar or low-osmolar mediums should be employed after optimization of hydration status. Clinicians should be aware of the accumulation of renally eliminated drugs and associated metabolites in the presence of reduced GFR. Conversely, accelerated clearance occurs during the recovery phase of AKI. It is also important to keep in mind that measured GFR is often an inaccurate estimation of renal clearance in AKI and should not be used by itself to guide drug dosing, without taking into account the serum creatinine trend. Therefore, close monitoring of treatment response and drug toxicity is required in addition to appropriate dosage adjustment. Where available, therapeutic drug monitoring assays can be used to guide dosing schedules, especially in those undergoing renal replacement therapy (RRT) support, where drug elimination is further complicated by dialytic removal.

Fluid management

In the setting of AKI, volume depletion must be corrected to prevent further ischemia and facilitate renal recovery. Over the past two decades, the type of intravenous fluid employed to reverse hypovolaemia has been much debated. Colloid solutions have a theoretical advantage by achieving rapid intravascular expansion while crystalloids equilibrate between the intravascular and extravascular space. However, studies comparing albumin administration to isotonic saline in patients with AKI, albeit in an intensive care setting, found no renal or survival benefit. Limited data exists for the use of gelatin, and hyperoncotic hydroxyethyl starch preparations have been demonstrated to be nephrotoxic. Recent research has focused on the use of physiologically balanced salt solutions for resuscitation in patients with AKI to prevent hyperchloraemic metabolic acidosis. Based on the above findings, KDIGO recommends the use of isotonic crystalloids for volume expansion in the initial management of patients with or at risk of AKI (https://kdigo.org/guidelines/acute-kidney-injury/; accessed 9 March 2021). An exception to this is the clinical scenario of end-stage liver disease, where there is data to support the use of albumin.

More often than not, the majority of patients with AKI tend to be volume overloaded. This is due to the development of oligo-anuria and is associated with worse clinical outcomes. The management of hypervolaemia is crucial to preventing the life-threatening complication of pulmonary oedema. Loop diuretics had once been considered to carry a therapeutic advantage by reducing the metabolic demand of medullary tubules and thus abrogating ischaemic injury. However, this is unfounded and the only rationale for using loop diuretics in AKI lies in their potential ability to manage volume overload by augmenting urine output.

Electrolyte and acid–base management

The most important and pressing electrolyte abnormality encountered in AKI is hyperkalaemia, which may occur due to AKI itself or its underlying aetiology such as massive haemolysis or tumour lysis syndrome. Similarly, metabolic acidosis from the underlying cause of AKI, such as profound sepsis, may contribute to the hyperkalaemia of AKI by shifting intracellular potassium into the extracellular space. The treatment principles of severe hyperkalaemia are two-fold. Firstly, the stabilization of cardiomyocyte excitability takes precedence to prevent fatal arrhythmias. Secondly, prompt lowering of extracellular and total body potassium should be achieved by various means including dextrose-insulin infusion, correction of acidosis, potassium-binding resins and use of diuretics. Severe metabolic acidosis can be corrected by the administration of intravenous sodium bicarbonate. However, this can only be entertained in the absence of hypervolaemia, hypernatraemia, and hypocalcaemia, in which case, dialysis should be instituted.

Nutritional support and glycaemic control

AKI often constitutes a catabolic state fuelled by uraemia, acidosis, and other metabolic derangements that result in hyperglucagonaemia and insulin resistance. The excessive catabolism may be further exacerbated by the underlying disease process of AKI and modulated by the type and intensity of RRT. As such, appropriate nutrition should be initiated early and tailored to prevent hyperkalaemia, hyperphosphataemia, and volume overload in oligo-anuric individuals. While increased nitrogenous waste generation is expected when instituting nutritional therapy, protein restriction in an attempt to avoid RRT is not advisable.

KDIGO guidelines recommend providing 0.8–1.0 g/kg per day of protein in non-catabolic patients with AKI. The protein goals for patients requiring RRT are increased to 1.1–1.5 g/kg per day, and a maximum of 1.7 g/kg per day in hypercatabolic patients undergoing continuous RRT. The basis of such recommendation is the need to compensate for the profound amino acid and nutrient losses from the extracorporeal circuit. Enteral nutrition is the preferred route to support the nutritional demands of patients with AKI, aiming to achieve a total energy intake of 20–30 kcal/kg per day. Where this is not possible, or inadequate, parenteral nutrition should be considered. Often, the parenteral route of administration is necessary and can be incorporated into the dialytic therapy, so as to supplement existing enteral nutrition. Hyperglycaemia in AKI also requires close attention. The potential goals of stringent glycaemic control must be balanced against the heightened risk of hypoglycaemia in this cohort. In critically ill patients, KDIGO guidelines suggest targeting plasma glucose of 6.1–8.3 mmol/L, with the use of insulin (https://kdigo.org/guidelines/acute-kidney-injury/).

Role of renal replacement therapy

Severe and prolonged AKI often necessitates RRT support to prevent death from severe complications. The urgent indications for RRT in patients with AKI are clear and include the development of uremic complications, fluid overload refractory to diuretic therapy, severe hyperkalaemia, and metabolic acidosis. In addition, certain drug intoxications will necessitate urgent removal via RRT, even in the absence of AKI; these are covered in Chapter 19. However, in clinical scenarios lacking these urgent indications, the timing and modality of RRT initiation have not been well defined. Trials comparing early and delayed RRT initiation have yielded conflicting results, yet considerations must be made regarding factors such as the need for volume removal in individuals requiring nutritional support or reduction of the uremic and inflammatory milieu in patients with sepsis. There are a variety of RRT modalities available to support patients with AKI. While each modality has specific advantages, none have yet been proven superior in achieving renal recovery or survival benefit. Often, the choice between continuous and intermittent haemodialytic therapies is determined by the haemodynamic stability of the individual. In conclusion, the timing and modality of RRT initiation at present rely heavily on clinical context and judgement.

Outcomes and Prognosis

Due to the heterogeneity of the underlying causes of AKI, the outcome and prognosis of AKI are highly variable. Nevertheless, even modest reductions in kidney function are associated with increased short- and long-term morbidity and mortality, irrespective of aetiology. In particular, the risk of chronic kidney disease (CKD) is heightened following an episode of AKI, with the risk being accumulative for each subsequent episode. Predictors of new onset or worsening CKD include older age, severity of AKI, presence of proteinuria, and pre-existing renal impairment at presentation of AKI. Patients should therefore be followed-up by renal specialists even after resolution of AKI.

6

Urinary Tract Infection and Urogenital Tuberculosis

Zi Chan and Sunny Wong

Introduction

Infection of the urinary system is a commonly encountered clinical problem. This chapter provides an overview of the causes, clinical presentations and management of urinary tract infection (UTI) and urogenital tuberculosis. UTIs can be classified as uncomplicated and complicated, while there are a few special patterns that require attention (Table 6.1).

Pathogenesis of Urinary Tract Infection

UTI predominantly affects females and is uncommon in males except in the two extremes of life. The higher risk of UTI in women than men is related to the shorter distance from the anus to the urethra. The risk factors of UTI in an otherwise healthy woman include sexual intercourse and the use of spermicides. The ability of bacteria to adhere to the uroepithelium is an important determinant of their capability to cause clinical infections. The majority of cases of uncomplicated cystitis are caused by *Escherichia coli*. Other species of Enterobacteriaceae, such as *Klebsiella pneumoniae* and *Proteus mirabilis*, and other bacteria, such as *Staphylococcus saprophyticus* and group B *Streptococcus*, are also causative organisms for UTIs. For complicated UTI, resistant bacteria and polymicrobial infection are more common. Risk factors for complicated UTI include anatomical or functional abnormalities of the urinary tract (e.g. benign prostatic hyperplasia, neurogenic bladder, vesicoureteric reflux), the presence of foreign bodies and instrumentation (e.g. renal calculi, urinary catheter, ureteric stent), and immunocompromised states (e.g. diabetes mellitus, use of immunosuppressants).

Clinical Characteristics

The presentation of UTI varies from mild and transient symptoms to septicaemic shock. Classic manifestations of cystitis include dysuria, frequency, urgency, and suprapubic pain. Pyelonephritis may occur with or without symptoms of cystitis, and should be suspected in patients who present with fever, chills, flank pain, nausea, vomiting, or costovertebral angle tenderness. The urine may be cloudy, and contain traces of protein and blood. Gross haematuria is sometimes seen in cystitis.

Investigation

A urine dipstick can be used as a quick screening test to aid the diagnosis of UTI. The presence of leucocyte esterase (an enzyme released by leucocytes, reflecting pyuria) and nitrite (reflecting the presence of Enterobacteriaceae, which convert urinary nitrate to nitrite) is highly suggestive of UTI. Microscopy and culture of midstream urine is a more accurate test for UTI. White blood cell (WBC) $\geq$ 10/μL is considered abnormal. Positive urine culture > 10^5 cfu/ml with an isolated growth of uropathogen is considered significant. However, in symptomatic patients, especially those who are debilitated or immunocompromised, a urine culture yielding < 10^5 cfu/ml or mixed growth may still be clinically relevant and warrant treatment. Patients with pyelonephritis or complicated UTIs should be evaluated for underlying abnormalities of the urinary tract or factors leading to an immunocompromised state.

Table 6.1: Different clinical patterns of urinary tract infection and their definitions

Patterns	Definitions
Asymptomatic bacteriuria	• Presence of significant bacteriuria without symptoms.
Cystitis	• Infection localized to the urinary bladder.
Pyelonephritis	• Infection involving the kidneys and the collecting system.
Uncomplicated UTIs	• Acute lower (uncomplicated cystitis) and/or upper (uncomplicated pyelonephritis) UTI, limited to non-pregnant women with no known relevant anatomical and functional abnormalities within the urinary tract or comorbidities.
Complicated UTIs	• All UTIs which are not defined as uncomplicated (i.e. all men, pregnant women, patients with relevant anatomical or functional abnormalities of the urinary tract, indwelling urinary catheters, renal diseases, and/or with other concomitant immunocompromising diseases such as diabetes).
Recurrent UTIs	• Recurrences of uncomplicated and/or complicated UTIs, with a frequency of at least three UTIs per year or two UTIs in the last six months.
Catheter-associated UTIs	• UTIs occurring in a person whose urinary tract is currently catheterized or has had a catheter in place within the past 48 hours.
Urosepsis	• Sepsis caused by infection originating from the urinary tract.

UTI, urinary tract infection

Management

Asymptomatic bacteriuria

Asymptomatic bacteriuria is common in women and elderly people of both sexes, and corresponds to commensals colonization. Routine screening of asymptomatic bacteriuria is not recommended in patients without risk factors, and treatment is generally not indicated except in pregnant women or patients undergoing invasive urological procedures.

Uncomplicated cystitis

Oral nitrofurantoin and amoxicillin-clavulanate (given for 5–7 days) are preferred empirical treatments for uncomplicated cystitis. Fluoroquinolones and trimethoprim-sulfamethoxazole can be used as alternatives if first-line agents are contraindicated.

Uncomplicated pyelonephritis

Patients with high fever or pain, or inability to maintain oral hydration or take oral medications should be admitted. Intravenous amoxicillin-clavulanate is the preferred empirical treatment. Intravenous piperacillin-tazobactam and carbapenem should be considered in patients with risk factors for multidrug-resistant bacteria, such as those with prior history of hospitalization or recent use of antibiotics. The recommended duration of antibiotics for uncomplicated pyelonephritis is 14 days.

Recurrent UTI

For healthy women who have no risk factors for complicated UTIs, extensive work-up such as cystoscopy and renal imaging is not mandatory as the diagnostic yield is low. However, it should be performed if there is atypical symptoms suggestive of renal calculi, outflow obstruction, or urothelial cancer. Non-antimicrobial preventive strategies including increased fluid intake, post-coital urination, and avoidance of spermicides may help reduce UTIs. For post-menopausal women with recurrent cystitis, vaginal oestrogen may help to re-establish the normal vaginal flora and prevent bacterial colonization. While some small uncontrolled studies have suggested that cranberry products and probiotics may also prevent recurrent UTIs, more evidence are needed to recommend their routine use. When behavioural modifications and non-antimicrobial measures have been unsuccessful, antibiotics (e.g. nitrofurantoin and trimethoprim-sulfamethoxazole) may be given as continuous low-dose prophylaxis for longer periods (three to six months), or as post-coital prophylaxis.

Complicated UTIs

Complicated UTIs can be related to both upper or lower UTIs, and are frequently due to resistant bacteria or polymicrobial infections. Patients with septic manifestations should be treated initially with broad-spectrum antibiotics, with further modification after culture and susceptibility results are available. In general, a third-generation cephalosporin, piperacillin-tazobactam or carbapenem should be given for 7–14 days, but patients with underlying urological abnormalities might require a longer duration.

Catheter-associated UTIs

Catheter-associated UTIs are a common healthcare-related infection, with the duration of catheterization being the most important determining factor for this type of infection. A urine specimen should be obtained for culture prior to initiating antibiotics due to the wide spectrum of possible organisms and the increased likelihood of antimicrobial resistance. The recommended empirical antibiotics are the same as for complicated UTIs. Indwelling urinary catheters should be removed if possible. If a urinary catheter is still needed, it should be replaced at the start of antibiotics therapy. Avoidance of unnecessary catheterization, use of a sterile technique for insertion, and early removal are essential measures to prevent catheter-associated UTIs.

Urosepsis

Elderly and immunocompromised patients (e.g. diabetics, transplant recipients, and patients receiving cancer chemotherapy or corticosteroids) are at high risk of developing urosepsis. Local predisposing factors for urosepsis include urinary tract calculi, obstruction at any level in the urinary tract, congenital uropathy, neurogenic bladder disorders, or endoscopic manoeuvres. Patients who develop septic shock should receive fluid resuscitation and, if necessary, also vasopressor support. Empirical intravenous antibiotics should be initiated without delay, with carbapenems being the drug of choice for patients who show severe and rapid clinical deterioration. Urinary obstruction should be actively excluded because this is the most frequent cause of urosepsis. Drainage of obstruction and abscesses and removal of foreign bodies (e.g. urinary catheters or stones) are also important measures for the treatment of urosepsis.

Urogenital Tuberculosis

Pathogenesis of urogenital tuberculosis

Involvement of kidneys and the urological systems by tuberculosis (TB) can occur at the time of primary pulmonary infection, during reactivation, or in the case of miliary disease. Direct invasion of the renal parenchyma or the urinary collecting system (including renal pelvis, calyces, ureters, and bladder) is the most common form of urogenital TB, and unilateral involvement occurs more frequently than bilateral involvement. Renal TB can cause extensive destruction of kidney tissue, leading to the development of chronic kidney disease and, in bilateral involvement, may even cause end-stage renal disease. Less commonly, TB can induce interstitial nephritis or various forms of glomerulonephritis, but the pathogenic mechanisms for these renal abnormalities remain elusive. Acute interstitial nephritis can also arise from anti-TB medications, most notably rifampicin. Renal amyloidosis (AA type) due to chronic and poorly treated TB is rarely seen nowadays.

Clinical characteristics

TB infection of the urinary system is easily overlooked as it is usually asymptomatic. Urogenital TB should be suspected in patients who show symptoms of cystitis but do not respond to the usual antibacterial agents, or when urine examination reveals pyuria in the absence of a positive bacterial culture. Painless microscopic haematuria is also common. Other possible symptoms include back, flank and suprapubic pain, and gross haematuria. Systemic symptoms, such as fever, weight loss, and night sweats, are unusual.

Investigation

When genitourinary TB is suspected, at least three to six early-morning urine samples should be sent for acid-fast staining and mycobacterial culture. Urine for TB Polymerase Chain Reaction (PCR) is also a useful diagnostic test for genitourinary TB and is associated with high specificity. Computerized tomography (CT) with contrast, magnetic resonance imaging, and ultrasonography are all possible imaging modalities for urogenital TB. In this context, a CT scan can readily demonstrate the extent of the infection, presence of renal scars or obstruction, and distribution of calcifications in the affected kidney (Figure 6.1). Patients with atypical presentations such as elevated serum creatinine and proteinuria should be considered for renal biopsy. Patients should also be investigated for pulmonary and other organ involvements of TB.

Management

The common anti-TB regimen for urogenital TB is similar to that used in pulmonary TB, which comprises a four drug combination [isoniazid (H), rifampicin (R), pyrazinamide (Z), and ethambutol (E)] for two months, followed by H and R for another four months (Table 6.2). The dosages of anti-TB medications need to be adjusted according to the degree of renal impairment. Radiological or surgical interventions are indicated for ureteric obstruction. Relief of ureteric obstruction by stenting or percutaneous nephrostomy may aid functional recovery. In cases of advanced unilateral disease complicated by pain or haemorrhage, nephrectomy of the non-functioning or partially functioning kidney may be required.

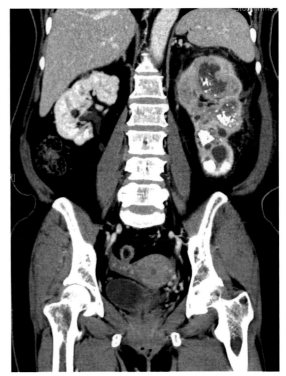

Figure 6.1: A computer tomographic image showing tuberculosis infection of the left kidney

Table 6.2: Dosage adjustment for common anti-TB medications in chronic kidney disease

Drugs/ Usual dose	CKD stages 1–3	CKD stages 4–5	PD	HD	Remarks
Isoniazid (H) 300 mg/D	No adjustment	No adjustment	No adjustment	No adjustment	• Increased risk of neurotoxicity in patients with renal disease and supplemental pyridoxine should be co-prescribed.
Rifampicin (R) 450–600 mg/D	No adjustment	No adjustment	No adjustment	No adjustment	• Can be used safely in renal disease. • Exercise caution with concomitant drugs due to potential for significant drug–drug interactions.
Pyrazinamide (Z) 1.5–2 g/D	No adjustment	25–30 mg/kg 3×/week	No adjustment	25–30 mg/kg 3×/week After HD if on HD day	• Main route of clearance is hepatic with active metabolites undergoing some renal clearance.
Ethambutol (E) 15 mg/kg/D	No adjustment	15 mg/kg 3×/week	15 mg/kg 3×/week	15 mg/kg 3×/week After HD if on HD day	• Mainly renal excreted. Ocular toxicity is an important concern in patients with renal disease and regular ophthalmological reviews are essential.

CKD, chronic kidney disease; HD, haemodialysis; PD, peritoneal dialysis; TB, tuberculosis

7

Tubulointerstitial Diseases and Kidney Fibrosis

Sydney Tang and Susan Yung

Introduction

The tubular and interstitial compartments of the kidney constitute over 90% of the kidney mass, and tubulointerstitial diseases represent a broad group of acute and chronic disorders with variable aetiologies and manifestations.

Renal tubules are important for the retrieval of filtered electrolytes, nutrients and small proteins, and for maintaining acid–base balance as well as control of total body sodium and water balance. Thus, tubular dysfunction may manifest as aminoaciduria or mild proteinuria together with glycosuria, phosphaturia and bicarbonaturia (defective reabsorption leading to Fanconi syndrome—see Chapter 4), increased urinary frequency and nocturia (defective urinary concentration—see Chapter 3), or renal tubular acidosis (defective urinary acidification—see Chapter 4).

The renal interstitium provides a structural matrix vested with a peritubular capillary network, dendritic antigen-processing cells, and fibroblasts that produce erythropoietin. Interstitial damage therefore results in relative erythropoietin deficiency that accounts for the anaemia observed in chronic tubulointerstitial disease.

Aetiology

Acute tubulointerstitial disease can be caused by toxic or ischemic tubular injury, as in acute tubular necrosis, or by inflammation, as in acute (allergic) interstitial nephritis (AIN) or pyelonephritis. Chronic interstitial nephritis (CIN) is the result of a persistent challenge from toxic, mechanical, infectious, immunologic, hereditary, or other aetiologies. Commonly encountered causes of AIN and CIN are listed in Table 7.1. In addition, CIN can also result from a prolonged episode of AIN that is not adequately resolved or from sustained proteinuria that induces tubular inflammation and damage, which is frequently seen in chronic glomerulonephritis. Indeed, secondary tubulointerstitial inflammation and fibrosis is the final common pathway of progressive glomerular diseases, regardless of aetiology, and the 'end-stage' kidney often displays extensive tubulointerstitial lesions that are more predictive of the overall renal outcome in patients with chronic kidney diseases (CKD).

Pathophysiology

The high metabolic demand of the tubulointerstitium makes it particularly susceptible to injury because any inflammation and the associated oedema compromise renal blood flow. Therefore, tubulointerstitial nephritis (TIN) is usually accompanied by variable degrees of acute kidney injury (AKI) (see Chapter 5). Interstitial oedema and infiltration of lymphocytes and plasma cells also cause tubular dysfunction and impair renal function. In chronic TIN, interstitial fibrosis (as opposed to oedema) causes a reduction in GFR. If prolonged, acute interstitial inflammatory reactions can lead to the accumulation of an extracellular matrix that causes irreversible attrition of renal function with interstitial fibrosis and tubular atrophy.

Table 7.1: Common causes of acute and chronic interstitial nephritis

Conditions	AIN	CIN
Drugs and exogenous toxins (see Chapter 19)	• Antibiotics (especially penicillins, cephalosporins, sulphonamides, rifampin) • NSAIDs, COX-2 inhibitors • Furosemide • Proton-pump inhibitors • Immune checkpoint inhibitors	• Lithium • Heavy metals (e.g., lead, cadmium) • Chinese herbs (e.g., tainted with aristolochic acid) • Calcineurin inhibitors (e.g. cyclosporine)
Infections (see Chapter 9)	• Bacterial: Streptococcus, Staphylococcus • Viral: CMV, EBV, BKV, Hantavirus • Others: Mycobacterium, • Toxoplasma, Mycoplasma, Rickettsia, Leptospira	
Autoimmune diseases (see Chapter 9)	• SLE • Sarcoidosis • Sjögren's syndrome • Inflammatory bowel disease • IgG4-related kidney disease • TINU (mostly in children)	
Neoplasms (see Chapter 9)		• Multiple myeloma or light chain cast nephropathy • Lymphoma
Metabolic causes		• Hypercalcaemia or nephrocalcinosis • Hyperuricaemia • Prolonged hypokalaemia
Obstruction		• Vesicoureteral reflux • Bladder outlet obstruction
Hereditary (See Chapter 13)		• Nephronophthisis • Polycystic kidney disease • Sickle cell disease • Hyperoxaluria • Cystinosis
Miscellaneous	• Idiopathic	• Chronic glomerulonephritis • Ischaemia

AIN, acute interstitial nephritis; BKV, BK virus; CIN, chronic interstitial nephritis; CMV, cytomegalovirus; COX2, cyclo-oxygenase 2; EBV, Epstein–Barr virus; SLE, systemic lupus erythematosus; TINU, tubulointerstitial nephritis with uveitis; NSAIDs, nonsteroidal anti-inflammatory drugs

Acute Interstitial Nephritis

AIN is an important cause of AKI. Antibiotics, non-steroidal anti-inflammatory drugs, and cyclooxygenase-2 inhibitors are currently the most common causative agents, although AIN can occur with almost any medication (see also Chapter 19). Proton pump inhibitors are also increasingly recognized as a cause of AIN. AIN can also develop in the setting of infection, malignancy or systemic disease, or as an idiopathic condition.

Clinical characteristics and diagnosis of AIN

A challenging feature of AIN is the non-specific nature of presentation, which often leads to delayed diagnosis that may portend worse outcomes. Very often, AIN is either unnoticed or presents with non-specific symptoms such as fatigue, myalgia, arthralgia, flank pain, and a low-grade fever. In drug-induced AIN, the latent period with first exposure may be several weeks long, though with re-exposure it usually occurs within 3–5 days. Notably, the risk is not dose-dependent. The classical hypersensitivity reaction including pruritic skin rash, fever, and eosinophilia is present in only about 10% of patients. In addition, as the symptoms are not specific to AIN and are associated with many other clinical conditions, a high clinical index of suspicion and thorough review of potential risk factors are needed for accurate identification and prompt diagnosis.

Urinalysis, in particular when revealing sterile pyuria and white cell casts, can provide a useful clue to suggest the possibility of underlying AIN. Eosinophiluria may be present but this test may not be readily available in many laboratories. Varying levels of dipstick-positive proteinuria ranging from trace to 1 or 2+ may be seen. Spot urine samples for the protein-to-creatinine ratio generally demonstrate protein concentrations < 1 mg/mg, consistent with 'tubular' proteinuria. Microscopic haematuria is a relatively common finding.

A kidney ultrasound should be part of the list of investigations for patients with AKI or CKD. In AIN, enlarged, swollen kidneys with increased echogenicity on ultrasound are seen; however, this finding is not specific to AIN and can be seen with ATN, glomerulonephritis, infiltrative diseases, and other aetiologies of AKI. Nevertheless, increased echogenicity of the renal parenchyma with loss of corticomedullary differentiation are notable sonographic features of AIN.

Kidney biopsy yields a definitive diagnosis of AIN that shows an interstitial inflammatory infiltrate dominated by lymphocytes, monocytes, and eosinophils, along with tubulitis and interstitial oedema (Figure 7.1). Drug-induced AIN is more likely to feature a significant number of eosinophils (Figure 7.2), but neither the presence nor absence of eosinophils is diagnostic. A higher density of neutrophils and plasma cells suggests a bacterial aetiology.

Management

There is no definitive treatment for AIN. Treatment is primarily guided by eliminating the underlying offending agent, if it can be ascertained. For instance, patients with drug-induced AIN may recover spontaneously with the cessation of the culprit medication, particularly if it is promptly identified. Likewise, appropriate and timely treatment of any secondary causes, such as infection or neoplasm, is important. Corticosteroids are widely used by many clinicians on the theoretical basis that early steroid treatment could prevent fibrosis by decreasing inflammatory infiltrates. However, an evidence-based therapeutic efficacy is lacking. In addition, no consensus has been established regarding the duration or dose of steroid treatment.

Tubulointerstitial Fibrosis

Progressive tubulointerstitial fibrosis is the final common pathway for all kidney diseases, and it is the best histological predictor of kidney function decline in patients with CKD. Tubulointerstitial fibrosis is characterized by the deposition of pathological fibrillar matrix components (e.g. collagen I and III) and constituents of the normal capillary basement membrane (e.g. collagen IV and V, fibronectin, laminin, and perlecan) between the tubular basement membrane and peritubular capillaries resulting in the expansion of the tubulointerstitium. It is considered a wound healing response to kidney injury that has not been resolved, and it is associated with leukocyte recruitment, activation and expansion of interstitial fibroblasts, tissue remodelling,

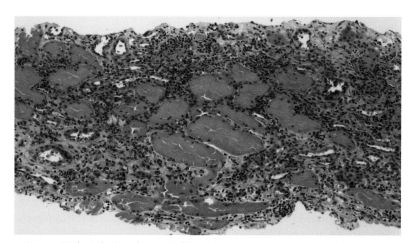

Figure 7.1: Acute interstitial nephritis. There is diffuse interstitial infiltrate comprising lymphocytes, plasma cells and eosinophils (H&E, ×100, Dr G. S. W. Chan).

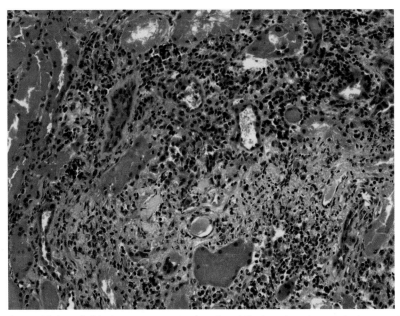

Figure 7.2: Acute interstitial nephritis. Large amounts of eosinophils, lymphocytes, and plasma cells are present in the interstitium. The presence of abundant eosinophilic infiltrates is commonly seen in drug-induced acute interstitial nephritis (H&E, ×400, Dr G. S. W. Chan).

tubular atrophy, and microvascular rarefaction, which ultimately results in the destruction of the kidney parenchyma and loss of kidney function. Tubulointerstitial fibrosis interferes with the normal function of tubules to secrete toxins from peritubular capillaries, and impairs tubular transport activity and exchange of nutrients from the circulation.

Activated fibroblasts, termed myofibroblasts, are the key effector cells that mediate tubulointerstitial fibrosis, and they are primarily derived from local stromal cells such as the resident fibroblasts or perivascular fibroblasts (pericytes). There is evidence that proximal tubular epithelial cells (PTEC) also contribute to myofibroblast recruitment through epithelial-to-mesenchymal transition (EMT), a process wherein, upon stimulation with mediators of fibrosis, PTEC lose their epithelial morphology and acquire an elongated, fibroblastic phenotype that endows them with high proliferative, migratory, and invasive properties. Characteristic features of EMT include a loss of epithelial markers such as E-cadherin, cytokeratin and tight junctions, and induction of mesenchymal markers such as vimentin, α-smooth muscle actin and collagen I and III. Myofibroblast activation, proliferation, and survival are mediated by cytokines, growth factors, and mechanical stress and/or stiffness.

Tubulointerstitial fibrosis can also be initiated through direct PTEC injury and their subsequent dedifferentiation upon exposure to albuminuria, high glucose concentration, repetitive AKI, chronic inflammation, defective fatty acid oxidation, growth factors, and reactive oxygen species. Epithelial cell injury may lead to cell senescence resulting in replicative arrest, DNA damage, telomere shortening, and oxidative stress. Senescent cells are resistant to apoptosis and they possess an inflammatory and fibrotic phenotype with increased production of TGF-β1, CTGF, and matrix metalloproteinases; the latter are enzymes that degrade basement membrane components. Although inflammation is an integral part of the host defence mechanism in response to injury, dysregulated innate and adaptive immune responses are major contributors to kidney fibrosis. Macrophages release numerous soluble factors that contribute to tubulointerstitial fibrosis, although subsets of macrophages possess antifibrotic properties and can phagocytose matrix protein fragments and apoptotic cells. A critical role for CD4+ T cells in kidney fibrosis has also been proposed since mice that lack CD4 but not CD8 cells are protected from interstitial expansion and collagen deposition following ureteric obstruction. Recent advances in the understanding of how tubulointerstitial fibrosis is initiated may offer new therapeutic approaches for the treatment of kidney fibrosis.

8

Glomerulonephritis

*Desmond Yap, Sydney Tang, Kar Neng Lai, Alex Tang, Kwok Wah Chan,
and Tak Mao Chan*

Introduction

Glomerulonephritis (GN) is an important cause of various forms of renal dysfunction including nephritic syndrome, nephrotic syndrome, and chronic kidney disease (CKD). This chapter provides an overview of the clinical characteristics, pathophysiology, and management of important primary GNs.

Immunoglobulin A Nephropathy

Clinical characteristics

In 1968, the French pathologists Jean Berger and Nicole Hinglais first described 25 patients with recurrent haematuria and mesangial IgA deposits that surmounted IgG deposits. The eponym 'Berger's Disease' was introduced in 1973, and by 1975 the defining features of this condition became apparent and the term IgA nephropathy (IgAN) was commonly used thereafter.

IgAN is still the most common primary glomerulonephritis worldwide. The prevalence of IgAN also differs across populations and geographic locations. IgAN is most common in East Asia, less prevalent in Europe, and infrequent in Africa. In Hong Kong, IgAN accounts for approximately 30% of all primary glomerular diseases. Within Europe, IgAN is most prevalent in the northern countries. The prevalence and genetic risk increase for native populations as the distance from Africa increases northwards and eastwards. Prevalence rates are much lower in the United Kingdom, Canada, and the United States. In North America, the disease is twice as common in males as in females, whereas in Asia the gender ratio is roughly equal. The spectrum of presentation is highly variable and ranges from asymptomatic urine abnormality such as microscopic haematuria, to episodic gross haematuria, to CKD with proteinuria and hypertension.

The incidence of IgAN is highest in the second and third decades of life. The first episode of macroscopic haematuria generally occurs between 15 and 30 years of age. Not infrequently, patients may first present with macroscopic haematuria complicating mucosal infection (respiratory or gastrointestinal), and the former is often described as 'synpharyngitic macrohaematuria'. Macrohaematuria occurs shortly (within 12–72 hours) following the pharyngitic episode and is sometimes accompanied by loin pain. The urine colour is red or brown, but seldom contains clots. Asymptomatic microscopic haematuria is a more common presentation than macrohaematuria, especially in Asian populations, and is often detected with health screening. Urine microscopy reveals dysmorphic red blood cells and red cell casts.

Proteinuria, when present, tends to fluctuate within a narrow range for most patients. Proteinuria is usually not heavy and < 30% have proteinuria exceeding 1 g/day. A transient increase of proteinuria occurs with gross haematuria complicating mucosal infection or urinary tract infection. In a small group of patients, proteinuria reaches the nephrotic range (> 3.5 g/24 hours) and kidney histology typically shows ultrastructural features of minimal change disease but with mesangial IgA deposits. This is referred to as 'an overlapping syndrome of IgAN and minimal change disease (MCD)'. This entity occurs more frequently in children and clinically resembles MCD, responding well to corticosteroids.

Acute kidney injury (AKI) is an uncommon presentation and the pathology is frequently associated with extensive crescent formation. Around 15% of patients have significant renal impairment (CKD stage 3 or higher) at first presentation. Occasionally, IgAN may present with advanced CKD that requires prompt initiation of renal replacement therapy.

A subset of patients, particularly children, manifest a vasculitic form of illness. IgA vasculitis (IgAV), formerly Henoch-Schönlein purpura, is a form of vasculitis marked by IgA deposition within the blood vessels of affected tissues. IgAV commonly affects the small blood vessels of the skin, joints, intestines, and kidneys, leading to a tetrad of palpable purpura mostly in the lower extremities without platelet or coagulation disorder, arthralgia, abdominal pain, and kidney disease. Rarely, it can affect the lungs and central nervous system. It is the most common form of vasculitis in children. When IgAV occurs in children younger than 16 years, it is often self-limiting. Adults may have more severe and relapsing disease. Kidney involvement in IgAV is histopathologically indistinguishable from that seen in the kidney-limited disease of IgAN.

The prognosis of IgAN is variable. Some patients have only a single haematuric episode, others have repeated exacerbations. Overall, IgAN pursues a slow but relentless clinical course with consequent kidney failure in 30–40% of patients within 20–30 years after clinical presentation. The percentage of patients who will go into renal failure is roughly the same as the duration of the disease in years from the time of diagnosis. Overall, however, there is a wide range of interindividual variability in the disease course, and specific factors that affect progression to end-stage kidney disease (ESKD) are poorly understood. Even among patients with apparently good prognostic markers, such as normal renal function, blood pressure, and minimal proteinuria on presentation, up to one-third could develop significant proteinuria and CKD upon prolonged follow-up in Chinese cohorts, whereas only 4% of similar low-risk patients progressed over a 15-year period in a Spanish cohort, highlighting a genetic difference in disease progression.

As such, predicting clinical outcomes for IgAN remains an imprecise process. There are clinicopathological features that are generally, but not universally, accepted as indicating a less favourable prognosis in patients with preserved renal function at diagnosis (Table 8.1).

Table 8.1: Commonly accepted indicators of a worse prognosis in IgA nephropathy

Demographic
  Male sex
  Older age at diagnosis
  Obesity

Clinical
  No history of macroscopic haematuria
  Persistent microscopic haematuria
  Persistent hypertension

Biochemical
  Proteinuria persistently > 1 g/day
  Hyperuricaemia

Histological (light microscopy):
  Mesangial hypercellularity
  Focal segmental glomerular sclerosis
  Endocapillary cellular proliferation
  Capillaritis
  Interstitial fibrosis/tubular atrophy
  Crescents
  Thrombotic microangiopathy
  Loss of podocytes

Pathogenesis and histopathological features

Accumulating evidence suggests a strong heritable component to IgAN. This includes numerous reports of familial aggregation of IgAN from the 1980s, and more recently the observation that with increasing distance from Africa, there is increasing genetic predisposition to IgAN, with significant west-to-east and south-to-north risk gradients. Genome-side association studies have been performed in Caucasian and Chinese populations, revealing different risk alleles of IgAN, including those involved in adaptive and innate immunity, glycosylation of IgA1, the renin-angiotensin system, and the human leukocyte antigen (HLA) molecules HLA-DQ and HLA-DR.

The primary defect of IgAN seems to lie in the structure of the IgA molecule, rather than in the kidney. Human IgA may be monomeric (mIgA) or polymeric (pIgA, in which two or four IgA molecules are joined by the bridging protein J chain that is essential for pIgA assembly). There are two subclasses, IgA1 and IgA2, whose functional distinctions are not well understood. The mucosal immune system produces both pIgA1 and pIgA2, which reach mucosal surfaces as secretory IgA (pIgA + secretory component) by transepithelial transport. Serum IgA is mostly marrow-derived monomeric IgA1.

A working hypothesis is that patients with IgAN have inherited defects in B cells producing galactose-deficient pIgA1 that escapes hepatic clearance, thus leading to increased serum IgA1 concentrations. Indeed, mesangial IgA in IgAN is mostly pIgA1. In addition, under-galactosylated IgA1 molecules are prone to self-aggregate and to form complexes with IgG antibodies. With increased immune-complex formation and its decreased clearance, IgA1 (mainly polymeric) binds to glomerular mesangium and triggers the local production of cytokines and growth factors, leading to mesangial cell proliferation and complement activation.

To date, there are no reliable diagnostic laboratory tests for IgAN. The condition can only be diagnosed with a kidney biopsy. In many centres, this will only be performed in patients with significant proteinuria or otherwise unexplained kidney function impairment. The defining histological hallmark is the presence of dominant or codominant deposition of IgA in the glomerular mesangium by immunofluorescence (IF) study (Figure 8.1). Light microscopy (LM) typically shows an increase in mesangial cells with matrix expansion (Figure 8.2) and normal glomerular basement membranes. However, the LM findings can be highly variable in different cases of IgAN, ranging from normal or minimal lesions in the glomeruli, to diffuse mesangial proliferative changes, focal segmental glomerulosclerosis, endocapillary proliferation and rarely focal segmental necrotizing lesions with crescent formation. Electron microscopy (EM) typically show electron-dense deposits over the mesangial area (Figure 8.3).

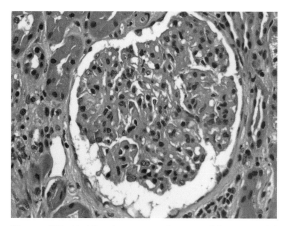

Figure 8.2: Light microscopy shows mild mesangial matrix expansion and increase in mesangial cellularity (H&E, ×400, Dr A. H. N. Tang)

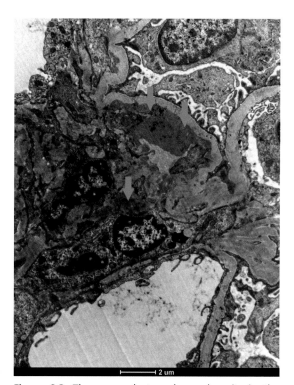

Figure 8.3: There are electron-dense deposits in the mesangial area (arrows) in electron microscopy study (transmission electron microscopy, ×5000, Dr G. S. W. Chan)

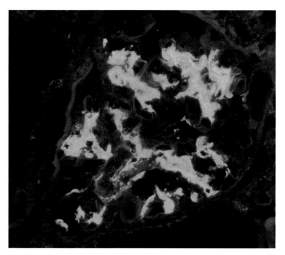

Figure 8.1: Direct immunofluorescence study shows dominant or codominant granular IgA staining in the mesangium (anti-IgA immunofluorescence, ×400, Dr A. H. N. Tang)

Due to the high variability of LM findings, the 'Oxford Classification of IgA Nephropathy', first developed in 2009, showed that four glomerular and parenchymal parameters possess reproducible and independent predictive values on renal outcomes: mesangial hypercellularity (M), endocapillary proliferation (E), segmental glomerulosclerosis (S), and tubular atrophy/interstitial fibrosis (T). The histologic classification was further refined to MEST-C scores with the incorporation of C (crescents) lesions for crescentic IgAN. Nowadays, kidney histology reports across the world use this classification.

Management

There has been no approved specific therapy for IgAN and treatment is largely symptomatic, aiming at control of blood pressure to < 125/75 mmHg, proteinuria, and preservation of renal function. Lifestyle measures, including a low-salt diet, weight reduction, smoking cessation, and avoidance of nephrotoxins, are important initial approaches.

Treatment is based on the use of angiotensin-converting enzyme inhibitor or angiotensin receptor blocker for patients with proteinuria with or without elevated blood pressure control. The addition of aliskiren (a direct renin inhibitor) on top of losartan has a further antiproteinuric effect, though the development of hyperkalaemia limits this combination in patients with moderate CKD. The addition of high-dose corticosteroids to supportive care in selected patients with risk factors for CKD progression has been shown to confer at best marginal benefits, but was associated with significant treatment-related adverse events. There is little convincing evidence for additional benefits from cytotoxic or other immunomodulatory agents, except for CYC in crescentic IgAN. Mycophenolate mofetil (MMF) has been reported to be efficacious only in Chinese patients, and could be considered for steroid-sparing for patients in whom high-dose corticosteroids are to be commenced. Tonsillectomy, with or without corticosteroids, was associated with improved kidney survival and/or haematuria/proteinuria in Japanese studies.

For patients who progress to kidney failure, transplantation offers the best potential for full rehabilitation. After transplantation, mesangial IgA deposition has been shown to recur in 20–60% of grafts. Recurrent IgAN is associated with progressive loss of allograft function in about 10%.

Minimal Change Disease

Clinical characteristics

MCD is an important cause of nephrotic syndrome. MCD is the most common cause of nephrotic syndrome in children, accounting for over 90% of all cases. It is also responsible for 10–25% of nephrotic syndrome in adults. MCD patients usually present with bilateral lower limb or even generalized oedema (e.g. peri-orbital swelling, scrotal swelling, or anasarca in severe cases). Proteinuria in MCD is typically heavy and rapid-onset, patients generally do not show overt renal dysfunction. Nonetheless, acute kidney injury can occur in some older adults with MCD. Due to heavy proteinuria, most MCD patients have hypogammaglobulinaemia (especially IgG) and severe dyslipidaemia. MCD shows association with viral illness (e.g. upper respiratory infections), drugs (e.g. non-steroidal anti-inflammatory drugs) or haematological disorders (e.g. non-Hodgkin's lymphoma) (Table 8.2). Relapses are common in adult patients with MCD. Prognosis of MCD is generally favourable, with low risk of progression to CKD or ESKD.

Table 8.2: Common clinical conditions that are associated with minimal change disease

	Examples
Infections	• Upper respiratory infection, syphilis, HIV
Drugs	• NSAIDs, lithium, bisphosphonates
Malignancy	• Non-Hodgkin's lymphoma, leukaemia

HIV, human immunodeficiency virus; NSAIDs, nonsteroidal anti-inflammatory drugs

Pathogenesis and histopathological features

The pathogenesis of MCD remains obscure and is postulated to be related to aberrant T-cell responses. LM typically shows normal glomerular morphology (Figure 8.4), which is accompanied by a negative IF staining. The pathognomonic EM features include extensive effacement of foot processes, vacuolation, and the appearance of microvilli in the podocytes (Figure 8.5).

Management

Since MCD is the most common cause of nephrotic syndrome in children, empirical high-dose corticosteroids (60 mg/m²/day) can be initiated without the need for kidney biopsy. Kidney biopsy, however,

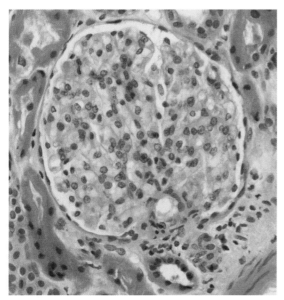

Figure 8.4: Minimal change disease. The glomerulus is unremarkable by light microscopy (H&E, ×400, Dr A. H. N. Tang).

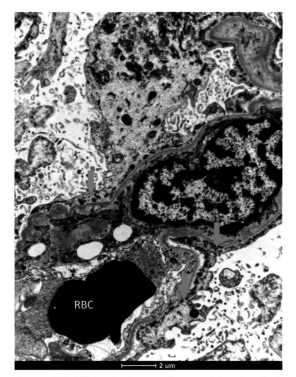

Figure 8.5: Minimal change disease. Extensive foot process effacement (arrows) and microvillous transformation of podocytes are present (transmission electron microscopy, ×5000, Dr G. S. W. Chan).

should be considered in children with clinical features atypical of MCD (Table 8.3). Children tend to show better and more rapid response to corticosteroids compared with adults. In this context, many children with MCD can be tapered off from corticosteroids after approximately six months. For children with steroid-dependent or frequently relapsing MCD, second-line treatments such as alkylating agents (e.g. cyclophosphamide [CYC] or chlorambucil), calcineurin inhibitors (CNI), or levamisole can be considered. Growth retardation remains an important concern in children receiving high doses or repeated courses of corticosteroids. Alkylating agents should also be used with caution in children due to their long-term toxicities. Side effects of levamisole include neutropenia, skin rashes, and hepatotoxicity.

Table 8.3: Clinical features atypical of minimal change disease in children

- Age of onset < 1 year old or > 12 years old
- Steroid resistance or subsequent failure to respond to corticosteroids in steroid-sensitive nephrotic syndrome
- Family history of nephrotic syndrome
- Presence of other extra-renal manifestations (e.g. skin rash, joint pain)
- Presence of features suggestive of nephritic syndrome (e.g. active urine sediments, hypertension, renal insufficiency)

Compared with children, adults have a much wider spectrum of diseases that can cause nephrotic syndrome and therefore a kidney biopsy is required to confirm a diagnosis of MCD. In general, the dosage of corticosteroids used for adults is lower than that for children. Corticosteroids are commenced at 0.8–1 mg/kg/day (up to 80 mg/day) and are slowly tapered over six months. Appropriate prophylaxis for pneumocystis jiroveci (e.g. cotrimoxazole) and hepatitis B virus (HBV) (e.g. antiviral in those at risk of HBV reactivation), and gastroprotective agents (e.g. proton pump inhibitors) should be initiated in patients who receive high doses of corticosteroids. In patients who show poor response to corticosteroids, a repeat kidney biopsy should be performed to exclude focal segmental glomerulosclerosis. Up to 50% of adult MCD patients relapse after being completely weaned off corticosteroids. Adult MCD patients with a partial response or relapse can be managed with a course of CYC or prolonged CNI treatment. CYC has the advantage of conferring more sustained remission in steroid-dependent or frequently relapsing MCD, but long-term treatment-related side effects such as ovarian failure and increased risk of malignancy remain important concerns. Cyclosporin A (CYA) or tacrolimus (TAC) are both viable choices of CNI in MCD. Chronic CNI nephrotoxicity and the considerable rates of relapse upon drug withdrawal are potential problems of CNI treatment. Careful monitoring of CNI exposure and renal function can help lower the risk of nephrotoxicity of long-term CNI administration. There is also data to suggest that mycophenolate may be used for steroid-sparing and reducing disease relapse. Emerging evidence also shows the efficacy of anti-CD20 treatment in patients with refractory or frequently relapsing disease. Hepatitis B viral status must be checked prior to anti-CD20 administration and the appropriate prophylaxis given as stated above.

Focal Segmental Glomerulosclerosis

Clinical characteristics

Focal segmental glomerulosclerosis (FSGS) is an important cause of nephrotic syndrome and renal failure in children and adults. Histological features of FSGS can be detected in 30–40% of kidney biopsies performed in patients with proteinuria or nephrotic syndrome. The majority of children with FSGS present with nephrotic-range proteinuria, while adult FSGS patients may show either nephrotic- or subnephrotic-range proteinuria at the onset of disease. Hypertension is observed in 30–50% of patients with FSGS. Up to 20–30% of patients with FSGS also show evidence of renal impairment at presentation, and about 25–75% have microscopic haematuria at the time of diagnosis. FSGS is associated with a significantly higher risk of ESKD compared with other primary nephrotic glomerular diseases, and the risk of progression to ESKD is influenced by the severity of renal disease at presentation, ethnicity, histological variants, and response to treatments. Only a small proportion of patients have spontaneous remission while the majority of primary FSGS patients will experience a progressive increase in proteinuria and renal function decline. Up to half of the children and adult FSGS patients who do not respond well to treatment will develop ESKD after five years of diagnosis. FSGS can recur after kidney transplantation, with recurrence rates of around 30% after the first kidney transplantation and 85%–100% after the second kidney transplantation. Recurrent FSGS manifests as nephrotic syndrome early after transplantation (usually within one month) and is associated with rapid allograft loss.

Pathogenesis and histopathological features

FSGS can be classified as primary or secondary, depending on the underlying aetiology (Table 8.4). The pathogenesis of primary (idiopathic) FSGS remains unclear, though some evidence suggests that it might be related to a circulating factor (CF). Proposed candidates for this CF include the serum urine-type plasminogen activator receptor, cardiotrophin-like cytokine factor 1, apoA1b (an isoform of ApoA1), and anti-CD40 antibodies. Secondary FSGS can be related to genetic defects, infections, drugs, or maladaptive structural–functional responses. Typical LM findings are segmental solidification involving any portion of a glomerular tuft (Figure 8.6). The glomerular capillaries are obliterated by matrix substances, often accompanied by hyalinosis, endocapillary foam cells, and wrinkling of the glomerular basement membrane. IF is usually negative or with limited IgM and C3 staining in sclerotic areas. EM shows wrinkling or retraction of the glomerular basement membrane and extensive podocyte foot process effacement, with no electron-dense deposits. FSGS has different histological variants (Table 8.5) and each is associated with its distinct clinical behaviour and prognosis. The collapsing variant is highly resistant to immunosuppressive treatments and is associated with rapid progression to ESKD. The tip-lesion variant is more responsive to immunosuppressive treatments and has relatively low risk of ESKD. Similarly, the cellular variant is also responsive to immunosuppression and shows intermediate outcomes compared to the tip-lesion and collapsing variants. The perihilar variant is often seen in FSGS patients due to reduced nephron mass, and is frequently associated with glomerulomegaly. While classic FSGS (also known as 'FSGS not otherwise specified') is the most common histological variant, its prognostic significance remains undefined.

Table 8.4: Primary and secondary causes of FSGS

Primary (idiopathic) FSGS
• Postulated to be related to circulating factor
Secondary FSGS
• Genetic causes (e.g. APOL1)
• Maladaptive responses (e.g. reduced nephron mass such as low birth weight, single kidney, reflux disease, morbid obesity, cyanotic heart disease)
• Infection (e.g. HIV, parvovirus B19)
• Drugs (e.g. pamidronate, lithium)

FSGS, focal segmental glomerulosclerosis; HIV, human immunodeficiency virus

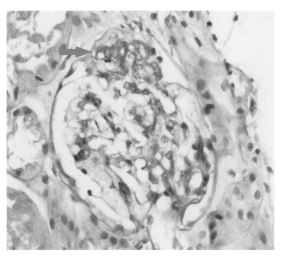

Figure 8.6: Focal segmental glomerulosclerosis (FSGS). There is segmental sclerosis of the glomerulus (arrow) with hyalinosis and adhesion to the Bowman's capsule (PASD, ×400, Dr A. H. N. Tang).

Table 8.5: Clinical behaviour and prognosis of different histological variants of focal segmental glomerulosclerosis

Histological variants	Clinical behaviour and prognosis
Classic FSGS (NOS) variant	• The most common form of FSGS • The prognostic significance remains undefined
Tip lesion variant	• More responsive to immunosuppressive treatments • Relatively lower risk of progression to ESKD
Cellular variant	• Responsive to immunosuppressive treatments • Intermediate renal prognosis between tip lesion and collapsing variants
Perihilar variant	• Often seen in FSGS due to reduction in nephron mass
Collapsing variant	• Association with HIV infection • Highly resistant to immunosuppressive treatments • Rapid and high rates of progression to ESKD

ESKD, end-stage kidney disease; FSGS, focal segmental glomerulosclerosis; HIV, human immunodeficiency virus; NOS, not otherwise specified

Management

Patients with primary FSGS and subnephrotic-range proteinuria should be treated with renin-angiotensin-aldosterone systems (RAAS) blocking agents. Immunosuppressive therapies are indicated in primary FSGS patients with nephrotic syndrome. The mainstay of treatment is high dosage of oral corticosteroid (1 mg/kg/day) for an initial period of 4–8 weeks, with subsequent tapering of the dosage. The cumulative remission rates range between 40 and 60%. Alkylating agents (chlorambucil or CYC) can be considered in steroid-resistant FSGS. There is evidence to show that the use of corticosteroids combined with CNI is superior to corticosteroids alone in preserving renal function. Corticosteroids and MMF have also been reported to be effective in the treatment of FSGS. Plasma exchange is indicated in patients with recurrent FSGS after transplantation. There are also anecdotal reports on the efficacy of biologics (e.g. anti-CD20) in refractory FSGS and recurrent FSGS, but data from prospective randomized clinical trials are still lacking.

Membranous Nephropathy

Clinical characteristics

Membranous nephropathy (MN) is a common cause of nephrotic syndrome in adults, and can be detected in up to 30% of kidney biopsies from adult patients who present with proteinuria or nephrotic syndrome. MN is relatively uncommon in children, accounting for 2–12% of cases that present with nephrotic syndrome. MN is characterized by the insidious onset of nephrotic- or subnephrotic-range proteinuria. About 80% of patients show overt nephrotic syndrome at the time of presentation. MN patients occasionally show microscopic haematuria and exhibit variable degrees of renal impairment. MN patients can also suffer from complications of nephrotic syndrome such as thromboembolic events or abnormal lipid profiles. Other systemic features may be present in patients with secondary MN due to autoimmune or neoplastic disorders. Approximately 25% of MN patients have spontaneous complete remission, but this can take quite a long time—several months or even years. Another 25% of patients have persistent proteinuria without loss of renal function. Of patients with nephrotic syndrome who are left untreated, up to 50% will have a progressive decline in renal function and eventually develop ESKD. Roughly a quarter of MN patients who achieve complete remission will experience a relapse of nephrotic syndrome. De novo and recurrent MN after kidney transplantation can occur, but are relatively uncommon.

Pathogenesis and histopathological features

MN can be classified as primary or secondary, depending on its causes (Table 8.6). About 70–80% of cases are primary MN and 20–30% are secondary MN. The initiating pathogenic event for both primary and secondary MN is the formation of an immune complex on the outer surface of the glomerular capillary wall. Compelling evidence suggests that the formation of the immune complex is a local or *in situ* process, and the antigens involved can be endogenous or exogenous. In this context, circulating IgG, which recognizes the endogenous autoantigens expressed on podocytes, can cause immune-complex formation and deposition. The discovery of autoantibody against the M-type phospholipase A2 receptor (anti-PLA2R) has provided significant insights into the pathogenic mechanisms of primary MN. Anti-PLA2R antibody is present in up to 70% of primary MN cases, but only in 15–30% of cases with secondary MN. Anti-PLA2R also shows clinical correlations with disease activity and has prognostic value in primary MN. Another antibody called anti-thrombospondin type 1 domain-containing 7A (anti-THSD7A) was also discovered though in a much smaller proportion (2–3%) of patients with primary MN. For secondary MN, circulating IgG can bind to exogenous antigens that localize at the subepithelial surface of the

podocytes and form immune complexes. For both primary and secondary MN, the deposition of immune complexes at the outer podocytic surface is followed by activation of the complement cascade to form the membrane attack complex (C5b-9), leading to further glomerular injury and non-selective protein loss through the glomerular capillary wall.

During the earliest stage of MN, the LM findings can appear relatively normal. The classical LM findings of MN are characterized by thickening of the capillary wall, and 'spikes' or 'bubbly' appearances seen on methenamine silver staining (Figures 8.7 and 8.8). IF typically shows granular IgG and C3 staining (Figure 8.9), and in primary MN cases the staining for PLA2R is often positive (Figure 8.10). Membranous lupus nephritis has to be suspected when the IF staining appears full-house. EM shows predominantly

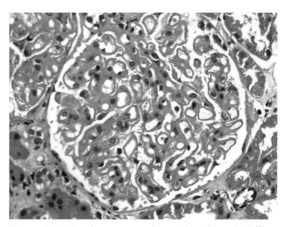

Figure 8.7: Membranous nephropathy. There is diffuse thickening of the glomerular capillary loops (H&E, ×400, Dr A. H. N. Tang).

Table 8.6: Causes of primary and secondary membranous nephropathy

Primary	
Autoantibody against podocytic antigens (e.g. PLA2R or THSD7A)	
Secondary	
Infection	HBV, HCV, syphilis, malaria, schistosomiasis
Malignancy	Lung, colon, and breast cancers
Drugs	NSAIDs, gold, penicillamine
Autoimmune conditions	SLE, RA, Sjogren syndrome, IgG4 disease

HBV, hepatitis B virus; HCV, hepatitis C virus; NSAIDs, non-steroidal anti-inflammatory drugs; PLA2R, phospholipase A2 receptor; RA, rheumatoid arthritis; SLE, systemic lupus erythematosus; THSD7A, thrombospondin type 1 domain-containing 7A

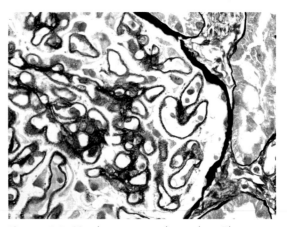

Figure 8.8: Membranous nephropathy. There are numerous epimembranous spikes and 'holes' along the capillary loops, representing the basement membrane reaction to the subepithelial immune complex deposits (PASM, ×1000, Dr A. H. N. Tang).

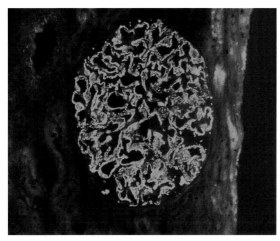

Figure 8.9: Membranous nephropathy. There is global granular staining along the capillary loops of glomerulus (anti-IgG immunofluorescence, ×400, Dr A. H. N. Tang).

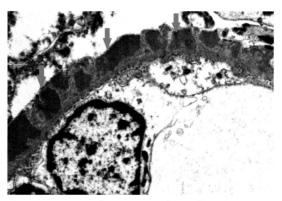

Figure 8.11: Membranous nephropathy. There are abundant subepithelial electron-dense deposits (arrows) with glomerular basement membrane reaction (Transmission electron microscopy, ×8000, Dr G. S. W. Chan).

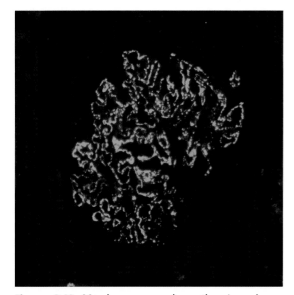

Figure 8.10: Membranous nephropathy. In primary membranous nephropathy, a significant proportion of patients will show global granular staining along the capillary loops for phospholipase A2 receptor (PLA2R) in immunofluorescence study (PLA2R immunofluorescence, ×400, Dr A. H. N. Tang).

subepithelial electron-dense deposits, accompanied by variable degrees of podocyte foot process effacement (Figure 8.11).

Management

In patients with histological evidence of MN, efforts must be made to exclude secondary causes of MN. Autoimmune and tumour markers, VDRL test, viral

hepatitis status, chest radiography, and stool occult blood can serve as screening investigations for secondary causes. PET-CT can be considered in patients whose initial screening tests were negative but have a high index of suspicion for secondary causes. Secondary MN should be managed with RAAS blockers and proteinuria usually resolves when the underlying aetiology is properly treated. HBV-related MN should be treated with antiviral therapy that readily induces remission. Primary MN patients with subnephrotic-range proteinuria can be treated with RAAS blockades. Immunosuppressive treatments are reserved for patients with heavy proteinuria or those who do not respond to RAAS blockades. The standard immunosuppressive treatments for primary MN are corticosteroids combined with an alkylating agent. The classical Ponticelli protocol comprises alternate cycles of pulse corticosteroid and chlorambucil. The modified Ponticelli regimen consists of corticosteroids and CYC, and is associated with better tolerability than the classical regimen. Corticosteroids in combination with CNI (CYA or TAC) can effectively reduce proteinuria in MN patients, but as in other glomerular diseases, the use of CNI is associated with long-term renal toxicity and high rates of relapse upon treatment discontinuation. Also, results from a large randomized controlled trial demonstrated that cytotoxic treatments in primary MN are associated with better preservation of long-term renal function compared with CNI or corticosteroids alone. Accumulating data demonstrates that anti-CD20 treatment is efficacious and well-tolerated in primary MN patients. The high drug costs, however, limit the widespread use as a first-line treatment in many localities, such as low- to middle-income countries.

Membranoproliferative Glomerulonephritis and C3 Glomerulopathy

Clinical characteristics

Membranoproliferative glomerulonephritis (MPGN), previously known as 'mesangioproliferative glomerulonephritis', is a relatively rare glomerular disease. MPGN accounts for less than 5% of all primary glomerulonephritis, and approximately 4–10% of all primary nephrotic syndromes in children and adults. In fact, MPGN refers to histological morphology rather than a distinct clinical entity. Patients with MPGN show protean clinical presentations, which may include microscopic haematuria and subnephrotic-range proteinuria, nephrotic syndrome with relatively mild renal impairment, slowly progressive renal impairment, and rapid deterioration in renal function with active urine sediments. MPGN in children and adolescents is usually idiopathic and manifests as primary renal disease without systemic involvement. Occasionally, some of these patients may have partial lipodystrophy affecting the face and the upper body. MPGN in adults is also limited to the kidneys but sometimes can be associated with systemic cryoglobulinaemia (especially in those with chronic hepatitis C virus [HCV] infection). Patients with MPGN due to cryoglobulinaemia can also have systemic manifestations such as joint pain, purpuric skin rash, and digital infarcts. Very often, decreased serum complement levels are observed in patients with MPGN. MPGN in both children and adults shows an unfavourable renal prognosis. Without any treatment, approximately 40–50% of children with MPGN progress to renal failure over 10 years. As for adult MPGN patients, about 50% develop ESKD at five years after diagnosis. MPGN can recur after kidney transplantation, with recurrence rates of 20–30% for immune-complex-mediated MPGN and 80–90% for complement-mediated MPGN.

Pathogenesis and histopathological features

The previous classification of MPGN into type I, II, or III by histological features has become obsolete. The updated reclassification of MPGN in 2015 is largely based on disease pathogenesis, categorizing it into immune-complex- or complement-mediated MPGN (Table 8.7). In immune-complex-mediated MPGN,

Table 8.7: Causes of immune-complex-mediated and complement-mediated membranoproliferative glomerulonephritis

Immune-complex-mediated MPGN
• Infections (e.g. HCV, HBV, cryoglobulinaemia)
• Autoimmune disorders (e.g. SLE)
• Monoclonal gammopathies (e.g. multiple myeloma)

Complement-mediated MPGN
• C3 dense deposit disease
• C3 glomerulopathy
• C4 glomerulopathy

HBV, hepatitis B virus; HCV, hepatitis C virus; MPGN, membranoproliferative glomerulonephritis; SLE, systemic lupus erythematosus

immune-complex deposition occurs preferentially in the mesangial and subendothelial regions of the glomerulus, leading to activation of the classical complement pathway. Complement-mediated MPGN is characterized by aberrant activation of the alternative complement pathway occurring in the fluid phase and in the glomerular microenvironment, which results in prominent glomerular C3 deposition and injury. Dense deposit disease and C3 glomerulopathy are the two major subtypes of complement-mediated MPGN, and show overlapping clinical and pathological features suggestive of a disease continuum. Complement-mediated MPGN is often related to acquired autoantibodies that target the C3 or C5 convertases, which prolong the half-life of these normally short-lived enzymes and thus results in overactivation of the alternative complement cascade. Genetic defects in complement-related genes are rare in Chinese patients. The typical LM features include hypercellularity (due to the infiltration of immune cells and proliferation of mesangial cells) and an increase in the mesangial matrix, which together give rise to a 'lobular' pattern in the glomeruli (Figure 8.12). Crescents can also be seen in patients who present with severe renal dysfunction. The methenamine silver or PASM stain reveals a 'double contour' (also known as 'tram-track') appearance due to the interposition of mesangial cells, immune-reactive cells, and endothelial cells in the capillary wall, accompanied by the synthesis of new basement membrane materials (Figure 8.13). IF for immune-complex-mediated MPGN usually shows granular IgG, IgM, and C3 (Figures 8.14 and 8.15) while complement-mediated MPGN shows only C3 staining, without other immunoglobulins. The

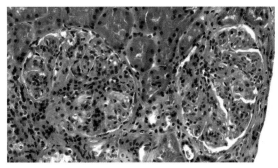

Figure 8.12: Membranoproliferative glomerulonephritis. The glomeruli show accentuation of lobular architecture with mesangial and endocapillary proliferation. Occasional neutrophils are present in the capillary lumen (H&E, ×200, Dr G. S. W. Chan).

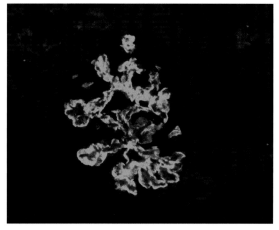

Figure 8.15: Membranoproliferative glomerulonephritis. Irregular, chunky deposits are present in the capillary loops and mesangium of the glomerulus (anti-C3 immunofluorescence, ×400, Dr G. S. W. Chan).

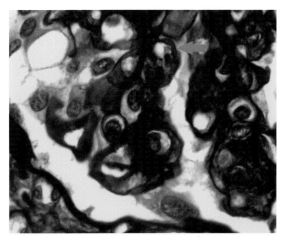

Figure 8.13: Membranoproliferative glomerulonephritis. The capillary wall shows double contour appearance (arrow), representing the reduplication of glomerular basement membrane (PASM, ×400, Dr G. S. W. Chan).

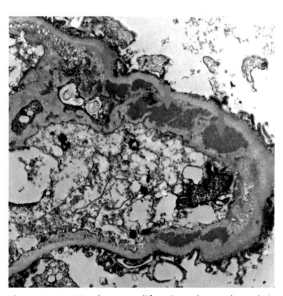

Figure 8.16: Membranoproliferative glomerulonephritis. There are a large number of subendothelial electron-dense deposits (arrows), which are associated with the formation of new underlying glomerular basement membrane (transmission electron microscopy, ×8000, Dr G. S. W. Chan).

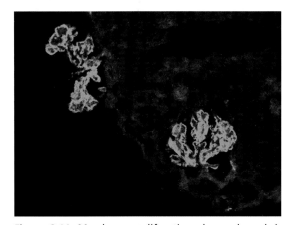

Figure 8.14: Membranoproliferative glomerulonephritis. Irregular, chunky deposits are observed in the capillary loops and mesangium of the glomeruli (anti-IgG immunofluorescence, ×200, Dr G. S. W. Chan).

classical EM findings of immune-complex-mediated MPGN are electron-dense deposits detected predominantly in the subendothelial regions (Figure 8.16). Complement-mediated MPGN (e.g. dense deposit disease) show highly electron-dense bands of homogenous substances occupying the glomerular basement membrane.

Management

Patients with a histological diagnosis of MPGN should be examined for underlying causes, such as chronic viral hepatitis infection, autoimmune diseases, or monoclonal gammopathies. More detailed investigation of the complement cascade should be considered in very young patients, those with significant family histories, or histological features suggestive of complement-mediated MPGN. Patients with chronic hepatitis B- or C-associated MPGN should receive antiviral therapies, while those with autoimmune disorders or monoclonal gammopathies should be managed accordingly. Patients with HCV-associated cryoglobulinaemia and MPGN may also benefit from anti-CD20 treatment. All MPGN patients should have optimal blood pressure and proteinuria control by RAAS-blocking agents. Children or adult idiopathic MPGN patients with nephrotic syndrome and progressive decline in renal function can be treated with corticosteroids and CYC or MMF for not more than six months. Pulse corticosteroids can be used when patients show rapidly deteriorating renal function or crescentic formations in the kidney biopsy. The efficacy of eculizumab (anti-C5b monoclonal antibody) has been reported, but there is insufficient data overall to recommend these biologics as first-line treatments in complement-mediated MPGN.

9

Systemic Diseases and the Kidneys

*Desmond Yap, Gary Chan, Sydney Tang, Harry Gill, Chik Cheung Chow,
Siu Ka Mak, Alex Tang, Gavin Chan, and Tak Mao Chan*

Introduction

The kidneys are often a target of injury in systemic conditions, including metabolic diseases, autoimmune disorders, infections, and malignancy. This chapter highlights the various important systemic diseases that affect the kidneys, focusing on their clinical characteristics, pathophysiology and management. Timely identification and appropriate management of these systemic causes are pertinent to improving renal and patient outcomes.

Diabetic Kidney Disease

Clinical characteristics

The global burden of diabetes mellitus (DM) is expected to reach 6.8%, affecting 578 million of the world's population by 2030, and diabetic kidney disease (DKD) is estimated to affect one-third to 40% of individuals with DM.

Individuals with DKD usually present with albuminuria, with or without renal impairment. There may be associated micro- and macro-vascular complications, especially when the diagnosis of DKD may be delayed for years in asymptomatic type 2 diabetics. Historically, DKD was thought to have a uniform and unidirectional natural history. Gradual disease progression from microalbuminuria to overt macro-albuminuria and renal insufficiency was expected. With increased understanding of this clinical entity in the past decade, DKD is now recognized to have a variable clinical course. In fact, the regression of macro-albuminuria to normo-albuminuria has been demonstrated to occur in contemporary studies for both type 1 and 2 DM. In the setting of persistent macro-albuminuria, glomerular filtration rate (GFR) decline is accelerated such that progression to ESRD is noticeably faster when compared with the non-diabetic kidney disease population.

Diagnosis of DKD is usually straightforward. Kidney sizes may be preserved on ultrasonography in spite of CKD. However, it is prudent to consider an alternative aetiology in the presence of atypical features, such as the presence of active urinary sediment with dysmorphic red blood cells and casts, onset of significant albuminuria shortly after or pre-dating the recognition of DM, a sudden increase in the magnitude of albuminuria, or an abrupt change to the trajectory of renal decline. Where diagnostic doubt exists, a confirmatory renal biopsy should be performed.

Pathogenesis and histopathological features

The pathogenesis of DKD is multifaceted and complex. Insulin resistance and persistent hyperglycaemia results in the generation of advanced glycation end-products and reactive oxygen species, which drives proinflammatory and profibrotic pathways in the kidney. Renal injury is further mediated by aberrant glomerular haemodynamics, characterized by persistently raised intra-glomerular pressure, which incites progressive glomerulosclerosis. The multiple mediators involved in this process are summarized in Figure 9.1. The varying contributions of these processes likely account for the differing natural histories of DKD in different individuals.

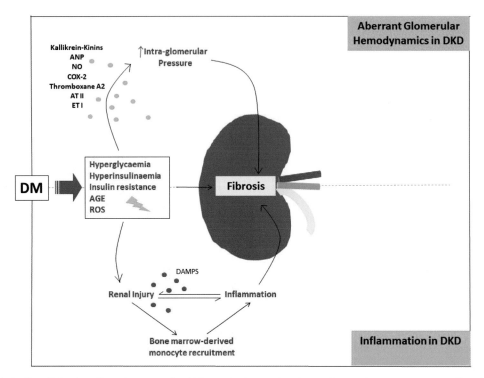

Figure 9.1: The diabetic milieu damages the kidneys by increasing intra-glomerular pressure as well as inducing inflammation and fibrosis. Reduced afferent arteriolar resistance is mediated by nitric oxide (NO), COX-2 prostanoids, atrial natriuretic peptide (ANP), Kallikrein-kinins, and hyperinsulinaemia. Raised efferent arteriolar resistance is mediated by angiotensin (AT) II, thromboxane A2, and endothelin (ET) I. Hyperglycaemia and advanced glycation end (AGE) products produces renal cell damage to leak damage-associated molecular patterns (DAMPS) to incite an inflammatory response within the kidney. In addition, cellular injury recruits bone marrow-derived monocytes, which differentiate into macrophages that home in on the injured renal parenchyma to amplify the inflammation. Hyperglycaemia on its own can also induce fibrosis.

The earliest renal histological changes on light microscopy (LM) in patients with DKD are glomerular hypertrophy, hyperplasia, and a thickened glomerular basement membrane (GBM). Subsequently, progressive mesangial matrix expansion occurs, resulting in nodular glomerulosclerosis (Kimmelstiel–Wilson nodules) (Figures 9.2 and 9.3). DKD is invariably accompanied by arteriolar hyalinosis with a variable degree of background tubular atrophy and interstitial fibrosis. These vascular and tubulointerstitial changes can be discordant with the degree of glomerulosclerosis, but become progressively pronounced as patients transit towards ESRD. Immunofluorescence (IF) may show linear IgG staining of the GBM, which is diffusely thickened on electron microscopy (EM). Additionally, marked podocyte foot process effacement is seen, with no evidence of immune-complex deposition in the expanded mesangial matrix.

Management

Although there is currently no cure for DKD, therapeutic options that can prevent or retard renal disease progression are available. The current armamentarium in the clinical management of DKD focuses on stringent glycaemic and blood pressure control.

Glycaemic control

Glycaemic optimization has been shown to delay the onset and progression of DKD in both type 1 and 2 DM cohorts. Early prospective data demonstrated a reduction in incident microalbuminuria. Subsequently, a significant risk reduction for ESRD in those with macro-albuminuria was also shown. However, the rigorous diabetic control required to achieve these favourable renal outcomes is offset by the risk of hypoglycaemia. The current American

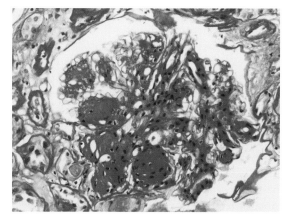

Figure 9.2: Diabetic nephropathy. There is significant increase in mesangial matrix with formation of multiple nodules (PAS, ×400, Dr A. H. N. Tang).

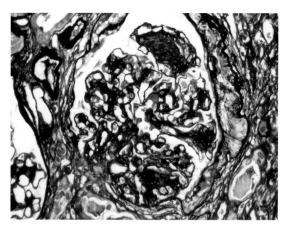

Figure 9.3: Diabetic nephropathy. A Kimmelstiel-Wilson nodule is shown at the 12 o'clock position of the glomerulus. The nodule displays a lamellated appearance (PASM, ×400, Dr A. H. N. Tang).

Diabetes Association recommendations target HbA1c < 7% for this population, but more stringent HbA1c goals should be employed where they can be achieved safely without significant hypoglycaemia, for the clear benefit of renoprotection.

In the 2010s, two new classes of antidiabetic agents have altered the prognostic landscape of DKD, above and beyond that offered by their glycaemic-lowering properties. Selective inhibitors of sodium-glucose cotransporter 2 (SGLT-2) are able to harness the kidney's ability to regulate glucose homeostasis by blocking the reabsorption of filtered glucose in the proximal convoluted tubules. Moreover, SGLT-2 inhibition concomitantly reduces tubular sodium reabsorption and increases sodium delivery to the macula densa. As a result, afferent arteriolar vasoconstriction via tubuloglomerular feedback reduces intra-glomerular pressure to confer renoprotection. Clinically, SGLT-2 inhibitors have been shown to reduce adverse renal (doubling of serum creatinine and ESRD incidence) and CV outcomes in individuals with DKD. Furthermore, this class of drugs is able to promote an attractive CKD portfolio, which includes blood pressure and body weight optimization by way of its natriuretic properties. To date, SGLT-2 inhibitors have been approved for patients with type 2 DM, with the latest data from a large multicentre randomized controlled trial (RCT) demonstrating their efficacy in patients with GFR ≥ 30 ml/min/1.73 m^2. It should be noted that SGLT-2 inhibitors are associated with urogenital infections and may be associated with a higher risk of lower limb amputations. Thus, caution should be exercised in individuals with these risk factors.

Another class of antidiabetic agents, which have shown renoprotective promise, are the glucagon-like peptide-1 (GLP-1) receptor agonists. These incretin-mimetics stimulate the release of glucose-dependent insulin, regulate post-prandial glucagon secretion and delay gastric emptying to achieve glucose control and beneficial weight reduction. Data from large multicentre RCTs suggest that GLP-1 receptor agonists retard GFR decline and reduce the composite outcomes of new-onset proteinuria, doubling of serum creatinine, ESRD, and death from renal disease in type 2 diabetics. As yet, the underlying mechanisms for the observed renal benefits conferred by GLP-1 receptor agonists have not been fully elucidated.

Blood pressure control

Hypertension is a prevalent comorbidity in diabetic individuals, and is an independent modifiable risk factor for the development and acceleration of micro- and macro-vascular complications. There is no doubt that the achievement of stringent blood pressure control, irrespective of the agent used, retards the onset and progression of DKD to confer a survival benefit. Inhibitors of the renin-angiotensin system (RAS) including angiotensin-converting enzyme (ACE) inhibitors and angiotensin II receptor blockers (ARB) are widely employed to control the blood pressure of diabetic patients. They are superior to other antihypertensive agents in DKD by virtue of their capacity to reduce intra-glomerular pressure and hence proteinuria by preferentially dilating the efferent arteriole. Attempts to achieve a more profound RAS blockade, by treating DKD patients with a combination of ACE inhibitors with ARBs, however, did not produce a clear renal benefit.

Instead, it was associated with an increased propensity for hyperkalaemia and acute kidney injury, emphasizing that RAS manipulation should be confined to a single agent in DKD. To date, available evidence from clinical trials recommends targeting a blood pressure of < 125/80 mmHg for patients with DKD. Of note, the data for RAS blockade have been established only in secondary prevention trials. Henceforth, the clinical practice guidelines of the National Kidney Foundation's Kidney Disease Outcomes Quality Initiative have not enforced the implementation of ACE inhibitors or ARB for the primary prevention of DKD in normotensive individuals with normo-albuminuria.

General management

The general management of DKD parallels that of CKD due to any other aetiology. However, it should be noted that individuals with DKD are at an even higher risk of adverse CV outcomes. As such, lifestyle modifications and stringent management of dyslipidaemia and hyperuricaemia should be instigated to reduce CV morbidity and mortality in DKD patients.

Renal replacement therapy in DKD

The consideration for renal replacement therapy (RRT) in patients with DKD is largely similar to patients with CKD from other aetiologies. RRT should be discussed and initiated in a timely manner, taking into account of the rapid decline in renal function in many DKD patients. Renal transplantation represents the optimal form of RRT for eligible patients, and in centres of expertise, the options of simultaneous pancreas-kidney transplantation or sequential pancreas-after-kidney transplant may be considered in selected patients.

Lupus Nephritis

Clinical characteristics

Lupus nephritis (LN) occurs in approximately 60–70% of Asian patients with systemic lupus erythematosus (SLE) and is an important cause of acute and/or chronic renal impairment. The presence of renal involvement is a significant risk factor for patient morbidity and mortality in SLE. Patients with LN can also experience other lupus manifestations such as fever, arthralgia, alopecia, aphthous ulcers, serositis, haematological abnormalities, and cerebral involvement. Isolated LN, however, can often be the first clinical presentation in Chinese SLE patients. LN

is characterized by repeated episodes of disease relapse interspersed with periods of disease quiescence. Changes in serological parameters, such as increases in anti-dsDNA titres and drops in serum complement levels, often precede or coincide with LN flare-ups. Lupus activity usually decreases as CKD progresses, but flare ups can occur in patients on dialysis or after kidney transplantation. Consequent to improvements in immunosuppressive management and general medical care, the clinical outcomes of LN patients have improved substantially over the past few decades and the reported patient and renal survival rates were over 90% and 70–80% respectively in different series.

LN can be categorized into different histological classes, and each class of LN is associated with distinct clinicopathological characteristics and prognoses (Table 9.1). Class I or II LN usually present with no or at most low-grade proteinuria or renal impairment, and generally show favourable renal prognoses unless they transform to other classes of LN. Proliferative (i.e., Class III [focal] or Class IV [diffuse]) LN is the most common forms of LN and patients usually present with significant proteinuria, active urinary sediments and renal dysfunction. Repeated flare-ups of proliferative LN will result in attrition of nephrons and thus progression to CKD. Class V (i.e. pure membranous) LN runs a relatively more indolent course than its proliferative counterparts. Class V LN patients usually present with significant proteinuria (often in the nephrotic range), but with relatively less severe renal impairment. Class V (membranous) changes can also coexist with other classes of LN. Patients with Class VI (advanced sclerosing) LN have poor renal prognoses and a high risk of developing ESRD.

Pathogenesis and histopathological features

The pathogenesis of LN is highly complex. Genetic predisposition, aberrant B- and T-cell responses, dysregulated cytokine milieu, abnormalities in the complement cascade, and the presence of pathogenic autoantibodies all contribute to the pathogenesis of LN. Kidney biopsies provide useful diagnostic and prognostic information to guide clinical decisions in LN management. Classes of LN are categorized according to LM findings (Table 9.1). In addition, the histological activity and chronicity indices are also scored during the assessment of the kidney biopsy samples. Typical LM features of proliferative LN are endocapillary proliferation, mesangial hypercellularity, and evidence of immune-complex

Table 9.1: The International Society of Nephrology/Renal Pathology Society (ISN/RPS) classification of lupus nephritis and its clinic-pathological correlations

Class of LN	Salient Histological Features	Clinical Characteristics and Prognosis
Class I	**Minimal mesangial LN** Normal glomeruli by LM, but mesangial immune deposits by IF	• Proteinuria and renal impairment are usually mild • Renal prognosis generally favourable unless transformed into other classes of LN
Class II	**Mesangial proliferative LN** Purely mesangial hypercellularity of any degree or mesangial matrix expansion by LM, with mesangial immune deposits	
Class III	**Focal LN** Mesangial, endocapillary and/or extracapillary GN involving < 50% of all glomeruli, typically with focal subendothelial ± subepithelial deposits	• Proliferative LN is the commonest form of renal involvement in SLE patients • Typically present with significant proteinuria, active serological markers and urine sediments ± renal dysfunction
Class IV	**Diffuse LN** Mesangial, endocapillary and/or extracapillary GN involving > 50% of all glomeruli, typically with diffuse subendothelial immune deposits ± subepithelial deposits	• Patients with crescents or TMA changes on biopsy often show severe renal impairment • Poorly managed or repeated flares of Class III or IV LN flares will result in CKD and ESKD
Class V	**Membranous LN** Global or segmental subepithelial immune deposits or their morphologic sequelae by LM and by IF or EM, with or without mesangial alterations	• Typically present with significant proteinuria, and occasionally mild renal impairment • Generally shows a relatively more benign disease course than its proliferative counterparts
Class VI	**Advanced sclerosing LN** ≥ 90% of glomeruli globally sclerosed without residual activity	• Unfavourable long-term renal prognosis with high risk of progression to ESKD

CKD, chronic kidney disease; EM, electron microscopy; ESKD, endstage kidney disease; GN, glomerulonephritis; IF, immunofluorescence; LM, light microscopy; LN, lupus nephritis; SLE, systemic lupus erythematosus; TMA, thrombotic microangiopathy

Modified from the ISN/RPS 2003 Classification for Lupus Nephritis and the 2018 Revision (Weening et al., 2004; Bajema et al., 2018).

deposition (Figure 9.4). Crescents or thrombotic microangiopathy can sometimes be seen in patients with severe LN. IF classically shows full-house staining (Figure 9.5). EM usually shows predominantly subendothelial electron-dense deposits (EDD) (Figure 9.6), with variable degrees of EDD over the subepithelial and mesangial regions. Pure Class V LN shows typical membranous features on LM, with predominantly subepithelial deposits on EM.

Management

The management of LN is generally guided by the severity of renal disease and histopathological findings. Patients with active severe LN (i.e. Class III or IV LN, or pure Class V LN with nephrotic-range proteinuria) should receive immunosuppressive treatments, which can be broadly divided into the induction and maintenance phases (Table 9.2). General measures such as antimalarials and RAS

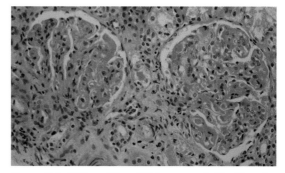

Figure 9.4: Diffuse (Class IV) lupus nephritis. The glomeruli show lobulation of the capillary loops. The capillary wall is thickened with 'wire-loop' appearance. The capillaries contain so-called hyaline thrombi. Both conditions are caused by the presence of massive subendothelial deposits (H&E, ×200, Dr G. S. W. Chan).

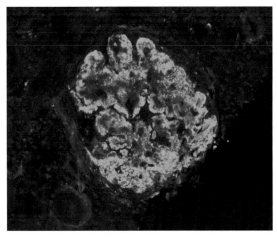

Figure 9.5: Diffuse (Class IV) lupus nephritis. There are chunky and granular deposits in both capillary loops and mesangium. C1q staining is typically prominent in lupus nephritis (anti-C1q immunofluorescence, ×400, Dr G. S. W. Chan).

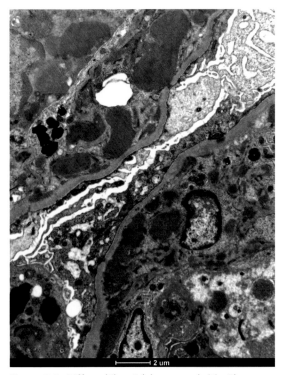

Figure 9.6: Diffuse (Class IV) lupus nephritis. There are massive subendothelial electron-dense deposits (transmission electron microscopy, ×5000, Dr G. S. W. Chan).

blockades in patients with CKD should be also instituted unless contraindicated.

The induction phase entails the use of intensive immunosuppressive therapies for approximately four to six months, with the objective being to rapidly abrogate active renal inflammation and preserve nephron mass. Pulse corticosteroids for up to three days followed by a tapering regimen of oral corticosteroids, combined with either mycophenolate mofetil (MMF) or cyclophosphamide (CYC), constitutes the standard initial therapy for severe LN. CYC can be given via the intravenous or oral routes in LN patients. The short-term side effects of CYC include myelosuppression, hair loss and haemorrhagic cystitis, and patients with repeated CYC exposure are at increased risk of gonadal failure and malignancy. Reduced-dose IV CYC (the EURO-LUPUS regimen) achieves similar short- and long-term efficacy as standard-dose CYC, but with less treatment-related toxicities. While both CYC and MMF induction show comparable short-term renal remission rates in LN patients, MMF treatment is often preferred nowadays because of better treatment tolerability and preservation of fertility. Notwithstanding, MMF can also cause unwanted effects such as gastrointestinal disturbance, anaemia, and teratogenicity. Maintenance immunosuppression is also crucial for the management of LN as it serves to consolidate renal remission and prevent disease relapse. The commonly used maintenance regimens are low-dose corticosteroids in combination with MMF or azathioprine (AZA), and accumulating data suggests that MMF is more effective than AZA at preventing disease flare-ups. Based on the above evidence and considerations, the upcoming Kidney Disease: Improving Global Outcomes (KDIGO) 2020 guidelines recommend that corticosteroids in combination with MMF or reduced-dose IV CYC (the EURO-LUPUS regimen) be administered as induction therapy for severe LN and MMF be used as first-line maintenance agent after completion of initial therapy (https://kdigo.org/wp-content/uploads/2017/02/KDIGO-GN-GL-Public-Review-Draft_1-June-2020.pdf, accessed 26 April 2021). Other considerations in choosing maintenance treatment for LN patients include prior induction regimen, history of disease relapse, pregnancy plans, and drug costs.

Calcineurin inhibitors (CNI) such as tacrolimus can be used as a second-line treatment in LN patients who cannot tolerate standard therapies. TAC-containing induction regimens show renal responses that are at least comparable to standard treatments in active LN patients and are associated with earlier

Table 9.2: Standard and emerging treatments for lupus nephritis

Induction treatments (usually last for 4–6 months)

• Pulse corticosteroids for up to three days followed by a tapering regimen of oral corticosteroids, combined with either MMF or CYC, constitutes the standard initial therapy for severe LN

Induction Agents	Mechanism of Action	Remarks
CYC	• An alkylating agent with potent cytotoxic effects on different immune-reactive cell types	• Both IV and oral CYC are effective induction agents, and patients with very severe renal impairment or crescentic LN often require IV CYC
MMF	• Inhibits IMPDH to interfere with de novo purine synthesis in lymphoid cells, thereby selectively suppresses lymphocytes	• Long-term toxicities of CYC (e.g. gonadal failure and neoplasms) are important concerns; reduced-dose IV CYC achieved similar short- and long-term efficacy as standard-dose IV CYC but with fewer toxicities • CYC or MMF induction shows comparable short-term renal response rates, but MMF is associated with better treatment tolerability and preservation of fertility • MMF can be used as continuous induction–maintenance treatment, and confers relatively favourable long-term outcomes in Chinese patients

Maintenance treatment (usually begins after the initial 6 months)

• The commonly used maintenance regimens are low-dose corticosteroids (5–7.5 mg/day) plus either MMF or AZA

Maintenance Agents	Mechanisms of Action	Remarks
MMF	• Same as above	• Growing data supports the superiority of MMF maintenance over AZA in preventing relapse (MMF is the first-line maintenance treatment in the latest KDIGO guidelines)
AZA	• Inhibit GPAT to intervene with purine synthesis in lymphocytes	• MMF is teratogenic and relatively more costly, while AZA is safe for pregnancy and is more economical • The choice of maintenance agent should take into consideration of prior induction treatment, history of relapse, pregnancy, and financial issues

Alternative and emerging treatments

TAC	• Specifically inhibits IL-2 and thus T cell function and proliferation • Distinct anti-proteinuric effects on podocytes independent of its immunosuppressive action	• TAC induction shows at least comparable short-term renal response as standard treatments, and TAC-containing regimens show earlier proteinuria reduction • Careful monitoring of renal function and drug levels are needed to prevent chronic nephrotoxicity
Biologics	• Target specific cell surface molecules (e.g. CD20 or CTLA4) on immune-reactive cells or relevant cytokines (e.g. BAFF)	• Recent data showed that certain biologics (e.g. belimumab or obinutuzumab) when added on to standard induction treatments could enhance renal response rates • Other indications for biologics include refractory/frequently relapsing disease, severe extra-renal manifestations, or steroid minimization

AZA, azathioprine; CYC, cyclophosphamide; GPAT, glutamine-phosphoribosyl pyrophosphate amidotransferase; IMPDH, inosine monophosphate dehydrogenase; IV, intravenous; KDIGO, Kidney Disease: Improving Global Outcomes; LN, lupus nephritis; MMF, mycophenolate mofetil; TAC, tacrolimus proteinuria reduction. Chronic nephrotoxicity with prolonged TAC treatment, especially in patients with pre-existing CKD, remains a clinical concern and therapeutic drug monitoring may help minimize its renal side effects. Recent data shows that certain biologics (e.g. belimumab or obinutuzumab), when added to standard therapies, can enhance renal response rates, but one should note that the overall renal remission rates are relatively low in these clinical trials and long-term data is also lacking. Also, the criteria for selecting appropriate patients for these biologics remain undefined. Other indications for biologics include refractory or frequently relapsing LN, corticosteroid minimization, and severe extra-renal manifestations. Recently, the United States Food and Drug Administration approved belimumab and the CNI voclosporin for the treatment of active lupus nephritis, the latter in patients with eGFR >45 mL/min/1.73 m². For patients with Class V LN and nephrotic-range proteinuria, corticosteroids in combination with MMF, CNI, or cytotoxic agents are all viable therapeutic options.

Anti-glomerular Basement Membrane Disease

Clinical characteristics

Anti-glomerular basement membrane (anti-GBM) disease (also known as Goodpasture disease) is an immune-complex small-vessel vasculitis that affects glomerular capillaries, pulmonary capillaries, or both. Anti-GBM disease has an incidence of less than 2 per million population per year and a bimodal age distribution, with peak incidences in the third decade and in the sixth to seventh decades of life. Most patients with anti-GBM disease present with rapidly progressive glomerulonephritis (RPGN). Renal manifestations include microscopic or macroscopic haematuria, non-nephrotic proteinuria, and active urine sediment. About 30–60% of patients will have concurrent pulmonary haemorrhage, although some can present with isolated pulmonary haemorrhage. Systemic complaints such as fever, malaise, weight loss, or arthralgia can also occur.

Pathogenesis and histopathological features

Infections (e.g. influenza A), cigarette smoke and inhalation of hydrocarbons, treatment with alemtuzumab, and genetic predisposition (e.g. HLA-DR2 haplotype) have been implicated in the pathogenesis of anti-GBM disease. Anti-GBM disease is characterized by the presence of circulating and deposited antibodies directed against GBM antigens. The pathogenic antibodies are usually of the IgG class, with IgG1 and IgG3 subclasses predominating. The principal target of the autoimmune response in anti-GBM disease has been identified as the non-collagenous (NC1) domain of the α3 chain of type IV collagen (α3[IV]NC1, the 'Goodpasture autoantigen'). Crescent formation (usually affecting more than 50% of glomeruli) is the histopathologic hallmark of anti-GBM disease (Figures 9.7 and 9.8). There are

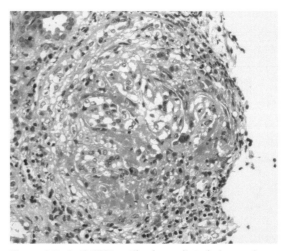

Figure 9.7: Anti-GBM antibody-mediated glomerulonephritis. Fibrinoid necrosis and karyorrhexis are present in the glomerulus. A cellular crescent is seen at the top (H&E, ×400, Dr A. H. N. Tang).

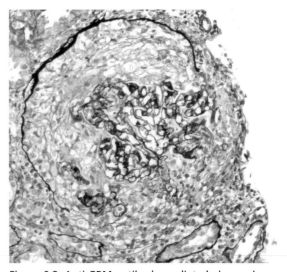

Figure 9.8: Anti-GBM antibody-mediated glomerulonephritis. A glomerulus displaying cellular crescent formation, ruptured glomerular basement membrane and Bowman's capsule, with surrounding periglomerular inflammation (PASM, ×400, Dr A. H. N. Tang).

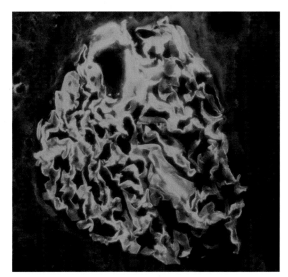

Figure 9.9: Anti-GBM antibody-mediated glomerulonephritis. Linear glomerular basement membrane staining pattern in direct immunofluorescence study for IgG is diagnostic of this disease (anti-IgG immunofluorescence, ×400, Dr A. H. N. Tang).

areas of fibrinoid necrosis in the glomeruli, sometimes with the rupture of Bowman's capsule and peri-glomerular inflammation. Linear ribbon-like deposition of IgG (usually polytypic, sometimes accompanied by C3 and C1q) can be demonstrated along the GBM under direct IF (Figure 9.9). EM usually reveals no EDDs.

Management

The mainstay of treatment is plasma exchange (PLEX) along with high doses of corticosteroids and CYC. The objective of PLEX is to rapidly remove anti-GBM autoantibodies, and the high doses of corticosteroids and CYC are to inhibit further autoantibody production. The recommended duration of plasmapheresis is 14 days or until anti-GBM antibody titre has become undetectable. Patients should be treated with intravenous pulse corticosteroids followed by oral corticosteroids, tapered over approximately six months. Oral CYC (2 mg/kg/day) is also given for approximately 2–3 months. Substitution with AZA or MMF may be considered if anti-GBM antibodies persist after three months of CYC.

Predictors of poor renal outcomes include severe renal dysfunction (serum creatinine > 500 μmol/L), dialysis-dependence at presentation, and a high proportion of glomeruli with crescents. Relapses are uncommon in anti-GBM glomerulonephritis,

although there may be a higher rate of recurrence in smokers or patients with occupational exposure to hydrocarbons. A period of months of sustained seronegativity for anti-GBM antibodies is recommended before consideration of renal transplantation.

Other variant forms of anti-GBM disease

Anti-GBM and ANCA dual-positive glomerulonephritis

Some patients with RPGN showed dual seropositivity for anti-GBM and antineutrophil cytoplasmic antibody (ANCA)-associated glomerulonephritis. ANCA-induced glomerular inflammation may be a trigger for the development of an anti-GBM response. The early disease course of these patients follows that of patients with anti-GBM disease, and during long-term follow-up they experience relapses similar to those in ANCA-associated vasculitis.

Atypical anti-GBM disease

Atypical anti-GBM disease is a rare clinical entity, accounting for only 10% of all anti-GBM cases. Compared with those with classical anti-GBM disease, these patients run a more indolent course and clinical outcomes are relatively more favourable. Lung involvement is uncommon and patients may be seronegative for anti-GBM antibodies. Unlike classical anti-GBM disease, atypical anti-GBM disease seldom shows diffuse crescentic lesions but up to 50% of cases exhibit linear monotypic Ig staining.

ANCA-Associated Vasculitis

Clinical characteristics

ANCA-associated vasculitis (AAV) is a necrotizing vasculitis primarily affecting small- to medium-sized vessels. AAV is a heterogeneous condition that includes three clinicopathologic conditions: granulomatosis with polyangiitis (GPA, formerly Wegener's granulomatosis), microscopic polyangiitis (MPA), and eosinophilic granulomatosis with polyangiitis (EGPA, formerly Churg-Strauss syndrome).

AAV has an incidence of about 20 per million population per year with a slight male preponderance at the age of 60–70 years. Patients may present with constitutional symptoms (fatigue, myalgia, and fevers—there is significant overlap in the clinical features of GPA and MPA; Table 9.3). GPA is characterized by the granulomatous manifestations and upper respiratory tract disease (e.g. rhinitis, sinusitis,

Table 9.3: Clinico-pathological features according to ANCA specificity

	PR3 ANCA	MPO ANCA
Demographics	• 50–70 years	• 60–80 years
Respiratory involvement	• Common: nodules, cavitation, nasal septal perforation	• Uncommon: pulmonary haemorrhage, peripheral reticulation, interstitial pneumonia
Renal presentation	• More acute presentation	• Relatively more indolent course compared to PR3 ANCA-associated GN • More chronic injury in biopsy
Histological features	• Necrotizing vasculitis with granulomatous inflammation; crescents	• Necrotizing vasculitis, crescents
Clinical outcomes	• More likely to have resistant disease and higher relapse rate	• Worse long-term renal survival and lower relapse rate

ANCA, anti-neutrophil cytoplasmic antibody; GN, glomerulonephritis; MPO, myeloperoxidase; PR3, proteinase 3
Adapted from Geetha D. and Jefferson JA. Am J Kidney Dis 2020.

otitis media, and nasal septal perforation or collapse). While patients with GPA may show pulmonary cavitation or nodular lesions, pulmonary haemorrhage is more common in patients with MPA. Similar to GPA, EGPA also shows granulomatous inflammation and necrotizing vasculitis but is distinguished from GPA by the presence of eosinophilia and asthma. Kidney involvement is common in AAV and is an important predictor of mortality. The typical renal presentation is a rapid decline in kidney function accompanied by subnephrotic-range proteinuria, microscopic haematuria, and hypertension over days to a few months. The ANCA serology pattern varies with different types of AAV (Table 9.4). The value of ANCA monitoring in predicting relapse is controversial, although in patients with renal involvement at presentation, a rise in ANCA level is predictive of relapse.

Pathogenesis and histopathological features

Infection with Staphylococcus *aureus*, exposure to silica and hydrocarbons, and medications (like hydralazine, propylthiouracil, minocycline, and anti–tumour necrosis factor agents) have been implicated in the pathogenesis of AAV. ANCA autoantigens (proteinase 3 [PR3] and myeloperoxidase [MPO]) are normally sequestered in the primary granules of neutrophils. Infection or other environmental stimuli result in neutrophil priming, with migration of PR3 and MPO to the cell surface. ANCA binds to these autoantigens, resulting in degranulation of neutrophils, which leads to the release of reactive oxygen species, proteases, and neutrophil extracellular

Table 9.4: Serological patterns of ANCA in different types of ANCA-associated vasculitis

	Seropositivity		
	PR3 ANCA	MPO ANCA	Remarks
GPA	75%	20%	Seronegative for ANCA in ~ 5%
MPA	30%	60%	Seronegative for ANCA in ~ 10%
EGPA	5%	45%	Seronegative for ANCA in ~50%
Renal-limited vasculitis	10%	80%	Seronegative for ANCA in ~ 10%
Drug-induced vasculitis	10%	90%	May have dual seropositivity for PR3 and MPO

ANCA, anti-neutrophil cytoplasmic antibody; EGPA, eosinophilic granulomatosis with polyangiitis; GPA, granulomatosis with polyangiitis; MPA, microscopic polyangiitis; MPO, myeloperoxidase; PR3, proteinase 3
Adapted from Geetha D and Jefferson JA. Am J Kidney Dis 2020.

traps (NETs), thereby damaging the endothelium. Chemokines and tissue deposition of PR3 and MPO further recruit autoreactive T cells and monocytes to perpetuate tissue injury. Typical LM features include crescents, necrotizing glomerulonephritis (GN), transmural arteritis, and active interstitial inflammation (Figures 9.10 and 9.11). IF staining is classically negative (i.e. pauci-immune) and EDDs are usually absent on EM.

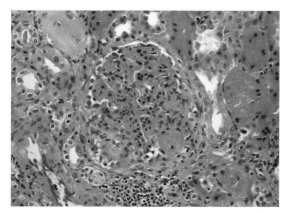

Figure 9.10: Granulomatosis with polyangiitis (Wegener's granulomatosis)/microscopic polyangiitis. A glomerulus displays near global necrosis, fibrin deposition, karyorrhexis, and a small cellular crescent at the 6 o'clock position (H&E, ×400, Dr G. S. W. Chan).

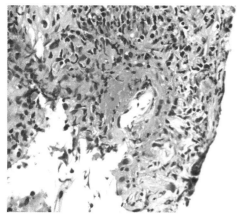

Figure 9.11: Granulomatosis with polyangiitis (Wegener's granulomatosis)/microscopic polyangiitis. An interlobular artery with focal transmural necrosis (H&E, ×400, Dr A. H. N. Tang).

Management

The recommended treatments for active ANCA-associated RPGN are high doses of glucocorticoids (intravenous pulse methylprednisolone followed by oral prednisolone), in combination with either CYC or anti-CD20 treatment. The use of PLEX in AAV remains controversial, but may be beneficial in selected patients, such as those with severe renal impairment, pulmonary haemorrhage, or concomitant anti-glomerular basement membrane disease. Methotrexate or MMF may be considered as alternative options in patients with mild diseases.

Approximately a third of patients will relapse by 18 months and less than a third will remain in relapse-free remission for more than a decade. While AZA maintenance was found to be superior to MMF for AAV, emerging data show that anti-CD20 maintenance was more effective than AZA in preventing disease relapse. The optimal duration of maintenance therapy in AAV remains undefined, but maintenance treatment for at least one year may be associated with a lower risk of relapse and ESRD. Disease activity usually become quiescent after patients have reached ESRD, and clinical remission for at least 12 months is a prerequisite for renal transplantation.

Polyarteritis Nodosa

Clinical characteristics

Polyarteritis nodosa (PAN) is an immune-complex-mediated necrotizing vasculitis that typically affects medium-sized arteries, and is associated with systemic organ involvement. Active vasculitis can result in arterial narrowing and tissue ischaemia, along with aneurysm formation through the weakened vessel wall, resulting in catastrophic bleeding. Apart from primary disease, PAN can present in patients with chronic hepatitis B virus (HBV) or hepatitis C virus (HCV) infection (especially in endemic areas) and hairy cell leukaemia. Systemic symptoms like fever, fatigue, weight loss, arthralgia, vasculitic skin changes, mononeuritis multiplex, and systemic organ involvements can occur. Renal involvement is common, presenting with hypertension, glomerular ischaemia, or even renal infarctions and perinephric haematoma from ruptured aneurysms.

Pathogenesis and histopathological features

The classical renal histologic findings are necrotizing vasculitis of renal, interlobar, and arcuate arteries at branch points with aneurysmal dilatation, fibrinoid necrosis, and neutrophilic infiltration of vessel walls, often accompanied by thrombosis. Features of necrotizing GN, seen in AAV, are absent. Diagnosis can be confirmed by a biopsy of the involved organ whenever applicable, or an arteriogram demonstrating aneurysms and irregular constrictions of involved arterial circulations.

Management

The mainstay of therapy for HBV- or HCV-associated PAN is antiviral therapy. The use of corticosteroids and other immunosuppressive drugs like CYC, methotrexate, or AZA, depending on the severity of the systemic vasculitis as in primary PAN, may also be required in these patients. PAN is a disease that can relapse, though at a lower rate when compared with other kinds of vasculitis.

Scleroderma

Clinical characteristics

Patients with scleroderma have a characteristic skin thickening as a result of uncontrolled deposition of normal collagen, and widespread thickening of the vascular wall and narrowing of the vascular lumen. The disease can be localized or systemic, and in the latter form, around 5–20% of cases involve internal organs, including the kidneys. Up to half of scleroderma patients have mild proteinuria, renal impairment, or hypertension, following a usually benign course. Approximately 5–20% of patients with diffuse cutaneous scleroderma (especially those with early stages of the disease with rapidly progressive skin involvement) develop a medical emergency known as scleroderma renal crisis (SRC). Patients with SRC present with abrupt development of accelerated or malignant hypertension and acute kidney injury (AKI). Full-blown features of malignant hypertension (retinopathy, encephalopathy, heart failure) with microangiopathic haemolytic anaemia may also be present. Corticosteroid treatment is a risk factor for SRC, and early identification is important for improving patient outcomes.

Pathogenesis and histopathological features

This is believed to involve a chemistry between immunological events and vascular damage, involving activated fibrogenic fibroblasts. Renal biopsies help predict prognosis but may not always be necessary, especially in patients with classical features. The main histopathologic changes in the kidney are intimal proliferation and 'onion-skin' hypertrophy of the small arcuate and interlobular arteries associated with narrowing or obliteration of the vascular lumen leading to diffuse intra-renal arterial stenosis.

Management

Patients with advancing skin involvement or severe inflammatory organ involvement are usually given immunosuppressive treatment. The principal management for SRC is to achieve timely blood pressure control with ACE inhibitors, with or without other agents like dihydropyridine calcium channel blocker (for Raynaud's phenomenon) and intravenous drugs for malignant hypertension. Despite these aggressive treatments, around 40% of patients with SRC require long-term dialysis.

Cryoglobulinaemia

Clinical characteristics

Cryoglobulinaemia refers to the presence of serum immunoglobulins that precipitate at temperatures below 37°C and redissolve on rewarming. These circulating immune complexes can be either monoclonal immunoglobulins (Type 1, usually IgG or IgM, from multiple myeloma or monoclonal gammopathy of undetermined significance [MGUS], Waldenstrom macroglobulinemia, or chronic lymphocytic leukaemia) or mixed (Type 2, typically monoclonal IgM against polyclonal Ig, often associated with chronic viral infections like HCV, presence of rheumatoid factor, and low complement C4 level); or Type 3 (polyclonal IgG against polyclonal IgM, commonly from autoimmune diseases). These patients present with arthralgia, palpable purpura and skin ulcers (or digital ischaemia, livedo reticularis), and hyperviscosity syndrome (high cryocrit level). They can have vasculitis involving small- and medium-sized vessels, as well as various organs, including the kidneys (30%), and peripheral neuropathy. Patients with renal involvement usually present with microscopic haematuria, proteinuria, and subsequently progressive CKD.

Pathogenesis and histopathological features

The exact pathogenesis of cryoglobulin-associated GN remains unclear, but is believed to be largely contributed by immune-complex deposition in the subendothelial regions and activation of the complement cascade. The typical renal histological finding is membranoproliferative glomerulonephritis (MPGN). Segmental necrosis or crescents may be observed in patients with severe renal disease. Methamine-silver staining often shows 'double-contouring' of GBM, and EM typically shows mesangial and subendothelial EDDs.

Management

Treatment is primarily targeted at the underlying lymphoproliferative, infectious, or autoimmune disorders. Immunosuppressive therapy with corticosteroids, CYC, or rituximab is warranted for organ threatening manifestations and plasmapheresis can be initiated in selected patients with hyperviscosity syndrome and crescentic GN requiring dialysis.

Rheumatoid Arthritis

Clinical characteristics

Rarely, patients with rheumatoid arthritis (RA) can develop GN such as mesangioproliferative GN or membranous nephropathy (MN). Renal disorders may also arise from the treatment of RA (e.g. MN related to the use of gold and penicillin, or nephrotoxicity associated with the use of non-steroidal anti-inflammatory drugs or NSAIDs). Patients with longstanding poorly controlled RA may develop secondary AA amyloidosis, but this has become less common with increasingly effective therapies for the disease.

Pathogenesis and histopathological features

Typical histologic findings of RA-associated GN are mesangioproliferative GN or MN. Immunohistochemical staining of AA protein can help distinguish renal AA amyloid from AL amyloidosis.

Management

RA is managed through the early use of effective treatment to achieve good disease control. Renal disorders arising from RA therapy may resolve themselves after treatment discontinuation.

Sjogren's Syndrome

Clinical characteristics

Sjogren's syndrome is characterized by dry eyes and mouth (sicca syndrome), and salivary and lacrimal gland enlargement, with or without systemic symptoms (fatigue and myalgia). It can be associated with other autoimmune diseases. The diagnosis relies on ocular and salivary function tests, labial biopsy, and the detection of anti-Ro and anti-La autoantibodies (60–80%). Extra-glandular involvements can include kidneys, affecting 5–27% of patients, in which chronic tubulointerstitial nephritis (CIN) is the most common presentation, followed by different forms of GN. Patients with CIN present with elevated serum creatinine levels or tubular dysfunctions (Fanconi syndrome, distal renal tubular acidosis, or nephrogenic diabetes insipidus).

Pathogenesis and histopathological features

The most common histologic finding is CIN. Various forms of GN, including MPGN and MN, have also been reported and are postulated to be related to the deposition of circulating immune complexes, sometimes with underlying cryoglobulinemia (with or without HCV).

Management

A short course of corticosteroids may be attempted. The best treatment of these glomerulopathies remains undefined, but the same treatment recommendations as for the primary counterparts have been tried.

Immunoglobulin G Subclass 4 Disease

Clinical characteristics

Immunoglobulin G subclass 4 (IgG4) disease is a rare autoimmune condition that affects isolated or multiple organ systems. Clinical presentations of IgG4-related kidney disease can be quite protean, which include AKI, subacute or chronic renal impairment, and subnephrotic- or nephrotic-range proteinuria. Common extra-renal manifestations include sialadenitis, dacryoadenitis, pancreatitis, and retroperitoneal fibrosis. Patients often show elevated serum IgG4 levels and abnormal image findings of the involved organs.

Pathogenesis and histopathological features

Accumulating evidence shows that abnormalities in the B-cell repertoire and Th2 response play crucial pathogenic roles in the development of IgG4-related diseases. Typical renal pathological changes are tubulointerstitial nephritis (TIN), MN, and occasionally nodular or patchy lesions in the kidney. The characteristic histopathological features of IgG4-related TIN are dense lymphoplasmacytic infiltrates (with prominent IgG4-positive plasma cells) accompanied by storiform fibrosis. IgG4-related MN may show IgG4 deposition in the GBM, either predominantly or along with other IgG subclasses.

Management

Corticosteroids are the mainstay of treatment for IgG4-related diseases, while AZA, MMF, or methotrexate can be used as steroid-sparing agents or in refractory cases. Mounting data shows that B-cell-depleting therapy (e.g. anti-CD20) may also be useful in IgG4-related diseases.

Chronic Liver Diseases and the Kidneys

Clinical characteristics

Chronic liver disease is an important local, regional and global health problem. The high incidence and prevalence of liver diseases in the Asia-Pacific region are related to the endemicity of chronic viral hepatitis (e.g. HBV or HCV). Renal impairment can occur in patients with severe liver dysfunction. The possible causes of renal dysfunction in patients with advanced cirrhosis include hypovolaemia (e.g. secondary to over-diuresis or excessive paracentesis), infection (e.g. spontaneous bacterial peritonitis), gastrointestinal bleeding, use of nephrotoxic agents (e.g. iodine contrast, NSAIDs), acute tubular necrosis (ATN) (e.g. hyperbilirubinaemia), and hepatorenal syndrome (HRS). HRS is the most severe form of renal dysfunction in patients with advanced liver diseases and can be broadly classified into type 1 or 2 HRS, depending on the tempo of renal function deterioration (Table 9.5). Type 1 HRS usually occur in patients who suffer from acute hepatic failure (e.g. fulminant hepatitis or drug toxicity) or acute decompensation with pre-existing cirrhosis. These patients typically present with features of advanced hepatic

failure and portal hypertension (e.g. ankle swelling, jaundice, clotting derangement, refractory ascites, and encephalopathy), and dilutional hyponatraemia. Patients with type 1 HRS generally show rapid deterioration in renal function and oligo-anuria, which often develop within 2 weeks. Type 2 HRS often shows more indolent renal function decline, and frequently occurs in decompensated cirrhotic patients with refractory ascites. The development of HRS in cirrhotic patients is associated with grave prognoses. Without liver transplantation, patients with type 1 HRS usually succumb within two weeks while those with type 2 HRS may survive up to 5–6 months.

Pathogenesis and histopathological features

The pathogenesis of HRS remains poorly understood, but is believed to be a functional renal disorder as a result of vasomotor dysregulation. This is inferred from autopsy findings that show unremarkable renal histology in kidneys from patients with HRS. Other supporting evidence includes the observations that HRS patients resume normal renal function after successful liver transplantation, and kidneys from individuals with HRS also function normally when transplanted to other patients. The more widely accepted view of the pathophysiology of HRS is the 'under-fill' theory. In patients with advanced cirrhosis and portal hypertension, there is an excessive splanchnic synthesis of vasodilators leading to overt vasodilatation of the splanchnic vasculatures and decreased effective circulating volume. Increased endogenous vasoconstricting mediators and exaggerated hepato-neural reflexes are also observed in patients with advanced liver failure. These mechanisms contribute to intense intra-renal vasoconstriction and thus a marked reduction in GFR in patients with HRS. Although patients with HRS generally show no structural abnormalities in

Table 9.5: Clinical characteristics of patients with type 1 or 2 hepatorenal syndrome

	Type 1 HRS	Type 2 HRS
Diagnostic criteria	• Doubling of the initial SCr to >221 μmol/L (2.5 mg/dL) in less than 2 weeks	• Increase in SCr to >133 μmol/L (1.5 mg/dL), which follows a steady or slowly progressive course
Clinical Presentations	• Usually precipitated by acute decompensation (e.g. fulminant hepatitis, infection, or GIB)	• Progressive decline in renal function • Patients usually have refractory ascites
Prognosis	• Usually succumb within 2 weeks if without liver transplantation	• Some patients may survive up to 5–6 months without liver transplantation

HRS, hepatorenal syndrome; GIB, gastrointestinal bleeding; SCr, Serum creatinine the kidneys, bilirubin casts and evidence of ATN may sometimes be observed in patients with severe hyperbilirubinaemia.

Management

It is important to look for reversible causes of renal impairment in patients with liver failure. Overzealous diuresis or paracentesis should be avoided in advanced cirrhotic patients. The volume of ascitic output should be limited to 5–6 L/day and intravenous albumin be administered during paracentesis. Clinicians should also actively exclude any infection (e.g. spontaneous bacterial infection) or gastrointestinal haemorrhage (e.g. peptic ulcers or variceal bleeding) and avoid the use of nephrotoxic agents (e.g. iodine contrast or NSAIDs). In patients with suspected pre-renal azotaemia, diuretics should be withheld and cautious volume expansion may be attempted. Urine sodium levels can sometimes help to differentiate between HRS and ATN in cirrhotic patients. HRS patients usually have urine sodium < 10 mmol/L, whereas those with ATN often have urine sodium > 20 mmol/L.

Patients with advanced liver disease and developed HRS should be assessed for the suitability of liver transplantation. Patients with established HRS who have the potential for liver transplantation often require intensive care unit support. Vasopressive agents (intravenous terlipressin 0.5–2 mg q4-12 h, in combination with albumin) can be used as a bridging therapy before a liver allograft is available. Other potentially useful pharmacological options include octreotide, midodrine, and noradrenaline. Extra-corporeal liver supportive therapy such as molecular adsorbents recirculating systems (MARS) have shown initial promise in HRS patients, but MARS has fallen out of favour due to lack of proven benefits and high resource implications. Continuous renal replacement therapy strategies are often employed to support HRS patients awaiting liver allografts. Transjugular intrahepatic portosystemic stent-shunting (TIPSS) can help relieve portal hypertension by deploying a metallic stent within the liver parenchyma to reinforce a shunt between the portal vein and the hepatic vein. Data from some small series have shown that the TIPSS approach in combination with pharmacological treatments may confer clinical benefits on HRS and ascites. Potential complications of TIPSS include shunt thrombosis, precipitation of liver function deterioration, and hepatic encephalopathy. Liver transplantation is the only definitive treatment for HRS, but is often limited by patients' comorbidities and shortage of organs. Previous studies have also demonstrated that HRS patients have comparable liver allograft outcomes but inferior long-term renal outcomes compared to patients without HRS.

Bacterial Infections and Glomerulonephritis

Clinical characteristics

Particularly in developed countries, the focus of bacterial infection-related GN has shifted from classical post-streptococcal glomerulonephritis (PSGN, group A beta-hemolytic *streptococcus* skin or throat infection in children) to other infection-related GN (IRGN) in adult, elderly, or immunocompromised patients (including diabetic patients). Endocarditis (20%), skin (20%), lung (15%), bone and joint (15%), and urinary tract (15%) infections are responsible for the bulk of cases, and *Staphylococcus* (60%) outnumbered *Streptococcus* (15%) as the causative organism. PSGN and IRGN share similar clinical (acute nephritic syndrome, low serum C3 level) and histological features. PSGN occurred after the infection has subsided and generally carries a favourable prognosis with resolution of nephritis within weeks, through supportive therapy alone (diuretics, antihypertensives). IRGN is diagnosed during ongoing infection and heralds less favourable outcomes, in which 20% of patients will end up with ESRD.

Pathogenesis and histopathological features

Both classical PSGN and adult IRGN show typical LM findings of endocapillary proliferation and exudative glomerular changes. Crescents and necrotizing lesions are often seen in severe cases, especially in those with classical PSGN. Classical PSGN usually exhibits strong C3 and IgG staining, while adult IRGN can show IgA predominance on IF. Subepithelial 'humps' are characteristic EM findings for both PSGN and adult IRGN.

Management

Treatment of IRGN is focused on the eradication of the infection and complications of nephritis. Corticosteroids have not been found to be useful, except in the rare occasion of crescentic and necrotizing GN with positive ANCA.

Leptospirosis and Renal Disorders

Clinical characteristics

Human infection of the spirochetes *Leptospira* species usually results from exposure to environmental sources, especially animal urine and contaminated fresh-water lakes and ponds, or soil, through the mucous membrane or breaks in the skin. Natural hosts include wild or domestic livestock, and rodents, residing in their renal tubules. Clinical manifestations occur after 5–14 days of exposure and include fever, myalgia, headache, conjunctival suffusion, cough, gastrointestinal upset, hepatosplenomegaly, lymphadenopathy, and skin rashes. This bacteraemic phase typically lasts for up to one week, would be followed after a few days of appearing well by an immune phase in which the bloodstream, as well as most organs and tissues, are cleared of *Leptospira* rapidly, except in specific sites. Weil disease is manifested as aseptic meningitis, jaundice, acute kidney injury, and pulmonary involvement. Hyponatremia, thrombocytopenia, and elevated serum creatinine levels are common and diagnosis is by serology, PCR, or culture.

Pathogenesis and histopathological features

The typical renal histologic finding in leptospirosis is acute interstitial nephritis (AIN).

Management

Antibiotics such as doxycycline and penicillin are the treatment of choice for leptospirosis.

Viral Hepatitis and Kidney Diseases

Clinical characteristics

Infection with HBV or HCV is associated with the development of various forms of glomerular pathologies. It is therefore apparent that patients with HBV or HCV infection should be assessed for renal function and urinary protein excretion. The reverse is also true that screening for viral hepatitis should be part of the investigation for these renal pathologies, especially in endemic areas. Patients with HBV- or HCV-associated glomerular diseases often present with proteinuria and variable degrees of renal impairment, with or without haematuria. In HBV-associated secondary MN, patients are more likely than primary MN to have microscopic haematuria and decreased complement levels.

Pathogenesis and histopathological features

Histopathological findings of HBV- or HCV-associated renal disorders include MN (HBV predominantly), MPGN (particularly with mixed cryoglobulinaemia in HCV) and PAN-related changes (see also Chapter 8 and previous sections). HCV RNA and HCV Ag-Ab complexes have been identified in cryoprecipitate and on top of the histological features of MPGN, vasculitis of small renal arteries can be evident. Patients with PAN typically have biopsies revealing necrotizing inflammation of small and medium arteries. Subepithelial deposit of HBeAg and anti-HBe Ab immune complexes has been suggested as a key pathogenic process in HBV-associated MN. Immune deposits can also be present outside the subepithelial region of GBM.

Management

The main focus of treatment for HBV- or HCV-associated renal diseases is antiviral therapies, though immunosuppressive therapies on top have a role in patients with RPGN, and severe manifestations of mixed cryoglobulinemia or PAN.

Human Immunodeficiency Virus and Renal Disorders

Clinical characteristics

Human immunodeficiency virus (HIV) is associated with a spectrum of kidney pathologies, including HIV-associated nephropathy (HIVAN), HIV-associated immune-complex kidney disease (HIVICK), minimal change nephropathy, and thrombotic microangiopathy. The antiretroviral medications used in HIV infection can also lead to various forms of renal disorders, such as AIN and Fanconi syndrome. Patients with HIVAN usually present with nephrotic-range proteinuria and progressive renal deterioration. The clinical manifestations in HIVICK vary from microscopic haematuria, to subnephrotic- or nephrotic-range proteinuria, to renal failure.

Pathogenesis and histopathological features

The typical histopathological finding in HIVAN is collapsing focal segmental glomerulosclerosis. Variable degrees of mesangial expansion, capillary loop thickening, or segmental sclerosis, with or without endocapillary proliferation and crescent formation, may be seen in HIVICK. Tubuloreticular aggregates within endothelial cells is a characteristic EM feature of HIVAN. Mesangial, subendothelial, and subepithelial deposits can be detected on EM in HIVICK.

Management

The use of highly active antiretroviral therapy in HIV-positive patients significantly reduces the risk of developing HIVAN and HIVICK, as well as the progression to renal failure.

Acute Viral Infection, Emerging Viruses, and Renal Disorders

Clinical characteristics

Kidney dysfunction may occur in various acute viral infections, and the clinical presentation is usually AKI with low-grade or absent proteinuria. Viruses that have been reported to cause AKI include influenza virus, hantavirus (see section below), dengue virus, and severe acute respiratory syndrome coronavirus 2 (SARS-CoV-2). SARS-CoV-2 is an emerging virus that causes pandemic infection, and the overall incidence of AKI related to it is reported to be around 11%, but can be up to 23–35% in critically ill patients. AKI in SARS-CoV-2 infection is often a consequence of acute respiratory distress syndrome (ARDS) or systemic inflammatory response syndrome (SIRS) in those with severe infection, but can also be a result of isolated tubulointerstitial nephritis. The presence of AKI in SARS-CoV-2 infection is an important risk factor for mortality.

Pathogenesis and histopathological features

AIN is a frequent finding in patients with AKI due to acute viral infections (see also Chapter 7). AKI due to ARDS/SIRS in SARS-CoV-2 often shows prominent features of acute tubular necrosis and interstitial inflammation.

Management

The AKI associated with acute viral infections generally resolves with supportive treatments. There is currently no specific therapy for SARS-CoV-2, and

critically ill patients who show oligo-anuria often require dialytic support.

Hantavirus and Renal Disorders

Clinical characteristics

Hantavirus infection can be transmitted to humans by inhalation of aerosolized particles of rodent excreta or by direct rodent contact. Manifestations can be haemorrhagic fever with renal syndrome (HFRS) or Hantavirus pulmonary syndrome (a form of non-cardiogenic pulmonary oedema), caused by different strains prevalent in different parts of the world. HFRS is primarily caused by the Hantavirus in Asia and Europe, with an incubation period of between two and four weeks. The illness typically begins with fever and non-specific symptoms, followed by hypotension, bleeding tendency, and renal failure. Thrombocytopenia, leucocytosis, or disseminated intravascular coagulation may be present and diagnosis is by serology.

Pathogenesis and histopathological features

The characteristic renal histologic features of HFRS are tubulointerstitial nephritis and haemorrhage in the medullary region.

Management

There is no specific treatment for Hantavirus and renal recovery is usually expected with supportive therapy.

Multiple Myeloma and Monoclonal Gammopathies

Clinical characteristics

Multiple myeloma is B-cell malignancy, characterized by the proliferation of a single clone of plasma cells that produce monoclonal proteins and the presence of end-organ damage (Table 9.6).

Each clone of antibody-secreting plasma cells only expresses either a kappa (κ) or a lambda (λ) light chain (LC), which have molecular weights of ~22.5 kDa and ~45 kDa respectively. Multiple myeloma is a disease of the elderly (median age of presentation at 65 to 70 years), with an annual incidence of 4 per 100,000. Other major forms of related monoclonal

Table 9.6: Myeloma-related end-organ damage ('CRAB')

Feature	Criteria
C: Hypercalcemia	Serum calcium > 0.25 mmol/L (> 1mg/dL) higher than the upper limit of normal or > 2.75 mmol/L (> 11mg/dL)
R: Renal insufficiency	CrCl < 40mL/min or SCr > 177 µmol/L (> 2mg/dL)
A: Anaemia	Haemoglobin > 2 g/dL below the upper limit of normal or < 10 g/dL
B: Bone lesions	One or more osteolytic lesions on skeletal radiographs, CT, or PET-CT
Others	Amyloidosis, recurrent bacterial infections, extra-medullary plasmacytomas, symptomatic hyperviscosity (rare)

CrCl, creatinine clearance; CT, computerized tomography; PET-CT, position emission tomography-CT; SCr, serum creatinine

gammopathies include MGUS and asymptomatic myeloma (or 'smouldering multiple myeloma'), in which end-organ damage is usually not present.

Approximately 20% of patients with multiple myeloma have kidney involvement. Common renal manifestations include cast nephropathy, immunoglobulin light chain deposition disease (LCDD), and renal amyloidosis (AL amyloidosis) (Table 9.7). In cast nephropathy, AKI occurs early during the course of the disease and proteinuria is usually mild. Proteinuria in cast nephropathy is selective and comprises mainly LCs. In LCDD and amyloidosis, nephrotic syndrome predominates at presentation before rapidly progressive renal failure reminiscent of GN sets in. Proteinuria in LCDD or amyloidosis is non-selective with albumin predominance. It is noteworthy that κ-LC multiple myeloma more commonly causes cast nephropathy, whereas renal amyloidosis is more frequently seen in λ-LC multiple myeloma. While patients with multiple myeloma often show reversed albumin-to-globulin ratios and abnormal serum immunoelectrophoresis (SIEP) results, the globulin levels in LC myeloma can be normal or low (because they do not form intact immunoglobulins), and conventional SIEP test may not be sensitive enough to detect LC myeloma. In this context, serum and urine free LC assays are more useful for diagnostic and disease-monitoring purposes. Direct infiltration of kidneys by myeloma cells or obstructive uropathy by soft plasmacytoma are exceedingly rare. In multiple myeloma with AKI, it is also important to exclude other precipitating factors such as dehydration, urinary tract infection, hypercalcemia, nephrolithiasis, and drug-induced AKI.

Pathogenesis and histopathological features

Under physiologic conditions, free LCs filter freely through the glomeruli and are reabsorbed in the proximal tubules by the megalin–cubulin complex and metabolized. In patients with multiple myeloma, the overt synthesis of free LCs overwhelms the megalin–cubulin system and excessive free LCs combine with the Tamm–Horsfall protein to form intra-tubular casts in the distal and collecting tubules. Myeloma casts are typically eosinophilic casts found within renal tubular lumens, frequently accompanied by surrounding giant cell reactions (Figure 9.12). Glomerular pathologies in LCDD can be quite heterogeneous, including nodular glomerulosclerosis (Figure 9.13) that are typically negative for Congo red staining and occasionally lesions that resemble MPGN. Monoclonal κ or λ staining can be demonstrated by immunohistochemical staining or IF in cast nephropathy (Figure 9.14) and LCDD (Figure 9.15). On EM, LCDD often shows a layer of dense granular deposits under the endothelium along the glomerular basement membrane (Figure 9.16). The pathogenesis and renal histological features of renal amyloidosis will be discussed in subsequent sections.

Management

The current standard treatment of multiple myeloma is the frontline use of a triplet regimen comprising a proteasome inhibitor (e.g. bortezomib), an immunomodulatory agent (e.g. thalidomide or lenalidomide), and corticosteroids. Novel agents such as carfilzomib, pomalidomide, and daratumomab (anti-CD38) are generally reserved for relapsed or refractory disease. Autologous haematopoietic stem cell transplantation (HSCT) is recommended for myeloma patients younger than the age of 70 who respond well to initial therapy. If treated early, cast nephropathy is rapidly reversible with the standard chemotherapeutic regimen. The benefit of (PLEX) or high cut-off dialysis in cast nephropathy remains controversial. In LCDD, glomerular damage is less reversible and the main objective of treatment is to retard the ongoing production of monoclonal LCs.

Table 9.7: Renal manifestations of multiple myeloma

Disease	Characteristics and Renal Manifestations	Extra-Renal Manifestations
Glomerular Lesions		
LCDD	• κ or λ LC-mediated • Proteinuria, microscopic haematuria, hypertension and CKD	• Common and often asymptomatic: heart, liver, and lungs
AL Amyloidosis	• Predominantly "amyloidogenic" λ LC • Proteinuria (usually nephrotic-range) and CKD • Hypertension and haematuria uncommon	• Frequent and symptomatic: heart, liver, peripheral nerve, and gastrointestinal tract
Type 1 cryoglobulinaemic vasculitis	• Rarely seen • Proteinuria (±nephrotic syndrome), microscopic haematuria, hypertension, and CKD • Occasionally nephritic syndrome and AKI	• Frequent: skin, peripheral nerves, and joints
GN with organized microtubular Ig deposits (or Immunotactoid GN)	• Rarely seen • Proteinuria (±nephrotic syndrome), microscopic haematuria, hypertension, and CKD	• Uncommon: peripheral nerve and skin
Proliferative GN with monoclonal Ig deposits	• Rarely seen • Proteinuria (±nephrotic syndrome), microscopic haematuria, hypertension, and CKD	• None
C3 glomerulopathy with monoclonal gammopathy	• Rarely seen • Proteinuria, nephrotic syndrome, microscopic haematuria, and hypertension	• None
Tubular lesions		
Cast nephropathy	• Predominantly κ LC-mediated • Tubular proteinuria, AKI, or progressive CKD	• None
Fanconi's syndrome	• Uncommon • Hypouricaemia, hypophosphataemia, normoglycaemic glycosuria, generalized aminoaciduria, low-molecular weight proteinuria, proximal (type 2) RTA, and slowly progressive CKD	• Bone: osteomalacia

AKI, acute kidney injury; AL amyloidosis, immunoglobulin light chain amyloidosis; CKD, chronic kidney disease; GN, glomerulonephritis; LC, light chain; LCDD, light chain deposition disease; RTA, renal tubular acidosis

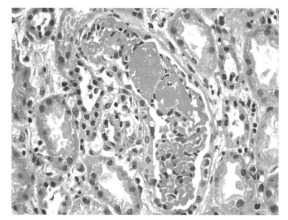

Figure 9.12: Cast nephropathy. Fractured casts which are rimmed by macrophages are characteristic of cast nephropathy (H&E, ×400, Dr A. H. N. Tang).

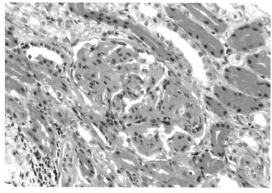

Figure 9.13: The glomerulus shows nodular appearance, which is characteristic of light chain deposition disease. Similar appearance can also be seen in nodular diabetic nephropathy (H&E, ×400, Dr A. H. N. Tang).

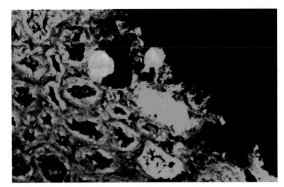

Figure 9.14: Cast nephropathy. Casts are stained positive in a monoclonal pattern with kappa or lambda light chains (anti-Lambda, ×400, Dr A. H. N. Tang).

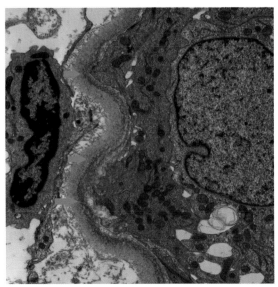

Figure 9.16: Light chain deposition disease (LCDD). The deposits in LCDD are finely granular (arrows) and are typically present in the internal aspect of the glomerular basement membrane (transmission electron microscopy, ×20000, Dr A. H. N. Tang).

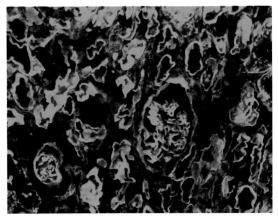

Figure 9.15: Characteristic linear staining of glomerular basement membrane and tubular basement membrane in a monoclonal light chain pattern is diagnostic for light chain deposition disease (LCDD). Monoclonal kappa light chain is more common in LCDD (anti-Kappa immunofluorescence, ×100, Dr A. H. N. Tang).

Amyloidosis

Clinical characteristics

Amyloidosis is a rare group of diseases of protein folding in where normally soluble proteins are deposited in the extracellular space as insoluble fibrils. Amyloid is a fibrillar material derived from various precursor proteins that self-assemble with highly ordered abnormal cross β-sheet conformations. Amyloidosis can be classified as systemic or localized, as acquired or hereditary, and based on the type of precursor protein (Table 9.8). AL amyloidosis is the most common form of acquired amyloidosis with renal involvement, with an incidence of three to five cases per million. AA amyloidosis is decreasing in incidence due to the remarkable improvement in the management of underlying inflammatory disorders.

Diagnosis of system amyloidosis requires careful history taking and physical examination, and evaluation for organ dysfunction, followed by histologic confirmation, fibril typing and delineation of the underlying disease mechanism (Figure 9.17). The pattern of presentation varies among the different diseases causing systemic amyloidosis. AL amyloidosis typically presents with prominent signs of multisystem tissue infiltration such as macroglossia, peri-orbital purpura, easy bruising and ecchymosis (due to perivascular connective tissue infiltration), nephrotic syndrome, heart failure, and peripheral neuropathy.

Pathogenesis and histopathological features

Amyloidosis occurs in clinical conditions which are associated with excessive production or impaired clearance of precursor proteins that have the propensity to form beta-pleated sheets (e.g. LC, serum amyloid A protein, or transthyretin). The classical LM appearance of renal amyloidosis is eosinophilic nodular lesions in the glomeruli (Figure 9.18). These lesions appear faintly red on a Congo red stain and

Table 9.8: Classification and clinical characteristics of amyloidosis

Subtype	Acquired vs. Hereditary	Underlying Pathogenesis	Precursor Protein	Organs Involved
AL	Acquired	Plasma cell disorder	Monoclonal LC	Heart, kidney, liver, soft tissue, gastrointestinal tract, peripheral, and autonomic nervous system
AA	Acquired	Underlying inflammatory disorder (e.g. RA, JIA, IVDU, FPS)	Serum amyloid A	**Kidneys** Rarely, liver, gastrointestinal tract, heart (late features)
ATTR	Acquired	Uncertain, probably aging	Wild-type TTR	Heart and carpel tunnel syndrome
	Hereditary	Mutations in TTR gene	Abnormal TTR	Heart, peripheral, and autonomic nervous system
AFib	Hereditary	Mutations in fibrinogen α-chain gene	Abnormal fibrinogen	**Kidneys**; rarely liver
ALect2	Acquired	Uncertain	Lect2	**Kidneys**, liver
AApoA1	Hereditary	Mutations in apolipoprotein A1 gene	Abnormal ApoA1	**Kidneys**, liver, rarely heart, peripheral nerves, testes
ALys	Hereditary	Mutations in lysozyme gene	Abnormal lysozyme	Liver, **kidneys**, gastrointestinal, skin
AGel	Hereditary	Mutations in lysozyme gene	Abnormal lysozyme	Peripheral nerves and cranial nerves. **Rarely kidneys**.
Aβ2M	Acquired or hereditary	Long-term dialysis	Aβ2M	Carpel tunnel syndrome, arthropathy Less commonly autonomic nervous system (only seen in hereditary form)

AA, Amyloid A; Aβ2M, β2-microglobulin-related; AFib, fibrinogen A α-chain; AGel, gelsolin amyloid; AL, amyloid light chain; ALect2, leucocyte cell-derived chemotaxin 2; ALys, lysozyme amyloid; ATTR, amyloid transthyretin; RA, rheumatoid arthritis; JIA, juvenile idiopathic arthritis; FPS, familial periodic fever syndrome; IVDU, intravenous drug use; LC, light chain; TTR, transthyretin

show a characteristic apple-green birefringence when examined under polarized light (Figures 9.19 and 9.20). Occasionally, the renal vasculatures and tubulointerstitium can also be affected by amyloidosis. Monoclonal κ or λ can be detected by immunohistochemical staining or IF in those with AL amyloidosis. On EM, AL amyloids appear as randomly oriented fibrils of 8–15 nm (Figure 9.21).

Management

Treatment of AL amyloidosis is similar to multiple myeloma, with the aim of eradicating the underlying plasma cell dyscrasia. The presence of severe peripheral neuropathy may preclude the use of bortezomib and thalidomide. Consolidation with autologous HSCT is recommended in patients without end-stage organ failure. The presence of heart failure in AL amyloidosis portends a worse prognosis. Management of hereditary amyloidosis is largely supportive and liver transplantation may offer a cure for fibrinogen, TTR, and Apo-A1 disorders. Novel therapies such as

tafamidis (a TTR stabilizer) and RNA inhibiting therapy are under development for ATTR amyloidosis.

Thrombotic Thrombocytopenia Purpura

Clinical characteristics

Thrombotic thrombocytopenia purpura (TTP) is a rare form of thrombotic microangiopathy (TMA) with an annual incidence of five cases per million. It is most commonly acquired due to autoantibodies that inactivate or bind A disintegrin and metalloprotease with thrombospondin 1 repeats member 13 (ADAMTS13). ADAMTS13 is a protease that is present in the plasma and platelets, and serves to cleave ultra-large multimers of von Willebrand factor (vWF) as soon as they are secreted from endothelial cells to the plasma. Various medical conditions are associated with acquired TTP (Table 9.9). Patients with TTP may first present with a platelet type of generalized bleeding tendency. Other typical features include neurological symptoms (seizures,

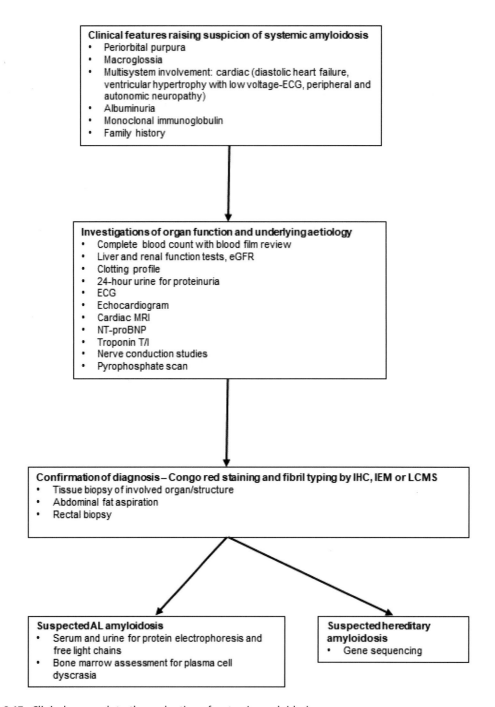

Figure 9.17: Clinical approach to the evaluation of systemic amyloidosis

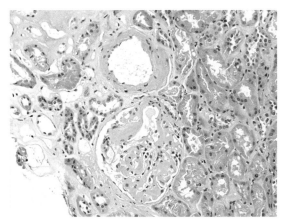

Figure 9.18: Amyloidosis. Amyloid deposits are present in the glomeruli and arterioles. The presence of extracellular, amorphous, eosinophilic material is characteristic of amyloidosis (H&E, ×200, Dr A. H. N. Tang).

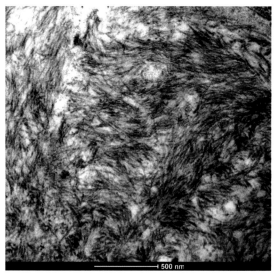

Figure 9.21: Amyloidosis. Amyloid fibrils are randomly distributed, non-branching fibrils ranging from 8–12 nm in diameter in electron microscopy (transmission electron microscopy, ×20000, Dr G. S. W. Chan).

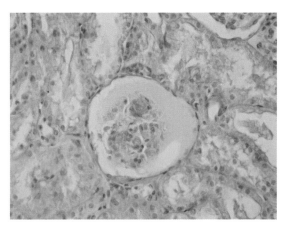

Figure 9.19: Amyloidosis. Congo red staining shows the presence of salmon-pink material in the glomerulus and arteriole, which are specific to amyloids (Congo red, ×400, Dr A. H. N. Tang).

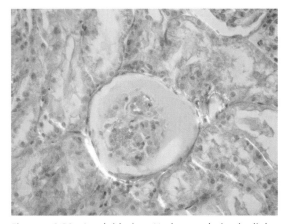

Figure 9.20: Amyloidosis. Under polarized light, amyloid gives a characteristic apple-green birefringence in Congo red staining section (Congo red, ×400, Dr A. H. N. Tang).

confusion, aphasia, dysarthria, diplopia, visual disturbances, and focal limb weakness), fever, and renal impairment. Microangiopathic haemolytic anaemia (MAHA) and consumptive thrombocytopenia are essential features for the diagnosis of TTP. Signs of MAHA include the presence of fragmented red cells (schistocytes) and reticulocytosis. Clotting profile is usually normal. Biochemical abnormalities include indirect hyperbilirubinaemia, a low or undetectable haptoglobin, and a markedly elevated lactate dehydrogenase (LDH) level (often > 1,000 U/L). Undetectable or low ADAMTS13 activity is a useful supportive feature, and anti-ADAMTS13 antibody assays can help delineate the underlying aetiology.

Pathogenesis and histopathological features

Defective ADAMTS13 activity due to autoantibodies binding or hereditary deficiency leads to impaired cleavage of large vWF multimers into small units. The increase in circulating vWF multimers enhances platelet adhesion to areas of endothelial injury, thereby resulting in widespread thrombi formation in capillaries of multiple organs, including those in the glomeruli. Red blood cells passing these microscopic thrombi are subject to shear stress to their cell membranes, resulting in MAHA. The LM features of renal TMA is characterized by diffuse microthrombi obliterating the capillary lumens (Figure 9.22), thickening

Table 9.9: Common conditions associated with acquired thrombotic thrombocytopenic purpura

- Autoimmune disorders (e.g. SLE, scleroderma)
- Pregnancy and post-partum
- Drugs (quinine, quinidine, ticlopidine, clopidogrel, cyclosporine)
- Chemotherapy (mitomycin, cisplatin, gemcitabine)
- Allogeneic haematopoietic stem cell transplantation
- Solid organ transplantation
- Cardiac surgery

SLE, systemic lupus erythematosus

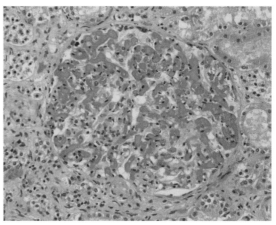

Figure 9.22: Thrombotic microangiopathy. There are numerous microthrombi in the glomerular capillary loops (H&E, ×400, Dr G. S. W. Chan).

of capillary walls due to endothelial cell swelling and accumulation of acellular materials between the endothelial cells and basement membrane. Double-contouring of GBM may also be observed on silver stain. Classical EM findings include swelling of endothelial cells and their detachment from the basement membrane and expansion of the subendothelial space by flocculent material (Figure 9.23).

Management

Daily PLEX should be initiated once a clinical diagnosis of acquired TTP is made. Adjunctive treatment with high doses of corticosteroids (e.g. prednisolone 1–2 mg/kg/day) is usually given. Red cell transfusion is given as required but platelet transfusion is generally contraindicated. Other therapeutic strategies for autoimmune-mediated or idiopathic TTP include the use of rituximab. Splenectomy may rarely be required in refractory autoimmune-mediated TTP. Recently, caplacizumab, a novel anti-von Willebrand nanobody, has been approved by the European Union and the US Food and Health Administration for the treatment of idiopathic TTP in adults. In the phase 3 HERCULES trial, caplacizumab, in addition to standard care, resulted in a shorter time to platelet normalization and reduction in the duration of PLEX and hospitalization.

Haemolytic Uraemic Syndrome

Clinical characteristics

Shiga-toxin mediated haemolytic uraemic syndrome

The classical and most frequent form of acquired haemolytic uraemic syndrome (HUS) is shiga-toxin mediated (STEC-HUS), which occurs acutely

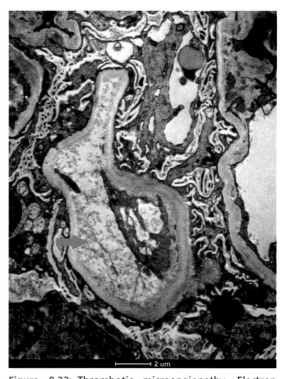

Figure 9.23: Thrombotic microangiopathy. Electron microscopy shows the presence of subendothelial lucency (arrow) in thrombotic microangiopathy (transmission electron microscopy, ×4000, Dr G. S. W. Chan).

following a sporadic gastrointestinal infection by toxin-producing bacteria. It typically occurs in infants and young children but may also occur in adults (especially the elderly). The most common bacterial agents associated with prodromal gastroenteritis in STEC-HUS include *Escherichia coli* serotypes 0157:H7 or O:104, and, less frequently, *Shigella dysenteriae* serotype I. Rarely, infectious agents that produce exotoxins (verocytotoxin), shiga toxin, or shiga-like toxins are also implicated in STEC-HUS. AKI is the predominant feature, and in some cases can be quite severe and require acute dialysis support. Up to a quarter of patients with STEC-HUS develop chronic renal impairment, and approximately 12% may even progress to ESRD. The peripheral blood film usually shows evidence of MAHA. ADAMT13 is normal or only mildly reduced in STEC-HUS.

Atypical HUS

Atypical HUS (aHUS) is a form of TMA caused by a dysregulated alternative complement pathway. aHUS can be sporadic or familial and is often triggered by infections, pregnancy, and drugs. Patients with aHUS frequently suffer from repeated episodes of HUS, and some may also have cardiac and neurological complications. Patients typically show low serum C3 levels. Many children with aHUS have their first episode of HUS at a very young age, often before the age of 6. Patients with aHUS generally show poor renal prognosis, with at least one-third progressing to ESRD. This can be as high as 60–70% in those with cofactor H mutations.

Pathogenesis and histopathological features

In STEC-HUS, the bacterial shiga toxin induces endoplasmic reticulum stress response and activates the inflammatory cascade within endothelial cells, thereby resulting in extensive endothelial injury and formation of microthrombi. Approximately half of aHUS patients have mutations in one of the complement regulatory proteins (factor H, factor I, MCP, or factor B), which leads to excessive activation of C3 convertase and partial consumption of C3 convertase. C3a and C3b deposit on the endothelial cell surface resulting in endothelial damage, and activation of platelet and leucocytes. The end-result is inflammation and thrombosis, particularly affecting the glomerular vessels although the brain, lungs, and gut can also be involved. The renal histological findings are indistinguishable between STEC-HUS and aHUS, with both showing features of renal TMA.

Management

In most patients, STEC-HUS is self-limiting. Patients with severe renal impairment may require dialysis support in the acute phase, but plasma exchange is not recommended. aHUS patients should be treated with plasma exchange. Eculizumab, a humanized monoclonal antibody that binds to C5, blocks the formation of the membrane attack complex and is an effective therapy recently approved for aHUS. Living-related kidney transplantation is generally contraindicated in aHUS due to the high risk of disease recurrence and allograft loss. Other possible treatment options include combined liver-kidney transplantation and isolated kidney transplantation with chronic eculizumab therapy.

Tumour Lysis Syndrome

Clinical characteristics

Tumour lysis syndrome is an oncological emergency characterized by the massive destruction of malignant cells and the release of their cellular contents into the bloodstream. Patients typically present with AKI and oligo-anuria after cytotoxic therapies in patients with high tumour loads (e.g. haematological malignancies). Biochemical abnormalities include raised blood levels of urea, creatinine, LDH, hyperuricaemia, hyperkalaemia, hypocalcaemia, and hyperphosphataemia.

Pathogenesis and histopathological features

The widespread deposition of uric acid and calcium phosphate crystals in the renal tubules causes intratubular obstruction and hence AKI. Diagnosis is clinical and renal biopsy is rarely required.

Management

Prophylactic xanthine oxidase inhibitors (e.g. allopurinol or febuxostat) and aggressive hydration should be given to patients who are scheduled to receive chemotherapeutic therapies for cancers with high cellular turnover (e.g. lymphoma or leukaemia). Rasburicase can be considered an alternative to xanthine oxidase inhibitors to lower blood uric acid levels. Concomitant electrolyte disturbances should be managed accordingly and haemodialysis should be commenced in patients who develop oligo-anuria or life-threatening electrolyte abnormalities.

Rhabdomyolysis

Clinical characteristics

Rhabdomyolysis refers to the breakdown of skeletal muscles caused by various medical conditions (Table 9.10). Patients may present with muscle pain and dark red discolouration of urine, and even oligo-anuria. Biochemical abnormalities include raised levels of blood urea, creatinine, creatine kinase, LDH, aspartate aminotransferase, hyperkalaemia, hypocalcaemia, and hyperphosphataemia. Urine myoglobin is usually positive.

Table 9.10: Common causes of rhabdomyolysis

Causes	Clinical examples
Primary muscle injury	Crush injury, pressure necrosis, polymyositis, dermatomyositis, burns
Tissue ischaemia	Arterial embolization, septicaemia
Excessive energy consumption	Status epilepticus, strenuous exercise, tetanus, malignant hyperthermia
Decreased energy production	Hypokalaemia, hypothermia, myxoedema, diabetic ketoacidosis
Infections	Gas gangrene, Legionnaire's disease, virus myositis
Drugs	Statins, fibrates, cocaine, amphetamines

Pathogenesis and histopathological features

The release of myoglobin from damaged skeletal muscle accumulates in the renal tubules, which combines with Tamm–Horsfall protein to cause intra-tubular obstruction. This disease process is often complicated by ATN. Diagnosis is usually established by compatible clinical history and features, and renal biopsy is rarely required. Typical histologic features show widespread intra-tubular myoglobin casts.

Management

The precipitating cause of rhabdomyolysis should be treated. Patients should be given generous amounts of intravenous normal saline, but this must be administered with caution in patients with reduced urine outputs. Electrolyte abnormalities should be corrected accordingly. The use of alkaline diuresis (keeping urine pH at 7–8) may be considered, although the overall clinical benefit remains controversial. Haemodialysis should be initiated in patients who develop oligo-anuria or life-threatening electrolyte disturbances.

10

Hypertension and the Kidneys

Gary Chan and Bernard Cheung

Introduction

Hypertension is the leading modifiable risk factor for cardiovascular (CV) disease and premature death. Its global prevalence is rising and is projected to exceed 30% by 2025, largely due to an ageing worldwide population. Hypertension can be classified as primary or secondary. Primary hypertension accounts for the majority of cases and is related to a multitude of genetic and environmental factors. Secondary hypertension arises most commonly from renal parenchymal disease, renovascular abnormalities, and endocrine disorders.

The Renin-Angiotensin System

The kidney is critical for blood pressure regulation by virtue of its capacity to handle sodium and water. The renin-angiotensin system (RAS) is instrumental in this process and comprises a systemic cascade of peptides, which form a circulating endocrine system. A simplification of this cascade begins with renin cleaving the hepatic precursor protein angiotensinogen to yield angiotensin I, which is then converted to angiotensin II by endothelial angiotensin-converting enzyme (ACE) in the lungs. Angiotensin II mediates vasoconstriction and stimulates adrenal aldosterone release to facilitate sodium retention. Systemic blood pressure is thus regulated by RAS and interrupting this pathway at various levels by ACE inhibitors, angiotensin II receptor blockers (ARBs), and mineralocorticoid receptor antagonists (MRAs) represents a major method of blood pressure control.

Diagnosis of Hypertension

The cut-off point for diagnosing hypertension varies somewhat according to different authorities (Table 10.1). Nevertheless, there is consensus towards initiating drug treatment for persistently raised blood pressure that exceeds 140/90 mmHg. In patients with blood pressure values 130–139/80–89 mmHg, the prevailing level of CV risk dictates the necessity for drug therapy. No matter which guideline is applied, accurate measurement and interpretation of blood pressure are crucial for the diagnosis and management of hypertension. Instead of using an auscultatory method, an oscillometric blood pressure device is recommended for the office setting. In patients found to have elevated office blood pressure, the diagnosis of hypertension should be confirmed with out-of-office measurements. This is preferably via ambulatory blood pressure monitoring (ABPM), which can help to exclude white-coat and masked hypertension. ABPM has been demonstrated to better predict both target-organ damage and CV events, when compared with office blood pressure readings. Where ABPM is unavailable, mean home measurements via an automated oscillometric device can be used to detect the presence of hypertension.

Evaluation of the patient aims to assess the presence of target-organ damage, concomitant CV risks, and contributory lifestyle factors. Furthermore, it is important to assess clinical clues that may suggest secondary hypertension in order to identify patients for further evaluation (Table 10.2).

Table 10.1: Definition of hypertension

	ACC/AHA Guidelines 2017	ESC/ESH Guidelines 2018
Office	≥ 130/80	≥ 140/90
Mean HBPM	≥ 130/80	≥ 135/85
Mean daytime ABPM	≥ 130/80	≥ 135/85
Mean night-time ABPM	≥ 110/65	≥ 120/70
Mean 24-Hour ABPM	≥ 125/75	≥ 130/80

ACC/AHA: American College of Cardiology/American Heart Association; ABPM: Ambulatory blood pressure monitoring; ESC/ESH: European Society of Cardiology/European Society of Hypertension; HBPM: Home blood pressure monitoring

Renal Aetiologies of Secondary Hypertension

Primary kidney disease

Hypertension is a frequent finding in patients with acute kidney injury (AKI) and chronic kidney disease (CKD). Often, the serum creatinine concentration is elevated and urinalysis is abnormal with renal disease. AKI resulting from acute glomerulonephritis is characterized by avid sodium retention resulting in volume expansion. The putative mechanisms that contribute to these changes include RAS activation and relative resistance to atrial natriuretic peptide. In patients with CKD, there are many factors at play that result in hypertension (Figure 10.1). The prevalence of hypertension increases as the glomerular filtration rate decreases, such that over 90% of individuals with stage 5 CKD are hypertensive.

Table 10.2: Clinical features to suggest secondary hypertension

Aetiology		Suggestive Clinical Features
	General	• Young age of onset • Severe or resistant hypertension • Acute sustained elevation in blood pressure
Renal	Primary kidney disease	• Raised serum creatinine/reduced creatinine clearance • Abnormal urinalysis
	Renovascular disease	• Abdominal bruit and bilateral kidney size discrepancy • Renal deterioration after instituting ACE inhibitor or ARB • Recurrent episodes of flash pulmonary oedema • Background history of generalized atherosclerosis
	Hyperaldosteronism	• Metabolic alkalosis • Hypokalaemia due to urinary potassium wasting
Non-Renal	Cushing's syndrome	• Cushingoid features
	Phaeochromocytoma	• Paroxysmal elevations in blood pressure • Classical triad (palpitations, headache and sweating)
	Obstructive sleep apnoea	• Overweight • Snoring and apnoeic episodes during sleep • Daytime somnolence
	Coarctation of aorta	• Blood pressure discrepancy between limbs • Radial–radial or radial–femoral pulse delay
	Hypothyroidism	• Symptoms of hypothyroidism
	Primary hyperparathyroidism	• Raised serum calcium
	Drugs	• Careful drug history (e.g. ESA, corticosteroids, NSAIDs, CNI, and any over-the-counter medications)

ACE, angiotensin converting enzyme; ARB, angiotensin II receptor blocker; CNI, calcineurin inhibitors; ESA, erythropoiesis stimulating agents; NSAIDs, non-steroidal anti-inflammatory drugs

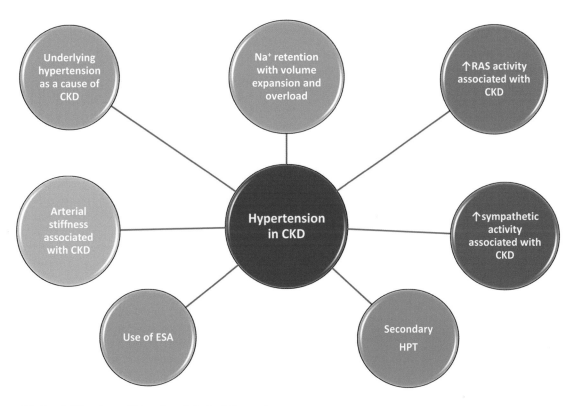

CKD: Chronic kidney disease; ESA: erythropoiesis stimulating agent;
HPT: hyperparathyroidism; RAS: Renin-angiotensin system

Figure 10.1: Factors contributing to hypertension in chronic kidney disease

Renovascular hypertension

This is an important and potentially reversible cause of secondary hypertension in which the RAS pathway is activated to increase both vascular tone and sodium retention. It usually occurs in the context of generalized atherosclerosis in patients over the age of 50 years with concomitant CV disease. A sudden deterioration in renal function after instituting ACE inhibitors or ARBs, a disparity in kidney sizes of greater than 1.5 cm, and recurrent episodes of acute (flash) pulmonary oedema are suspicious features in a vasculopath with uncontrolled hypertension. A thorough clinical examination may reveal a lateralizing abdominal bruit. With time, there is a loss of renal function from prolonged ischaemia that results from poor parenchymal perfusion. Rarely, renovascular hypertension may arise in young females due to fibromuscular dysplasia (FMD).

Reasonable non-invasive methods for initial testing include duplex Doppler ultrasonography (USG), computed tomographic (CT), and magnetic resonance (MR) angiography. USG is operator dependent and technically difficult in obese patients.

Both CT and MR angiography have high sensitivity and specificity, only to be limited by potential complications arising from iodinated and gadolinium contrast. However, the false negative rate of these non-invasive tests increases in the setting of intrarenal vascular stenotic lesions, commonly seen in FMD, and conventional angiography may be required to delineate the vascular lesion.

Hyperaldosteronism

Primary hyperaldosteronism has been reported to occur in up to 10% of the hypertensive population. It is associated with metabolic alkalosis and potassium wasting, but serum potassium concentrations are frequently normal. The most common causes of primary hyperaldosteronism are aldosterone-producing adenomas and bilateral adrenal hyperplasia. Rarely, it may be the result of glucocorticoid-remediable aldosteronism. Pathophysiologically, hyperaldosteronism increases sodium reabsorption at the cortical collecting tubule and induces extracellular fluid expansion to give rise to hypertension.

Primary hyperaldosteronism can be screened by evaluating the ratio of plasma renin activity/concentration (PRA/C) to that of plasma aldosterone concentration (PAC). The test is performed in the morning, after the patient has been ambulatory for at least two hours. In the absence of interfering medications (MRAs, ACE inhibitors, ARBs, diuretics), a reduced PRA/C associated with an inappropriately raised PAC is suggestive of primary hyperaldosteronism and should prompt referral to an endocrinologist for further work-up. Secondary hyperaldosteronism due to malignant hypertension and renin-secreting tumours is considered when both PRA/C and PAC are elevated.

Occasionally, genetic (syndrome of apparent mineralocorticoid excess [AME]) and acquired (chronic ingestion of liquorice or liquorice-like compounds) deficiencies of 11-beta-hydroxysteroid dehydrogenase (11-beta-HSD) will masquerade as hyperaldosteronism. This enzyme is responsible for the conversion of cortisol to cortisone. Cortisol has mineralocorticoid activity and in the absence of 11-beta-HSD, even usual levels of cortisol production can manifest as mineralocorticoid excess. A state of mineralocorticoid excess similarly occurs in Cushing's syndrome due to ectopic ACTH release, where the metabolic capacity of 11-beta-HSD is overwhelmed by uncontrolled cortisol secretion. These disorders are characterized by low PRA/C and PAC levels.

Liddle's syndrome is a rare autosomal dominant disorder characterized by a gain in function of the aldosterone-sensitive epithelial sodium channels (ENaCs) in the cortical collecting tubule. This results in manifestations akin to primary hyperaldosteronism, with the exception that most patients present at a young age. The measured PRA/C and PAC are concomitantly low in Liddle's syndrome and genetic testing is available for definitive confirmation.

Effects of Hypertension on the Kidneys

Prolonged suboptimally controlled hypertension can lead to renal insufficiency and varying proteinuria. In patients with an underlying renal disease, the presence of hypertension accelerates the rate of renal decline. Microscopically, vascular wall medial thickening and afferent arteriolar hyaline deposits are evident. These are associated with ischaemic glomerular changes with variable glomerular basement membrane wrinkling, glomerulosclerosis, tubular atrophy, and interstitial fibrosis. In malignant hypertension, arteriolar lesions are more pronounced with endothelial cell swelling and fibrinoid necrosis, which may obliterate the vascular lumen.

Management

Principles

The therapeutic paradigm aims to control blood pressure to target levels to prevent adverse CV outcomes and preserve renal function. Management must take into account the clinical context, which dictates the rapidity with which blood pressure should be lowered. Patients with severe hypertension complicated by acute and ongoing target-organ damage may need more aggressive blood pressure control. Even then, the choice of agent and blood pressure target varies according to the specific hypertensive emergency. In the chronic setting, the blood pressure target would depend on the absolute CV risk of the individual. Higher-risk populations, which require a lower blood pressure goal, include those with known atherosclerotic CV disease, heart failure, diabetes mellitus, CKD, age ≥ 65 years, or a 10-year CV event risk >10%. However, patients with significant cranial artery stenosis will require less stringent blood pressure control. Similarly, elderly patients with a high burden of comorbidity, postural hypotension, or a diastolic blood pressure < 60 mmHg will require treatment individualization.

Primary hypertension

Lifestyle modifications should be prescribed to all patients with elevated blood pressure, which should include instituting dietary salt restriction, enhanced dietary potassium, aerobic exercise, weight loss, moderation in alcohol intake, and following dietary approaches to stop hypertension. Each of these components has independently been found to reduce systolic blood pressure by 4–6 mmHg. The decision to initiate pharmacological therapy will depend upon the severity of hypertension and the individual level of CV risk. If single-agent therapy is unable to control blood pressure adequately, combination therapy with different classes of drugs may be employed. Multiple meta-analyses have shown that CV risk reduction is determined by the degree to which blood pressure is lowered rather than the choice of antihypertensive agent. However, certain classes of antihypertensive agents may be indicated for diseases unrelated to hypertension. Thus, the therapeutic regimen should be individualized according

Table 10.3: Common clinical conditions and the preferred anti-hypertensive agents

Clinical Condition	Antihypertensive Drug Class (Survival Benefit Independent of Blood Pressure Control)	Antihypertensive Drug Class (Symptomatic Treatment)
Post myocardial infarction	ACE inhibitors ARBs Beta-blockers	Diuretics
Heart failure	ACE inhibitors ARBs Beta-blockers MRAs	Diuretics
Atrial fibrillation/flutter	–	Beta-blockers Non-dihydropyridine CCBs
Non-dialysis CKD	ACE inhibitors ARBs	Diuretics
Polycystic kidney disease	ACE inhibitors ARBs	–
ESKD on RRT	ACE inhibitors ARBs	–
Post ischaemic cerebral vascular accident	ACE inhibitors	–
Post subarachnoid haemorrhage	Dihydropyridine CCB	–
Liver cirrhosis	Beta-blockers	Diuretics MRAs
Benign prostatic hypertrophy	–	Alpha-blockers
Essential tremor	–	Beta-blockers
Migraine	–	Beta-blockers

ACE, angiotensin converting enzyme; ARB, angiotensin II receptor blocker; CCB, calcium channel blocker; CKD, chronic kidney disease; ESKD, end stage kidney disease; MRA, mineralocorticoid receptor antagonist; RRT, renal replacement therapy

to patient characteristics to control hypertension and achieve additional survival benefits independent of blood pressure control (Table 10.3). If the target blood pressure cannot be achieved with three classes of antihypertensive drugs that encompass a diuretic at maximally tolerated dosages, hypertension is defined as resistant. In this case, white-coat hypertension and non-adherence should be excluded, with causes of secondary hypertension sought and managed. In the absence of a secondary cause, intensified diuretic therapy is often tried in resistant hypertension, unless there is overt evidence of hypovolaemia. Subsequently, an MRA or potassium-sparing diuretic can be introduced if blood pressure control remains suboptimal. Further combinations utilizing centrally acting agents, alpha-1 antagonists, or direct vasodilators will depend on patient characteristics and tolerance. Several experimental therapies for resistant hypertension have been tried, which include renal denervation and carotid sinus

baroreceptor stimulation. These methods have not demonstrated efficacy and are associated with significant procedure-related adverse events.

Secondary hypertension of renal aetiologies

In patients with secondary hypertension resulting from atherosclerotic renovascular disease, it is important to address the underlying CV risk. In addition to the aforementioned lifestyle modifications, diabetes mellitus and dyslipidaemia must be controlled. In the absence of overt bleeding risk, antiplatelet therapy is often instituted in patients with atherosclerotic renovascular disease. In addition, ACE inhibitors and ARBs are often employed, but not in combination, with proven renoprotective efficacy. The only caveat is the heightened risks of hyperkalaemia and AKI in cases of bilateral disease. In select cases, revascularization via percutaneous angioplasty and stenting may have a role. Patient selection for revascularization is crucial, since the restoration of extra-renal blood flow does not necessarily guarantee an improvement in blood pressure control or renal recovery. Significant improvements following intervention are not usually observed in cases with a high intra-renal vascular disease load or longstanding hypertension, which may partly be driven by established CKD. Indications for revascularization include a failure of optimal medical therapy to control blood pressure, progressive renal insufficiency, and recurrent flash pulmonary oedema. Surgery may be required in cases with complex anatomical vascular lesions.

Primary hyperaldosteronism requires specialist management by an endocrinologist. The optimal therapy for the syndrome of AME is unknown. MRAs have been used to halt potassium wasting, sodium retention, and thus hypertension. The treatment for Liddle's syndrome, however, requires potassium-sparing diuretics that block ENaC (amiloride or triamterene). MRAs in this scenario are ineffective since the ENaC gain in function is aldosterone independent.

11

Pregnancy and Kidney Diseases

Gary Chan and Noel Shek

Introduction

Pregnancy results in profound anatomical and physiological changes in the kidneys to accommodate for the demands of the foetus. While previously healthy individuals may develop renal complications during the course of gestation, women with pre-existing renal diseases are predisposed to a higher risk of maternal and foetal morbidity and mortality. The management of pregnant women with renal disease is challenging and a multidisciplinary approach is required to care for both the mother and the developing foetus.

Renal Adaptations in Pregnancy

Alterations in anatomy and physiology

Anatomically, the kidney volume expands by approximately 30%, resulting in a length increase of approximately 1 cm. Hormonal and mechanical forces cause the urinary collecting system to dilate and produce physiological hydronephrosis. This is usually more prominent on the right and peaks by 28 weeks of gestation. Physiologically, there is significant cardiovascular adaptation, which is characterized by a 30–50% increase in cardiac output associated with a concomitant fall in systemic and renal vascular resistance. This results in an increase in renal plasma flow to elevate glomerular filtration rate (GFR) by 50% above baseline, only for it to return to pre-pregnancy levels at 6–8 weeks post-partum. Additionally, a fall in systemic blood pressure by 5–10 mmHg below baseline occurs during pregnancy, reaching a nadir in the second trimester. By the third trimester, the systemic blood pressure gradually returns to pre-pregnancy values.

Alterations in solute handling

As a result of raised GFR, serum creatinine concentrations during pregnancy are markedly lower. The implicit corollary of this is that normal serum creatinine levels during pregnancy already indicate impaired renal function and signify the presence of underlying kidney disease. A better estimation of renal function can be obtained by performing a 24-hour urine collection for creatinine clearance. Similarly, uric acid clearance is increased and serum urate levels fall in early pregnancy. There is also increased excretion and reduced tubular reabsorption of glucose to produce glycosuria, in spite of normal plasma glucose concentrations. As a consequence, approximately 50% of pregnant women test positive for glycosuria by urine dipstick, rendering it a poor screening tool for diabetes mellitus (DM) in this setting.

Alterations in serum sodium and potassium concentrations

Osmoregulation is altered in pregnancy with a downwards adjustment of the plasma osmolality set point. As a consequence, there is a lower threshold for thirst and ADH secretion, which in combination with increased human chorionic gonadotropin production, results in plasma volume expansion by 30–50% and mild dilutional hyponatraemia. During the gestational period, the renin-angiotensin system also becomes hyperactive due to low prevailing blood pressures. Coupled with a supra-physiological GFR, this may result in hypokalaemia, especially in the context of pre-existing tubular pathology.

Proteinuria in pregnancy

There is a substantial increase in proteinuria during pregnancy as a result of elevated GFR and an increase in glomerular basement membrane permeability. The normal level of proteinuria may increase up to 300 mg per day. When significant proteinuria is detected, the common occurrence of urinary tract infection (UTI) in pregnancy should first be excluded.

Renal Impairment in Pregnancy

Renal diseases that occur in the general population can also be present in pregnant women. Additionally, there are specific renal conditions that only occur during pregnancy. In general, renal impairment in pregnancy can be divided into two cohorts: (1) pregnant women with pre-existing chronic kidney disease (CKD); and (2) pregnant women with acute kidney injury (AKI). These settings are not mutually exclusive and it is well recognized that pregnant women with pre-existing CKD have increased incidence of AKI.

Pregnant women with pre-existing kidney disease

Women with CKD are less likely to become pregnant. Putative mechanisms that contribute to subfertility in women with CKD include hormonal disturbances, which may result in anovulatory cycles and erratic menstruation. In patients who successfully conceive, there is an increased risk of adverse maternal and foetal outcomes (Table 11.1). The observed risk is increased as GFR deteriorates and is further elevated by hypertension and proteinuria, which are commonly present in CKD (Figure 11.1). A bi-directional relationship is present, such that the course of CKD is also adversely influenced by pregnancy. The raised intra-glomerular pressures and hyperfiltration, associated with the physiological adaptations of pregnancy, act to induce further renal injury and accelerate CKD progression. In this context, the levels of proteinuria and CKD stage at baseline are strong predictors of pregnancy-related GFR loss.

Autosomal dominant polycystic kidney disease (ADPKD) is a common hereditary disorder and

Table 11.1: Adverse maternal and foetal outcomes associated with chronic kidney disease

Maternal Risks	Foetal Risks
• Renal function deterioration	• Miscarriage
• Flare of underlying glomerulonephritis	• Foetal growth restriction
• Gestational hypertension	• Preterm labour and delivery
• Preeclampsia	• Stillbirth
	• Polyhydramnios

women who become pregnant with ADPKD need special attention. Generally, pregnancy in those with preserved renal function is not associated with adverse renal outcomes and cystic growth does not seem to be affected. However, cystic complications with UTI and haemorrhage resulting in haematuria and loin pain may occur during the gestational period. Appropriate genetic counselling should be offered to women with ADPKD, and screening for cystic liver disease and intracranial aneurysms should be performed prior to planned conception.

Unknown history of pre-existing kidney disease

Many women may not have undergone a medical assessment prior to becoming pregnant. As a result, a small proportion of women present with renal abnormalities characterized by haematuria, proteinuria, or renal impairment for the first time during antenatal care. A carefully elicited clinical history will help to determine whether this results from a pre-existing renal condition versus a de novo entity, with or without AKI. In addition, proteinuria documented in the early stages of pregnancy is an important clue that suggests pre-existing renal disease while its onset after 20 weeks of gestation is indicative of preeclampsia until proven otherwise.

Pregnant women with acute kidney injury

Pregnancy-associated AKI (P-AKI) is uncommon in developed countries. However, a rising trend has been observed in recent times due to several reasons. These include higher detection rates from meticulous modern-day antenatal care, breakthroughs in assisted reproductive techniques which facilitate women with pre-existing disease to conceive and

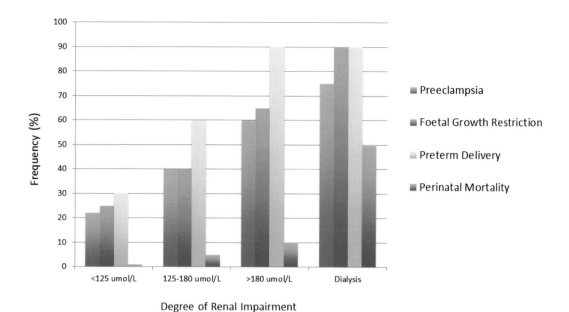

Figure 11.1: Correlation of maternal and foetal risks with degree of renal impairment

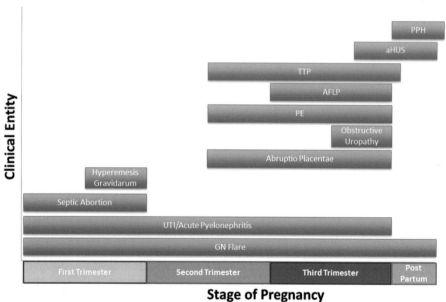

Figure 11.2: Causes of acute kidney injury according to the gestational period of pregnancy
AFLP, acute fatty liver of pregnancy; aHUS, atypical haemolytic uraemic syndrome; GN, glomerulonephritis; PE, preeclampsia; PPH, post-partum haemorrhage; TTP, thrombotic thrombocytopenic purpura; UTI, urinary tract infection

result in high-risk pregnancies, and a higher number of pregnancies from women of advanced maternal age. The clinical approach to P-AKI is guided by its timing of onset with respect to the gestational period (Figure 11.2), and appropriate investigations should be performed to aid the management of these patients.

Acute kidney injury before 20 weeks of gestation

AKI in early pregnancy is commonly due to pre-renal causes such as hyperemesis gravidarum. Women with pre-existing heart failure may decompensate under the physiological demands of pregnancy and give rise to pre-renal failure due to a decline in effective circulatory volume. If severe or prolonged enough, pre-renal causes of AKI can progress to ischemic acute tubular necrosis (ATN). Sepsis-related ATN might also arise from acute pyelonephritis and septic abortion.

Acute kidney injury after 20 weeks of gestation

Many causes of AKI in the later stages of pregnancy are typically intrinsic in nature. These include preeclampsia (PE), conditions characterized by thrombotic microangiopathy (TMA), and acute fatty liver of pregnancy (AFLP). Pregnancy-associated TMA can be due to the haemolysis, elevated liver enzymes, and low platelet count (HELLP) syndrome, atypical haemolytic uremic syndrome (aHUS), and thrombotic thrombocytopenic purpura (TTP). Often, it is challenging to differentiate between these clinical entities, as they present similarly and, at times, concomitantly. Renal cortical necrosis secondary to obstetric catastrophe (e.g. severe haemorrhage, placental abruption) and obstructive uropathy are also important causes of P-AKI in the latter stages of gestation.

Preeclampsia

PE complicates 3–5% of all pregnancies worldwide and remains the leading cause of maternal and foetal morbidity and mortality. It is the most common cause of P-AKI and accounts for 15–20% of all cases. Important risk factors include a previous history of PE, hypertension, DM, systemic lupus erythematosus (SLE), antiphospholipid syndrome, and CKD from any cause. The pathogenesis is epitomized by an abnormal utero-placental circulation, which elaborates a host of factors to cause systemic endothelial

dysfunction, and usually presents with hypertension and proteinuria after 20 weeks of gestation. In severe cases, PE is indistinguishable from other causes of TMA in pregnancy. Foetal delivery is the cornerstone of management, which usually leads to resolution with a good renal prognosis.

Thrombotic microangiopathies associated with pregnancy

HELLP syndrome occurs in approximately 1% of all pregnancies, and can occur in isolation or in association with PE. Although the exact pathophysiology remains elusive, the disease is characterized by TMA, which accounts for the haematological, hepatic, and renal manifestations. Most patients present with gastrointestinal symptoms in the third trimester, but late second trimester or early post-partum presentations are also common. When P-AKI is associated with HELLP syndrome, hypertension and proteinuria are invariably observed and is associated with a higher rate of placental abruption and obstetric haemorrhage. Many features of HELLP overlap with those observed in SLE, AFLP, aHUS, and TTP. Prompt delivery is the only effective treatment and generally carries a favourable renal prognosis.

Other disorders associated with TMA in pregnancy include aHUS and TTP. These conditions may occur *de novo* or relapse, with an incidence of 1 in 25,000 pregnancies. TTP is characterized by an acquired or constitutional deficiency in ADAMTS13 activity. It tends to occur in the late second and third trimesters due to a progressive decline in protease levels during gestation. In contrast, aHUS represents familial or sporadic mutations that result in unregulated complement activation and commonly occurs in the post-partum period. Both conditions are associated with P-AKI and diagnosis can be extremely challenging. Renal biopsy is often contraindicated in view of the bleeding risks and the late stage of gestation. The treatment of these conditions in pregnancy is the same as that in the general population (see Chapter 9), and the availability of plasma exchange and eculizumab has improved the prognosis of these disorders. Nonetheless, a significant proportion of women will end up with residual CKD, or less often, end-stage renal disease (ESRD).

Acute fatty liver of pregnancy

AFLP occurs with an approximate incidence of 1 in 7,000 to 20,000 pregnancies and is mainly characterized by liver dysfunction presenting with gastrointestinal symptoms in the third trimester. AFLP is associated with P-AKI in up to 60% of cases and central diabetes insipidus may occur due to reduced hepatic metabolism of vasopressinase. Multi-organ dysfunction can occur in severe cases and prompt delivery is required, irrespective of gestation, which usually leads to resolution within days to weeks.

Renal cortical necrosis

This historically important cause of P-AKI in patients suffering from obstetric catastrophes is now rare in the developed world. Patients typically present with severe flank pain, abrupt oliguria and gross haematuria. Hypoechoic regions in the kidney cortex are found on renal imaging. There is no effective treatment for this disorder with a poor prognosis, and a high proportion of patients are rendered dialysis-dependent.

Obstructive uropathy in pregnancy

Pregnancy predisposes women to several causes of post-renal AKI. Rarely, polyhydramnios can compress on the urinary system and result in AKI. Mechanical compression by the gravid uterus of twin pregnancy may also give rise to obstructive uropathy.

Causes of acute kidney injury in all stages of pregnancy

Asymptomatic bacteriuria is common in pregnancy and 40% of patients develop symptomatic UTI, which is associated with adverse pregnancy outcomes. Relative urinary stasis associated with physiological dilation of the urinary system further predisposes pregnant women to acute pyelonephritis. It is therefore prudent to screen and treat women for asymptomatic bacteriuria during antenatal check-ups. Patients with acute pyelonephritis will require admission for parenteral antibiotics.

Glomerulonephritis may also present for the first time or as a flare-up of pre-existing disease to cause AKI in any stage of pregnancy. The clinical presentation is characterized by hypertension and proteinuria, with or without AKI. Presentation after 20 weeks of gestation makes it extremely difficult to distinguish from PE, with the exception of lupus nephritis, where defining serology of SLE may aid diagnosis. Where diagnostic doubt exists, a renal biopsy may be considered, depending on the stage of gestation and risks involved. Corticosteroids, calcineurin inhibitors

(CNIs) and azathioprine (AZA) are safe immunosuppressants during pregnancy.

General Management

Given the profound effects of CKD on pregnancy and vice versa, women of childbearing age with renal impairment should receive contraceptive counselling to prevent unintended pregnancies. The decision to conceive should be made with knowledge of the individual maternal and foetal risks, and necessitates a thorough assessment tailored to the stage of CKD. A well-planned pregnancy in the setting of CKD is still considered high-risk and antenatal care must involve both nephrologists and obstetricians.

Blood pressure control before and during pregnancy is crucial. The majority of CKD patients are prescribed angiotensin-converting enzyme (ACE) inhibitors or angiotensin receptor blockers (ARB) to control their hypertension and proteinuria. These agents must be substituted by non-teratogenic medications in CKD women attempting to conceive. As conception is expected to take months or even years in women with CKD, individuals should be aware of their increasing maternal and foetal risk profile as CKD evolves. During this period, there may be changes in attitude towards family planning and it is important to resume renoprotective ACE inhibitors and ARB upon the decision to forgo pregnancy.

The diagnosis of pregnancy in women with CKD can be challenging. Commercial test kits and measurement of serum human chorionic gonadotrophin may be unreliable and ultrasonography is often required to confirm pregnancy. During the course of pregnancy, patients should be monitored closely for renal deterioration, and maternal and foetal complications. Pregnancy in women with CKD incurs a high risk of superimposed PE, and thus blood pressure should be meticulously managed with aspirin prophylaxis prescribed. Serial ultrasound scans are required to monitor foetal growth and liquor volume. In women who develop P-AKI, the causes should be promptly identified and treated accordingly. A renal biopsy is rarely undertaken during pregnancy in the absence of significant proteinuria or rapidly progressive renal deterioration. In particular, the bleeding risk from a renal biopsy is elevated in the third trimester and the gravid uterus during the latter stages of gestation makes the procedure extremely difficult. In stable patients, further investigations can be performed to establish the underlying renal pathology in the post-partum period if the abnormalities persist.

End-Stage Renal Disease and Pregnancy

Dialysis and pregnancy

Hormonal disturbances associated with ESRD render conception extremely rare among women on dialysis. Historically, it is also associated with high rates of maternal and foetal morbidity and mortality. Foetal growth restriction, pre-term delivery, low birth weight, and a complicated neonatal course becomes a rule rather than an exception.

Haemodialysis (HD) is the preferred dialysis modality in pregnancy. In those with CKD, timely initiation of dialysis is the key to circumventing very poor pregnancy outcomes. For those already on HD, the prescription must be substantially intensified to reduce maternal complications, prolong gestation and increase the chance of live birth. Volume assessment in pregnant women on dialysis is expectedly difficult and weight gains proportional to the stage of gestation must be accounted for. It is imperative to avoid intradialytic hypotension, which compromises the utero-placental circulation and thus foetal health. Close attention to the mineral and nutritional requirements of this population are also required, taking into account the foetal needs and the losses during intensified dialysis.

Renal transplantation and pregnancy

Successful renal transplantation usually restores menstrual cycles and fertility within six months. Comprehensive pre-pregnancy counselling should be provided for all women of childbearing age who have undergone transplantation. During pregnancy, renal allografts appear to adapt physiologically and anatomically in the same way as native kidneys. Although pregnancy outcomes are generally good in women with adequate allograft function, maternal and foetal risks remain high and thus multidisciplinary care and close monitoring by both nephrologists and obstetricians remains an absolute necessity.

Pregnancy should be planned and maintenance immunosuppression modified in advance. Mycophenolic acid (MPA) and mammalian target of rapamycin (mTOR) inhibitors are contraindicated, while corticosteroids, CNIs and AZA appear safe during pregnancy. The optimal timing to conceive following renal transplantation is unclear, and the general consensus to wait for a minimum of one year aims to navigate past issues pertaining to the heightened risk of early allograft rejection, when discontinuation of MPA and mTOR inhibitors are required for pregnancy. CNI levels should also be closely monitored because of the changes in pharmacokinetics during pregnancy. Long-term graft survival appears unaffected by pregnancy, but antibody formation via this sensitizing event may induce subsequent rejection.

12

Common Urological Problems

James Tsu

Introduction

Urological problems are important causes of urinary symptoms and renal impairment. This chapter will focus on some commonly seen urological problems in nephrology practice, namely benign prostatic hyperplasia (BPH), nephrolithiasis, and neoplastic conditions arising from acquired cystic disease.

Benign Prostatic Hyperplasia

The development of histologic BPH is a virtually inevitable process among all men with normal testicular androgens. Autopsy studies revealed that histologic BPH was present in 8%, 50%, and 80% in the 30s, 50s, and 70s age group respectively. Histologic BPH does not necessarily constitute clinical symptoms. The prevalence of 'BPH symptoms' (*vide infra*), together with an enlarged prostate, increases from 14% in the 40s to 24% in the 50s, and goes up to 40% in the 70s age group.

Pathophysiology

Histologic BPH refers to the proliferation in numbers of both epithelial and stromal cells in the transition zone of the prostate. The older term, 'benign prostatic hypertrophy', is thus incorrect. Two elements are essential to the development of histologic BPH: ageing and testicular androgens. The prostate maintains the ability to respond to androgens throughout life via a constant expression of androgen receptors (AR) in its tissue. Testosterone is converted to its active metabolite dihydrotestosterone, which binds to AR, causing hyperplastic prostate growth. In some

men, after years of slow hyperplastic growth starting from the 30–40s, obstruction to urine flow in the prostatic urethra ensues. However, it has been shown that the size of the prostate does *not* correlate with the degree of obstruction. The urinary obstruction by BPH has both a static and dynamic component. The former results from the sheer increase in the size of the prostate gland against a fixed capsule, while the latter arises from the tone of the smooth muscle in the prostate. Human prostate smooth muscle expresses abundant α_1-adrenergic receptors, which mediate its contraction and tone. The increase in urethral resistance to urine induces a compensatory change in bladder function, often at the expense of normal bladder storage function. The combination of impeded urine flow, obstruction-induced changes in detrusor function, compounded by age-related changes in the bladder and nervous system function, give rise to the symptoms we so often see in patients who are labelled 'BPH'.

Clinical characteristics

The older concept that 'BPH symptoms' or 'prostatism' is simply due to a mass-related increase in urethral resistance is now considered over-simplistic. It is now recognized that a significant proportion of these symptoms, the correct term of which should be lower urinary tract symptoms (LUTS), is due to age-related detrusor dysfunction and other pathologies such as polyuria, overactive bladder (OAB) and a variety of systemic medical conditions unrelated to the prostate. LUTS that are caused by BPH can be broadly classified into storage and emptying. The former includes frequency, urgency, and nocturia while the latter consists of weak stream, hesitancy, and sensation of incomplete emptying. In the majority of patients, LUTS demonstrate minimal or no progression over time. Only a minority experiences BPH progression events such as acute urinary retention (AUR), obstructive uropathy, and haematuria from prostate bleeding.

Evaluation and investigations

Clinical evaluation of patients presenting with LUTS starts when the patient walks in the clinic, noting any gait disturbance or uraemic appearances indicating underlying neurologic disorders and obstructive uropathy respectively. History should focus on his voiding pattern (including a history of AUR), previous genitourinary surgical procedures, and his current medications. Of note, any prior visible haematuria is an important red-flag symptom and thus necessitates further investigations to rule out bladder cancer. Voiding symptoms and how bothersome they are should be quantified with the International Prostate Symptoms Score (IPSS) and its Quality of Life question respectively. In some patients, a voiding diary covering a 24-hour period is needed to rule out the underlying polydipsia or nocturnal polyuria. Next, a focused physical examination of the abdomen and pelvis should be performed to look for any ballotable kidneys, distended bladder, and motor/sensory deficits in the lower extremities. Examination of the external genitalia and digital rectal examination (DRE) is a must in the clinical evaluation of these patients. The prostate gland should be palpated with respect to its approximate size, consistency, and the presence of hard nodules suggestive of cancer. Urinalysis and renal function tests should be performed. Serum prostate-specific antigen (PSA) may be performed after a detailed discussion with the patient (*vide infra*). Upper tract imaging and cystoscopy, however, are not routinely indicated. Uroflowmetry and post-void residual urine measurement should be conducted in selected patients with emptying LUTS, especially if invasive treatment is contemplated. In some patients, a urodynamic study, which is the only means to differentiate detrusor underactivity from bladder outlet obstruction (BOO) in patients with poor flow, may be indicated.

PSA and early case-finding of prostate cancer

PSA is a 33-kD serum glycoprotein secreted by the epithelial cells of the prostate and it functions as a serine protease in liquefaction of the ejaculate. For all practical purposes, the prostate is considered the only source of serum PSA and thus PSA is a prostate-specific biomarker. However, the expression of PSA is not cancer-specific as both benign and malignant prostate cells secrete PSA. Serum PSA is elevated in BPH, prostatitis, urinary tract infection, and after prostate biopsy, prostate surgery and AUR. DRE in the clinic setting can lead to an increase in PSA, but the change in PSA after DRE does not appear to be clinically significant, as the change has been shown to be within the error of the assay and rarely causes false positive tests. As such, PSA is not prostate cancer-specific and there is a substantial overlap in values of benign and malignant prostatic conditions.

The use of serum PSA as a screening tool for prostate cancer is controversial. There is conflicting evidence from two large-scale screening studies (PLCO and ERSPC) as to whether population PSA screening will reduce the mortality from prostate cancer. It is even more difficult to extrapolate the results of the screening trials, which were conducted on European and US men, to Asian men, in whom the incidence of prostate cancer is much lower. At present, PSA should only be used as a tool for opportunistic case-finding of prostate cancer, after a thorough discussion with the patient regarding the false positive rates of the PSA test and the false negative rate of its invasive confirmatory investigation, namely prostate biopsy.

Management

The objectives of management of LUTS due to BPH are to: (1) alleviate symptoms and improve quality of life; (2) reduce the incidence of BPH progression events; and (3) relieve BOO to prevent upper urinary tract damage.

Watchful waiting

Watchful waiting is appropriate for a proportion of men who experience no or low degree of 'bothersomeness' from their LUTS and have mild symptoms (IPSS <8). Lifestyle modifications including abstinence of bladder irritants and reduction of fluid intake before sleep are sufficient. These patients should be taught to monitor their own LUTS and any BPH progression.

Medical therapy

Medical therapy is indicated for patients who lack the indications for surgery but have symptoms that are severe and/or bothersome enough to require treatment.

Alpha-adrenergic receptor blockers

The prostate stroma as well as the bladder neck is richly innervated with α_1-adrenergic nerve endings and α_1-adrenergic receptors, the blockage of which pharmacologically (with prazosin, terazosin, doxazosin, alfuzosin, tamsulosin, or silodosin) will lead to the relaxation of smooth muscle and the subsequent reduction in urethral resistance. On average, treatment with alpha-adrenergic receptor blockers (AARB) increases urine flow rate by 2–3 ml/s and reduces IPSS by 3–6 points. Improvement often occurs within one week. Important side effects include asthenia, postural hypotension, and retrograde ejaculation in selected AARB. Despite symptomatic relief, AARBs do not reduce the risk of AUR or the future need for BPH surgery.

5α-reductase inhibitors

5α-reductase converts testosterone into its potent metabolite dihydrotestosterone, which promotes prostatic growth. Inhibitors of this enzyme (finasteride, dutasteride) induce a slight reduction in prostate volume and modest improvement in flow rate and symptoms. On average, 5α-reductase inhibitors (5ARIs) increase the flow rate by 2 ml/s and reduce the IPSS by 3 points. 5ARIs only work for bigger prostates (> 40 g), generally take 6–9 months to reach optimal effect, and reduce serum PSA by 50%. Common side effects include decreased libido, reduced ejaculate volume, and erectile dysfunction. 5ARIs have been shown to diminish the risk of AUR and future need for BPH surgery by 55%.

Combination therapy

In men with larger prostates (> 40 g), a combination of AARB and 5ARI has been shown in large-scale, placebo-controlled studies to be superior to either of the drugs alone in terms of symptomatic relief as well as a reduction in risk of AUR and future need for BPH surgery.

Surgical treatment

Patients with the following are indicated for BPH surgery:

1. Refractory AUR despite trial without catheter
2. Recurrent AUR
3. Renal insufficiency as a result of BOO (obstructive uropathy)
4. Recurrent gross haematuria from prostate
5. Bladder stone as a result of BOO
6. Recurrent urinary tract infection due to BOO

Surgery may also be considered in patients who find the response to medical treatment unsatisfactory. However, they should be made fully aware that surgery in general improves emptying LUTS significantly but alleviates storage LUTS less effectively. BPH surgery is a vast subject in its own right and will not be discussed in detail in this chapter.

Nephrolithiasis

Nephrolithiasis refers to the presence of stones within the pelvi-caliceal system of the kidney. Urinary tract stones (urolithiasis) have been described since antiquity. Historical evidence has shown a significant increase in kidney stones in the last century but in contrast the incidence of bladder stones decreased, but only in the developed world. The exact reason for this trend is unknown but postulated theories include Westernization of nutritional habits (food and alcoholic beverages), vitamin supplementation and reduction of urinary tract infections. In developed countries, over the last century, the site of stone formation has migrated from the lower to the upper urinary tract. It is also a disease with notoriously high recurrence rates, and as such its optimal management demands a clear understanding of its aetiology and pathophysiology.

Epidemiology

The prevalence of urolithiasis across the globe varies greatly, anywhere between 1 and 20%, depending on geographical location, ethnicity, climate, diet, and genetic factors. A recent meta-analysis revealed the prevalence of urolithiasis to range between 5.5–11.6% and 2.6–7.2% in the southern and northern parts of China respectively. Areas with hotter climates tend to have a higher prevalence of urolithiasis. In most countries, males are affected more (male-to-female ratio ranges between 1.3 and 5) although it appears that this gender preponderance is decreasing worldwide. Urolithiasis is uncommon in children and those below the age of 20, and its prevalence increases with age, peaking in the 30–50 age groups.

Pathophysiology

Urinary tract stones can be classified into: (1) infectious stones; (2) non-infectious stones; (3) stones due to genetic defects; and (4) stones due to adverse drug effects (drug stones). Common non-infectious stones include calcium oxalate, calcium phosphate, and urate stones. In general, urine must be supersaturated (above the thermodynamic solubility product) with a certain chemical before stones can form, but even at supersaturated concentrations, there are natural inhibitors (e.g. citrate and nephrocalcin) in urine that prevent crystal nucleation and aggregation. However, if the concentration of a certain chemical continues to rise in urine, there comes a point where crystal nucleation will occur despite the presence of stone inhibitors. For some chemicals such as urate, no known inhibitor of stone formation exists in urine.

Infectious stones

Infectious stones constitute about 10% of clinically encountered calculi. They are composed primarily of magnesium ammonium phosphate (struvite), which forms as a result of the infective process of urease-producing bacteria, such as *Proteus mirabilis*. Urea is split into ammonia and carbon dioxide, resulting in an alkaline environment that favours struvite formation.

Non-infectious stones

Calcium oxalate is the most common (60%) chemical composition of urinary tract stones. Causes of hyperoxaluria include excessive dietary oxalate intake, abnormal endogenous production (primary hyperoxaluria), and malaborptive states associated with small bowel resection and inflammatory bowel disease. Interestingly, hyperuricosuria associated with gout also promotes calcium oxalate stone formation in a phenomenon known as hyperuricosuric calcium nephrolithiasis. Among urinary tract stones, 20% contain calcium phosphate as the main constituent. Conditions predisposing to hypercalciuria include primary hyperparathyroidism and sarcoidosis. Urate stones constitute 10% of all stones, and acidic urine pH plays a pivotal role in its pathogenesis. At acidic pH, even a modest concentration of urate exceeds the solubility product, leading to urate stone formation. Of note, most urate stone formers are normo-uricosuric but almost invariably show a low urine pH. Low urine pH is commonly associated with gouty diatheses, excessive animal protein intake, type 2 diabetes mellitus, and/or metabolic syndrome.

Stones due to genetic disorders and adverse drug effects

These altogether constitute <1% of all urinary tract stones and are associated with rare conditions such as cystinuria, renal tubular acidosis, Lesch-Nyhan syndrome, xanthinuria, and the use of indinavir.

Clinical characteristics

The manifestations of renal calculi depend on the size and location of the stone. While small caliceal renal stones can be totally asymptomatic, these small calculi can also cause pain and bleeding despite staying in their calyces. Larger renal stones can obstruct the pelvi-ureteral junction, causing obstructive uropathy. In particular, struvite stones tend to grow to become staghorn-like and be associated with recurrent urosepsis and loss of kidney function. Renal stones can migrate into the ureter causing ureteral colic, which is characterized by excruciating loin pain that radiates to the suprapubic region, with or without haematuria and high fever.

Evaluation and investigations

Besides standard history, any systemic illness predisposing to stone formation, previous history of stone disease, prior stone surgery, and family history of urolithiasis should be elicited. A focused physical examination should be performed, noting any signs of azotaemia and scars from previous stone surgery. Urinalysis is essential, with an acidic pH pointing towards urate lithiasis and an alkaline pH indicating struvite stones. Urine should be cultured to look for any urease-producing bacteria. The blood levels of sodium, potassium, creatinine, calcium, phosphate, and urate should also be checked. A standard plain radiograph (KUB) can help evaluate the stone size and location. Of note, struvite and cystine stones are highly radio-opaque whereas urate and xanthine stones are completely radiolucent. Alternative imaging includes ultrasonography (USG) and non-contrast computer tomography (NCCT). USG is free from radiation, quick, and can accurately identify stones within the kidneys, but may have difficulty identifying ureteral stones. NCCT shows high sensitivity (93%) and specificity (97%) in detecting urolithiasis in every location. In addition, NCCT can measure the hardness of the stone by its Hounsfield unit and thus guide treatment decisions. NCCT also provides an objective assessment of hydro-ureteronephrosis and sometimes extra-urologic information. If surgery is contemplated and pelvi-caliceal anatomy imaging is needed, contrast excretory urography should be performed. Nowadays, CT urograms have virtually replaced intravenous urogram (IVU). Finally, any passed stone brought back by the patient should be sent for chemical analysis to elucidate any underlying reversible pathogenetic mechanisms.

Certain groups of patients, such as recurrent stone formers, children, and patients with malabsorptive states should be subjected to more extensive metabolic work-ups. This involves 24-hour urine quantification of calcium, phosphate, oxalate, and urate concentrations. An assay of citrate is also important for the evaluation of stone disease, but the test is not available in the Hong Kong public sector.

Management

Observation

Studies on the natural history of small (≤ 10 mm) asymptomatic calyceal renal stones showed that 33–75% of these stones progressed in size over time and a significant proportion of them became symptomatic and required treatment. Hence, the majority of asymptomatic calyceal stones should be offered active stone removal with surgical options (*vide infra*). However, observation is an option for patients with small (< 5 mm) asymptomatic renal stones, provided that reassessment for stone progression is feasible. In selected groups of patients, such as those with solitary kidneys, paediatric patients, and those in high-risk professions (e.g. pilots), active removal of such small stones is still indicated.

Medical treatment

Medical treatment (chemolysis or medical dissolution therapy) for formed stones is only available for urate stones and this involves alkalinizing the urine pharmacologically with oral sodium bicarbonate or potassium citrate. The objective is to keep the urine pH above 5.5 (preferably between 6 and 7) so that the formed urate stones will become soluble.

Surgical treatment

Surgical treatment options for renal stone removal include extra-corporeal shockwave lithotripsy, retrograde intra-renal surgery using flexible uretero-renoscope, and percutaneous nephrolithotomy. Nowadays, open surgery is virtually never necessary to manage renal stones. The choice of treatment should be individualized, taking into consideration the characteristics of the stone, patient factors, and the armamentarium or expertise available. Further discussion of surgical treatment options is beyond the scope of this chapter.

Prevention of renal stone disease

Urolithiasis has high recurrence rates and the risk is estimated to be 50% within 5–10 years after the first complete stone eradication. Although specific preventive strategies are available for some types of stones with respect to their distinct pathogenetic mechanisms (e.g. decreased dietary purine and/or oral allopurinol for patients with hyperuricosuric calcium nephrolithiasis), the general advice for all patients with urolithiasis is to increase fluid intake to achieve a daily urine output of 2 L. Other adjunctive general measures include a balanced diet, avoidance of excessive animal protein consumption, and moderate dietary calcium intake (calcium restriction leads to increased gut oxalate absorption and promotes stone formation).

Acquired Cystic Kidney Disease and Renal Cell Carcinoma

Clinical characteristics

End-stage renal disease (ESRD) patients have an increased risk of urinary tract cancer, especially renal cell carcinoma (RCC). One of the most important risk factors identified is the presence of acquired cystic kidney disease (ACKD). ACKD is a common finding in patients with ESRD and there is a strong linear relationship between ACKD and dialysis vintage, being present in 10–20% of patients on dialysis for up to 3 years, rising to > 90% of those having undergone 10 years or more of dialysis. Approximately 3–7% of ESRD patients with ACKD develop RCC in their native kidneys, meaning the risk is 100 times higher than in the general population. Almost any histologic variant of RCC can occur in the background of ACKD but the two most common types are clear cell papillary renal cell carcinoma and acquired cystic kidney disease-associated RCC (ACKD-RCC). The former can be seen in the general population while the latter is exclusively found in patients with ESRD.

ACKD-RCC, which has a unique histological appearance, was recognized as a distinct RCC variant in 2013. It is currently regarded as the most common form of RCC in ESRD patients. Patients with ERSD who develop RCC are often asymptomatic and RCC is frequently found incidentally during routine imaging, while a minority of patients present with microscopic/visible haematuria and flank pain. Studies have shown that ACKD-RCC tends to occur at a younger age, with a male predominance as compared with the sporadic type of RCC found in the general population. The incidence of RCC in ACKD increases with the duration of dialysis and interestingly, the risk remains high for patients who have undergone kidney transplantations.

Management

From a management perspective, standard RCC treatment applies to RCC found in ESRD patients, except that ESRD poses higher anaesthetic and bleeding risks. Nephron-sparing surgery is not required for tumours arising from non-functioning native kidneys and total nephrectomy is the rule. Owing to the need to preserve the peritoneum undisturbed for dialysis and anticipated adhesions from peritoneal dialysis, the retroperitoneoscopic approach is the preferred means of minimally invasive treatment in this group of patients, with the open retroperitoneal (loin) approach being the alternative. Published data regarding the prognosis of ACKD-RCC is limited, but in general, ACKD-RCC appears to be less aggressive than sporadic RCC in the general population. The value of a screening programme for ACKD-RCC in ESRD patients has been investigated, but to date, no evidence-based recommendation guidelines exist.

13

Hereditary Kidney Diseases and Paediatric Nephrology

Lorraine Kwan, Stella Chim, Alison Ma, Eugene Chan, and Wai Ming Lai

Introduction

Hereditary kidney diseases are important causes of chronic kidney disease (CKD) and end-stage kidney disease (ESKD). Inherited renal disorders can also lead to various electrolyte and acid–base disturbances. This chapter provides an overview of some important hereditary kidney diseases and also highlights key issues in managing children with CKD and ESKD.

Hereditary Kidney Diseases

Autosomal dominant polycystic kidney disease

Autosomal dominant polycystic kidney disease (ADPKD) is the most common hereditary renal disorder, occurring in 1 out of 1,000–2,500 individuals. It is the cause of ESKD in approximately 5% of the population initiated on dialysis. However, it is estimated that less than 50% of the cases are diagnosed. It is most commonly caused by mutations in the genes PKD1 (in 78% of disease pedigrees) or PKD2 (in 15% of disease pedigrees). PKD1, which is located on chromosome 16 (16p13.3), encodes polycystin-1 (PC1), and PKD2, which is located on chromosome 4 (4q21), encodes polycystin-2. Change in kidney volume (often expressed as height-adjusted total kidney volume) over time, is the strongest predictor of subsequent decline in renal function. The type of genetic mutation also influences the disease course. In this context, those with PKD2 develop fewer cysts and progress more slowly than those with PKD1 (the mean ages of developing ESKD are 54.3 years and 74.0 years for PKD1 and PKD2 respectively). Other important risk factors for progressive renal disease include hypertension, male sex, presence

of proteinuria, and early onset of symptoms. Kidney function remains relatively preserved up to forty years of age in many patients, as glomerular hyper-filtration in functioning nephrons compensates for the ongoing attrition of kidney tissue, until in their fifth decade, when approximately half develop ESKD. Haematuria, which is related to the rupture of a cyst into the collecting systems, occurs in approximately 35–50% of patients with ADPKD during their lifetime. Nephrolithiasis occurs in up to a quarter of patients with ADPKD, with uric acid stones present in more than half of these cases. Patients also have flank pain due to stretching of the renal capsule, haemorrhage into cysts, infection, or renal calculi. Hypertension is present in 50–70% of patients and is highly related to increased activity of the renin-angiotensin-aldosterone system (RAAS). ADPKD patients who reached ESKD invariably have hypertension. About 30–50% of patients have one or more episodes of urinary tract infection during their lifetime, which might be complicated by infected cysts and acute pyelonephritis. A urine culture may be negative in cases of infected cysts. A prolonged course of antibiotics of at least four weeks may be necessary for the treatment of infected renal cysts. Renal cell carcinoma is another important complication in patients with ADPKD.

Cerebral aneurysms are an important extra-renal complication in patients with ADPKD. The prevalence of intracranial aneurysms is estimated to be between 9 and 12%, which is four times higher than in the general population. The strongest risk factor associated with the development and rupture of cerebral aneurysms is a family history of intracranial aneurysms (> 20%), especially if complicated by subarachnoid haemorrhage. Screening with magnetic resonance angiography or computed

Table 13.1: Ultrasonographic criteria for the diagnosis of ADPKD in patients with positive family history

Diagnostic confirmation	Age	Ultrasound findings
	< 30	Total of ≥ 3 cysts
	30–39	Total of ≥ 3 cysts
	40–59	≥ 2 cysts in each kidney
Exclusion criteria		
	For PKD1	No kidney cyst by age of 30
	For PKD2	No kidney cysts by age of 40

ADPKD, Autosomal dominant polycystic kidney disease

tomographic angiography is recommended for: (a) ADPKD patients with a family history of intracerebral aneurysm; (b) ADPKD patients who work in high-risk occupations where loss of consciousness from a ruptured aneurysm would place the lives of others at risk; and (c) ADPKD patients who will be started on chronic anticoagulation. Patients with ADPKD can also have hepatomegaly with multiple hepatic cysts. The prevalence of liver cysts increases with age, with a prevalence of 10–20% in those below the age of 30 years and up to 50–70% in older than 60. Other extra-renal complications include pancreatic cysts, valvular heart disease (e.g. mitral valve prolapse and aortic regurgitation), colonic diverticulosis, abdominal wall and inguinal hernias, and seminal vesicle cysts.

The diagnosis of ADPKD can be established by renal imaging using ultrasonography, CT scans, or magnetic resonance imaging (MRI). The ultrasound-based criteria for diagnosis in patients with a positive family history are summarized in Table 13.1. The risk of disease progression can be predicted by MRI of kidneys using the Mayo classification system, which categorizes patients into five prognostic classes with the lowest to the highest risk for disease progression (1A, 1B, 1C, 1D, 1E) based on the patient's total kidney volume measurement at any given age. Genetic testing can be considered in the following scenarios: (1) patients with uncertain imaging but with the need for definitive diagnosis (e.g. live kidney donors); (2) patients with atypical presentations (e.g. early and severe ADPKD, kidney failure without significant enlargement of kidneys, marked discordant disease within family, marked asymmetry in disease severity between kidneys) or; (3) patients who require repro-ductive counselling.

Patients with ADPKD are advised to make life-style modifications including dietary salt restriction and increased fluid intake (> 3 L per day if esti-mated glomerular filtration rate or eGFR > 30 ml/min/1.73 m²). Compelling evidence has suggested the importance of stringent blood pressure control (target 110/70 mmHg). An angiotensin-converting enzyme (ACE) inhibitor or an angiotensin receptor blocker (ARB) is the drug of choice, because hyper-tension in ADPKD patients is greatly contributed by enhanced RAAS activity, increased sympathetic tone, and primary vascular dysfunction. Patients with a high risk of disease progression may be considered for tolvaptan treatment. Tolvaptan is a competitive vasopressin-2 receptor (V2R) inhibitor, which blocks V2R to decrease intracellular cAMP levels in cyst-lining tubular cells. Clinical studies have shown that tolvaptan can retard the rate of growth in total kidney volume and decline in eGFR in high-risk patients. The side effects of tolvaptan include thirst, polyuria, polydipsia, hypernatremia, and increased liver transaminases. Embolization or surgical interven-tions may be required in patients with complications such as severe haematuria. In patients with ESKD, peritoneal dialysis can sometimes be challenging due to reduced intra-abdominal space and increased risk of hernia. Nephrectomy may be needed prior to transplantation to provide space to accommodate the kidney allograft or in patients with recurrent and/or severe infections, symptomatic nephrolithiasis, recurrent and/or severe bleeding, uncontrolled pain, and suspicion of renal cancer.

Alport syndrome

Alport syndrome is an inherited progressive form of nephritis affecting the glomerular basement membrane (GBM). It is due to mutations of genes encoding the α-chain of the type IV collagen protein family. As type IV collagen α-chains are also basement membranes of the cochlea and the eyes, patients often also suffer from auditory and ocular abnor-malities. Up to 80% of patients with Alport syndrome show X-linked inheritance, while 15% of cases are autosomal recessive and only 5% show autosomal dominance. Patients usually have a positive family, with male relatives showing haematuria accom-panied by renal failure and deafness while female relatives sometimes also experience haematuria. Typical presentation is a boy with incidental finding of microscopic or occasional gross haematuria after upper respiratory tract infection symptoms. With time, proteinuria, hypertension, and progressive renal insufficiency develop. ESKD usually occurs between the ages of 16–35 years in patients with X-linked or autosomal recessive disease. Patients often also have bilateral sensorineural hearing loss (detected in up to 85% of affected boys), ocular manifestations (e.g. anterior lenticonus, retinal, or cornea changes), and leiomyomatosis.

The diagnosis can be established by molecular testing which demonstrates COL4A gene mutation. Electron microscopy (EM) shows the characteristic feature of longitudinal splitting of the lamina densa of the GBM (often described as 'weave-basket' appearance). There is no specific treatment for Alport syndrome. Renal transplantation is the best option for patients who have reached ESKD. However, in approximately 3% of affected males, anti-GBM disease can occur after kidney transplantation and cause allograft failure.

Fabry disease

Fabry disease is the most prevalent lysosomal storage disorder and is associated with renal dysfunction. The prevalence of classic Fabry disease is 1:22,000 to 1:40,000 in males, while the prevalence of atypical (late-onset) Fabry disease is 1:1,000 to 1:3,000 in males and 1:6,000 to 1:40,000 female respectively. Classic Fabry disease is caused by pathogenic variants in the alpha-galactosidase A (alpha-Gal A or galactosidase alpha) gene located in the long arm of the X chromosome, resulting in a deficiency or defect in the lysosomal hydrolase alpha-Gal A that catalyses the hydrolytic cleavage of the terminal galactose from globotriaosylceramide (Gb3). As an X-linked disorder, hemizygous males are more severely affected in classic Fabry disease and the disease course is more variable in females who are heterozygotes.

Fabry disease can affect different organ systems, including the kidneys. Proteinuria occurs in more than 80% of untreated male patients with a mean age of diagnosis of 35 to 40 years, and is an early sign of renal involvement. Patients may also present with polyuria and show progressive renal impairment. Cardiac involvement occurs in more than 80% of patients with classic Fabry disease, and these include concentric left ventricular hypertrophy, myocardial fibrosis, heart failure, coronary artery disease, aortic and mitral valve lesions, and conduction abnormalities. Gastrointestinal dysfunction is caused by the deposition of Gb3 in the autonomic ganglia of the

bowel and mesenteric blood vessels, leading to intestinal dysmotility, impaired autonomic function, vasculopathy, and bleeding. Dermatological lesions (e.g. telangiectasis and angiokeratomas) usually occur in the groin, hip and periumbilical areas, and can be present in up to 70% of patients with classic Fabry disease. Other clinical manifestations of classic Fabry disease include severe neuropathic or limb pain (acroparesthesias) and cornea verticillata (seen in almost all affected males and most females). Patients with atypical (later-onset) variants usually present later in life (third to seventh decades of life). They have residual alpha-Gal A activity (between 2 and 30% of the normal mean) and may not have Gb3 accumulation in capillaries and small blood vessels.

Diagnosis in males can be established by measurement of leukocyte alpha-Gal A activity followed by genetic testing, while diagnosis in females is usually by genetic confirmation. Patients with Fabry disease show characteristic changes of prominent vacuolation in glomerular cells (especially in the podocytes) on light microscopy (LM). EM reveals myeloid bodies which are pathognomonic of glycolipid storage disorders. Enzyme replacement therapy with recombinant human alpha-Gal-A aims to replace the missing or deficient enzyme in order to alleviate symptoms and reduce complications of Fabry disease. The high cost of treatment remains an important concern. The decision of whom to treat and the timing for initiation and discontinuation of treatment should take into consideration the symptom burden, clinical efficacy, and financial burden of treatment.

Tuberous sclerosis

Tuberous sclerosis complex (TSC) is an autosomal dominant genetic disease caused by mutations in either the TSC1 gene on chromosome 9 or the TSC2 gene on chromosome 16. TSC is characterized by the development of a variety of benign tumours in multiple organs, including the brain, heart, skin, eyes, kidney, lung, and liver. The prevalence of renal lesions in TSC increases with age, eventually affecting up to 80% of patients. Angiomyolipoma (AML) is the most common renal lesion and is detected in 49–60% of TSC patients. The number and size of renal AMLs also increase with age. Symptoms of AML are due to haemorrhage or the mass effect of AML. Patients may develop haematuria, flank pain, hypertension, or renal insufficiency. Renal AMLs larger than 4 cm are frequently symptomatic and are more likely to grow and develop aneurysms. The risk of significant haemorrhage or rupture is related to the degree of vascularity, size of AML, and also the size of aneurysms within the lesion. Renal cystic disease is the second most common renal manifestation of TSC. TSC patients are also at increased risk for the development of renal cell carcinoma, most often the clear cell type. The development of CKD in TSC patient can be related to: (1) nephrectomy for life-threatening haemorrhage from AML; (2) destruction of renal tissue related to extensive bilateral renal AML or cystic disease; and (3) focal segmental glomerulosclerosis (FSGS), with chronic interstitial disease thought to be a secondary disorder induced by nephron loss. Up to 81 to 95% of patients with TSC have dermatological involvement, which includes hypopigmented macules (ashleaf spots), angiofibromas typically involving the malar regions of the face, and Shagreen patches over the lower back. Patients can also have brain lesions such as glioneuronal hamartomas, subependymal nodules, and subependymal giant cell tumours. Up to 79 to 90% of patients may have seizures and around 44 to 65% of patients have cognitive disabilities. Other clinical manifestations include pulmonary manifestations (lymphangioleiomyomatosis), ophthalmic manifestations (e.g. retinal hamartomas), and cardiovascular manifestations (e.g. rhabdomyoma).

The diagnosis of TSC is usually established by clinical criteria and genetic confirmation. Patients also require investigations of multiple organ systems such as renal and neural imaging, electroencephalography, echocardiography, ophthalmological and dermatological assessments, and CT of the thorax. A multidisciplinary team approach is often required as TSC affect multiple organ systems. The mammalian target of rapamycin (mTOR) inhibitor everolimus is an approved treatment for TSC-related tumours in the brain (subependymal giant cell astrocytoma) and the kidneys (renal AML).

Glomerular and Tubular Disorders in Children

Nephrotic syndrome in children

The most common form of nephrotic syndrome in children is primary idiopathic nephrotic syndrome. The majority of these patients have histologic findings of minimal change disease and are steroid-sensitive (see also Chapter 8). Around 10–20% of patients have steroid-resistant nephrotic syndrome (SRNS), with worse prognoses and kidney survival rates. Some of

them have genetic mutations of podocyte proteins, including *NPHS1*, *NPHS2*, *PLCE1*, and *WT1* genes. Patients with a genetic form of SRNS are usually unresponsive to immunosuppressive therapy. These patients are usually treated with ACE inhibitors or ARBs, aiming to decrease proteinuria and slow the progression of chronic kidney disease. Congenital nephrotic syndrome (CNS) refers to a disease presenting during the first three months of life with marked oedema and massive proteinuria. When the onset of disease comes between three months and one year of age, it is called infantile nephrotic syndrome. Congenital or infantile nephrotic syndrome has a genetic basis and most patients have poor outcomes. Mutations in five different genes are responsible for over 80% of patients with CNS. *NPHS1*, encoding nephrin, is responsible for the Finnish-type CNS. *NPHS2*, encoding podocin, is responsible for familial FSGS. *NPHS3* (*PLCE1*), encoding phospholipase C epsilon, is responsible for isolated diffuse mesangial sclerosis. *WT1*, encoding the transcription tumour suppressor, is responsible for diffuse mesangial sclerosis with Denys-Drash syndrome. *LAMB2*, encoding laminin beta 2, is responsible for the Pierson syndrome with diffuse mesangial sclerosis. Genetic causes of CNS do not respond to steroid or immunosuppressive therapy. Conservative treatment includes regular albumin infusion and diuretics, replacement of gamma globulin, nutritional support with a high-protein and low-salt diet, vitamins and thyroxine supplements, and prevention of infections and thrombotic complications. Patients eventually require dialysis and kidney transplantation, which is commonly preceded by nephrectomy to control hypercoagulability and hyperlipidaemia due to the persistent nephrotic state.

Bartter syndrome

Bartter syndrome (BS) is an autosomal recessive disorder generated by a primary defect in sodium chloride reabsorption in the thick ascending limb (TAL) of the loop of Henle. It mimics the chronic use of a loop diuretic. Clinical manifestations include renal salt wasting, hypokalaemia due to renal potassium wasting, hypochloraemic metabolic alkalosis, polyuria, impaired urinary concentrating ability, hypercalciuria, hyperreninaemic hyperaldosteronism with normal blood pressure, hyperplasia of juxtaglomerular apparatus, and growth and mental retardation. Antenatal Bartter syndrome (type I & II BS) is also known as hyperprostaglandin E syndrome. This is characterized by antenatal presentations with polyhydramnios due to foetal polyuria and prematurity. After birth, patients may have life-threatening salt and water loss, nephrocalcinosis, and secondary elevation of prostaglandin level. Type II BS patients may also have transient hyperkalaemia with metabolic acidosis during the first days of life. Type I BS is caused by mutations in the *SLC12A1* gene located on chromosome 15q21, encoding the Na^+-K^+-$2Cl^-$ cotransporter NKCC2 in the TAL of the loop of Henle. Type II BS is caused by mutations in the *KCNJ1* gene located on chromosome 11q24, encoding the K^+ channel ROMK in the TAL. Classic Bartter syndrome (type III BS) is caused by mutations in the *CLCNKB* gene located on chromosome 1p36, encoding the Cl^- channel ClC-Kb. Patients have heterogeneous presentation as suspected antenatal BS, classic BS, or Gitelman-like syndrome. This is attributed to the distribution of the ClC-Kb channel throughout the nephron, particularly in the TAL and distal convoluted tubule (DCT). Acute management for BS patients with dehydration includes correction of fluid loss and electrolyte disturbance. Long-term treatment includes oral potassium supplements and prostaglandin inhibitors, such as non-steroidal anti-inflammatory drugs (e.g. indomethacin) or selective cyclooxygenase-2 inhibitors (e.g. celecoxib). In addition, a potassium-sparing diuretic such as spironolactone is usually administered, with monitoring of exacerbation of renal salt wasting and volume depletion. ACEI such as enalapril may be a useful adjunctive therapy. Thiazides should not be used to reduce hypercalciuria, as they interfere with compensation mechanisms in the DCT and further aggravate dehydration.

Gitelman syndrome

Gitelman syndrome (GS) is an autosomal recessive disorder characterized by hypokalaemia due to renal potassium wasting, metabolic alkalosis, hypomagnesaemia due to renal magnesium wasting, and hypocalciuria. It mimics the chronic use of a thiazide diuretic. Patients usually present in late childhood or adulthood with carpopedal spasm and tetany, muscle weakness or cramps, fatigue, thirst, nocturia, or incidental hypokalaemia in a routine blood test. Failure to thrive and polyuria are uncommon. GS is caused by mutations in the *SLC12A3* gene located on chromosome 16q13, encoding the Na^+-Cl^- cotransporter NCC in the DCT. Magnesium reabsorption is indirectly impaired in GS. Treatment is by magnesium and potassium supplements. Magnesium

chloride is recommended since it will also correct the urinary chloride loss. Potassium-sparing diuretics such as spironolactone and amiloride may be used. Monitoring of excessive diuresis and hypotension is required. Prostaglandin inhibitors such as indomethacin are less indicated in GS.

Cystinosis

Cystinosis is a rare multisystem genetic disorder characterized by lysosomal accumulation of cystine in different organs including the kidneys, eyes, bone marrow, muscles, thyroid, liver, pancreas, spleen, testes, and brain, resulting in subsequent dysfunction. It is of autosomal recessive inheritance, caused by mutations in the *CTNS* gene located on chromosome 17p13, encoding cystinosin, which is a lysosomal cystine transporter. The three distinct types are infantile nephropathic cystinosis, intermediate cystinosis, and ocular cystinosis. Infantile nephropathic cystinosis is the most common and most severe form. It is also the most common hereditary cause of renal Fanconi syndrome in childhood. Patients present in infancy with poor growth, renal Fanconi syndrome, and hypophosphataemic rickets. Cystine crystals are present in the cornea by the age of 2 years. Most untreated children will progress to ESKD by the age of 10 years. Diagnosis is established by one of the following three methods: identification of cystine crystals in the cornea on slit-lamp examination, elevated cystine content of peripheral blood leukocytes or fibroblasts, or confirmation of mutations of the *CTNS* gene. Pre-natal diagnosis is available by detecting elevated cystine levels or by genetic diagnosis from chorionic villus sampling or amniotic fluid cells. Management of cystinosis includes symptomatic therapy and administration of cysteamine, a cystine-depleting agent. Oral cysteamine and cysteamine topical eye drops should be prescribed. Renal Fanconi syndrome and rickets are treated by replacement of proximal tubular losses of water, electrolytes and bicarbonate, and phosphate and vitamin D supplements. Nutritional support is important and growth hormone therapy may be required. Dialysis and kidney transplantation are required when patients develop ESKD. Intermediate cystinosis usually presents in older children or adolescents, with milder forms of renal tubular and eye damage, and ESKD may occur later. Patients with ocular cystinosis have photophobia due to cystine crystals in the cornea, but usually do not have renal involvement or most of the other clinical features. They usually present in adulthood.

Hypophosphataemic rickets and vitamin D dependent rickets

Hypophosphataemic rickets is characterized by low serum phosphate levels and almost always caused by renal phosphate wasting. This can be isolated or part of a generalized renal tubular disorder such as Fanconi syndrome. X-linked hypophosphataemia (XLH) is the most common hereditary form of isolated renal phosphate loss. It is inherited as X-linked dominant manner due to mutations in the *PHEX* gene located on chromosome Xp22. The resulting overactivity of fibroblast growth factor 23 (FGF23) reduces phosphate reabsorption and vitamin D 1α-hydroxylation by the kidneys. Signs and symptoms usually begin in early childhood, and include bow legs and short stature. Laboratory findings include hypophosphataemia, hyperphosphaturia, normal serum calcium, elevated alkaline phosphatase (ALP), normal to high parathyroid hormone (PTH), and reduced $1,25(OH)_2$ vitamin D. Conventional treatment is with phosphate supplements and calcitriol or alfacalcidol. This is associated with the risk of secondary and tertiary hyperparathyroidism, as well as of nephrocalcinosis. The alternative therapy is burosumab, a humanized monoclonal anti-FGF23 antibody, which was approved in 2018 by the FDA in the United States and the European Medicines Agency for use in children one year or older. Burosumab is generally the treatment of choice for untreated children and for those who have limited benefits from phosphate and calcitriol therapy. Burosumab is given subcutaneously every two weeks and should not be given in combination with oral phosphate and calcitriol or alfacalcidol.

Vitamin D dependent rickets type 1A is an autosomal recessive disorder caused by mutations in the *CYP27B1* gene located on chromosome 12q14, resulting in a deficiency of the 1α-hydroxylase enzyme. 25OH vitamin D failed to be converted to the active $1,25(OH)_2$ vitamin D, leading to the clinical presentations of rickets and vitamin D deficiency in infancy. Laboratory findings include hypocalcaemia, elevated ALP, elevated PTH, normal or low phosphate, normal 25OH vitamin D, and low $1,25(OH)_2$ vitamin D. Lifelong treatment with $1,25(OH)_2$ vitamin D (calcitriol) should be offered.

Cystinuria

Cystinuria is an autosomal recessive disorder characterized by defective reabsorption of cystine and the dibasic amino acids ornithine, lysine, and arginine in the proximal renal tubule and gastrointestinal tract. Excessive urinary cystine excretion leads to the formation of cystine stones due to their low solubility in normal urinary pH. Cystine stones contribute to 4–5% of paediatric renal stones. Cystinuria is caused by mutations in two genes, *SLC3A1*, located on chromosome 2p21, and *SLC7A9*, located on chromosome 19q13. Clinical presentations are those related to renal stone formation, including stone passage, haematuria, flank pain, renal colic, obstruction, infection, and renal impairment. Cystinuria is diagnosed by the presence of renal stones and stone analysis showing cystine or pathognomonic hexagonal cystine crystals on urinalysis. It is confirmed by excessive urinary cystine excretion. Treatment includes high fluid intake aiming for 24-hour urine volume greater than 2 L/1.73 m^2 to reduce urinary cystine concentration, dietary sodium and methionine restriction, and urine alkalinization by potassium citrate to achieve a urine pH greater than 7.5 to increase cystine solubility. Cystine-binding agents such as tiopronin and D-penicillamine can be considered if conservative management fails. However, their use is limited by their significant side effects. Surgical treatment is warranted for patients with infected or obstructed kidneys. Family screening is suggested to identify high-risk patients and aim for the prevention of stone formation.

Hyperoxaluria

Hyperoxaluria is characterized by increased urinary excretion of oxalate. Primary hyperoxaluria is an autosomal recessive disorder, caused by enzymatic defects in glyoxylate metabolism that result in overproduction of oxalate. Excessive oxalate binds with calcium to form calcium oxalate stones in the kidneys and urinary tract. Recurrent stones formation, nephrocalcinosis, and accumulation of calcium oxalate in kidney tissue eventually lead to ESKD. Oxalate accumulation in various organs results in systemic oxalosis and organ dysfunction. Primary hyperoxaluria (PH) type 1 is the most common among the three types. This is caused by alanine glyoxylate aminotransferase (AGT) deficiency in the liver, due to mutation of the *AGXT* gene located on chromosome 2q37. Infantile oxalosis is most severe and infants usually present before six months of age and may progress to ESKD at a mean age of three years. Clinical diagnosis is suggested by recurrent renal stones with pure calcium oxalate monohydrate stones and markedly increased urinary oxalate excretion, together with increased urinary excretion of glycolate. The diagnosis is confirmed by mutation of the *AGXT* gene, or if no mutation is found, by a liver biopsy demonstrating a significant reduction in AGT activity. Pre-natal genetic diagnosis is possible. Medical management includes large fluid intake aiming at urine volume greater than 3 L/day/1.73 m^2 to decrease urine oxalate concentration. Potassium citrate should be given to increase the solubility of calcium oxalate. Avoidance of foods with high oxalate content is recommended. Around 20% of patients will respond to high-dose pyridoxine treatment. Dialysis is required when the patient reaches ESKD. Combined liver and kidney transplantation is the definitive treatment in children, while sequential liver-kidney transplantation should be considered in adults (especially those with high oxalate loads) to prevent early renal allograft loss. PH type 2 is caused by glyoxylate reductase/hydroxypyruvate reductase deficiency, due to mutation of the *GRHPR* gene located on chromosome 9p13. It is generally a milder disease than PH type 1.

End-Stage Kidney Disease in Children

End stage Kidney disease (ESKD) is uncommon in children. The common causes of ESKD in children include congenital abnormalities of the kidney and urinary tract, primary glomerular diseases, hereditary or other congenital disorders, and secondary glomerular diseases. The global prevalence of ESKD in children varies from 18 to 100 per million age-related populations. The figures vary around the world due to genetic, environmental, and economic factors. Renal replacement therapy (RRT) is indicated when the glomerular filtration rate is < 15 ml/min/1.73 m^2, and the options of RRT and related issues should be discussed with the family well before the child reaches ESKD.

Choice of renal replacement therapy in children

Kidney transplantation remains to be the best RRT in children with ESKD. It is associated with superior survival and quality of life compared with dialysis. Peritoneal dialysis (PD) or haemodialysis (HD) are the

two modalities of RRT bridging the child over until kidney transplant.

Peritoneal dialysis in children

PD is the preferred option in infants and small children with ESKD. It is cost-effective and avoids the need to utilize precious vascular access in young children. PD is undertaken at home, either manually or with the cyclers (automated PD). Automated PD is a popular option in children, where the exchanges are performed at night to facilitate schooling during the day. In contrast to the adults, prescriptions of PD in children are highly individualized and calculated according to their body surface areas. The fill volume, defined as the volume of dialysate to be instilled at each exchange is about 1,100–1,400 ml/m^2 in older children and 600–800 ml/m^2 for children under the age of two. The use of biocompatible dialysate with neutral pH is the preferred choice in children for the preservation of peritoneal membrane and residual renal function. With the advancement of remote patient management, clinical staff could access the children's dialysis profiles with ease and thereby facilitate early detection of ultrafiltration failure and PD related problems.

Haemodialysis in children

HD represents an alternative form of RRT for those who are not suitable for PD due to, for instance, a history of intra-abdominal surgeries or complicated anatomies. It is more commonly done in older children or adolescents whose vascular accesses are more available. HD is performed in the hospital 3–4 times per week, 4–5 hours per session. In children, the dialysers and blood lines must be size-matched, and the prescription of each treatment should be individualized. The HD circuit should be primed with either albumin or blood products if the extra-corporeal volume is estimated to be more than 10%. Arteriovenous fistula (AVF) is superior to central venous lines in children because of better blood flows and clearance. However, the creation of AVF is technically challenging in small children and therefore central venous catheters are still widely used in many places. There has been remarkable new developments in HD such as new HD strategies (haemodiafiltration), equipment catering for smaller patients, novel dialysers (with high flux properties) and nocturnal home HD. (see also Chapter 17).

Important aspects in the management of children on dialysis

The delivery of dialysis is only a part of management in children with ESKD. The management of growth, mineral bone disorder and psychosocial needs are also important issues in this group of patients.

Growth

Growth failure is common among children with ESKD. Apart from ensuring adequate dialysis, correction of anaemia, electrolytes and acid–base balance, and optimization of the nutritional intake are vital in the management of these children, especially in children younger than two years of age. Early implementation of enteral nutrition via gastrostomy may allow catch-up growth in young children with ESKD. The use of recombinant growth hormones should be considered in children who fail to demonstrate good weight gain despite optimization of nutrition and dialysis.

Chronic kidney disease and mineral bone disorder

Kidneys play an important role in maintaining the homeostasis of calcium and phosphate. In ESKD, the rise in phosphate levels result in increased FGF23 and PTH production, and thus bone demineralization and vascular calcifications. Reduction in 1,25-dihydroxyvitamin D (active vitamin D) results in hypocalcaemia, which also promotes bone demineralization via elevated PTH and FGF23. Such disturbed bone metabolism contributes to vascular calcifications and cardiovascular diseases in children on dialysis. While management of chronic kidney disease-mineral bone disorder in children is largely similar to that in adults, one should commence treatment early and ensure an adequate calcium level in a growing child.

Psychosocial aspect

Chronic dialysis is understandably associated with substantial psychosocial stress to the children and their family. A paediatric nephrologist could help coordinate multifaceted support for these children in an individualized manner to improve their quality of life. Inputs from nurses and allied health professionals including occupational therapists, physiotherapists, dietitians, clinical psychologists, clinical pharmacists, and social workers can facilitate effective communications with the family and thereby minimize the patient's concerns and promote adherence to the treatment.

Kidney transplantation in children

Kidney transplantation is the best form of RRT for children, and therefore clinicians should always explore any potential live kidney donors and the feasibility of pre-emptive transplantation in ESKD children. Detailed immunological, urological, medical, and psychological assessments prior to the surgery can help ensure favourable graft outcomes. Similar to adults, living-related kidney transplantation is associated with better overall outcomes compared to deceased donor kidney transplantation. Of note, in the paediatric population, graft survival is worst among adolescents due to non-adherence, so a well-structured transition program is crucial to empowering these patients for self-management. With the advances in surgical techniques and planning (e.g. 3D printing), and medical support, satisfactory clinical outcomes can be achieved even in young infants (~10 kg) receiving kidney transplantation.

The Way Forward

Recent advances in dialysis and transplantation have considerably improved the outcomes for children with kidney diseases. While awaiting further results from global registries to shed light on unanswered questions regarding various aspects of optimal RRT in children, a multidisciplinary approach would be beneficial in supporting children with ESKD.

14

Epidemiology of Chronic Kidney Disease: Global, Regional, and Local Perspectives

Kai Ming Chow, Chao Li, Xue-wang Li, Xue-mei Li, Chi Bon Leung, and Philip Kam Tao Li

Introduction

Chronic kidney disease (CKD) captures the essence of public health and epidemiology. This chapter lays out the concepts in applying epidemiology analysis in estimating the disease burden of CKD, expressed in terms of incidence and prevalence, mortality, and disability-adjusted life-years (DALYs) (Table 14.1). The global epidemic of CKD is a major public health problem, including the Asia-Pacific region. Students, practising clinicians, and public health epidemiologists can all benefit from recognizing several unique aspects of this non-communicable disease that affects more than 697 million people worldwide.

Estimating Incidence and Prevalence of Chronic Kidney Disease

The local, regional and global prevalence of CKD is rising steadily. Worldwide, it is estimated that the number of patients requiring renal replacement therapy (RRT) will cross 5 million by the year 2030. In terms of planning and allocating resources, the community and epidemiologists should compile data for risk assessments of the disease. While Hong Kong does not have a CKD registry, the burden of CKD can be inferred from the data of community-based studies and the end-stage kidney disease (ESKD) burden captured in the Hong Kong Renal Registry (HKRR). The HKRR is an electronic system that has captured the epidemiological and clinical data of all dialysis and kidney transplant patients from Hospital Authority-operated hospitals since 1995. According to a community-based survey in Hong Kong, 33% of subjects older than 60 years had either hypertension (HT) or urinary abnormalities, compared with 24%

in the 41–60-year-old group, and 9.7% in the 20–40-year-old group. Data from the HKRR showed that the incidence of ESKD in Hong Kong has also escalated steadily over the past two decades, with the number of incident RRT patients growing from approximately 600 in 1996 to more than 1,300 in 2019 (incidence rate of 180 per million population [pmp]). As of 2019, the total number of prevalent ESKD patients in Hong Kong was around 10,600 (a prevalence rate of 1,421 pmp).

As for mainland China, a national multicentre cross-sectional study in 2012 showed that the prevalence of CKD in adults was around 10%, using a definition of estimated glomerular filtration rate (eGFR) less than 60 mL/min per 1.73 m^2 or the presence of albuminuria (Table 14.2). The estimated overall number of adult CKD patients in China was 120 million, including approximately 2 million ESKD patients, with a male predominance. Besides, the proportions of advanced CKD in this national survey were lower than those reported in developed countries. The prevalence of stage 3 and stage 4 CKD is 1.6% and 0.1% respectively in China, compared with 7.7% and 0.35% in the United States. Considering that the prevalence of HT and diabetes mellitus (DM) have increased rapidly in the past 20 years in China, it may take another decade to demonstrate the impact of these diseases on the national prevalence rate of CKD. The prevalence of CKD also varies substantially among geographical regions in China. CKD prevalence reported in cross-sectional studies from different minority-populated areas in China ranged from 5.4% to 12.9%. This heterogeneity might be related to variability in genetic susceptibility, environmental factors, lifestyle, and economic development. Socio-economic status and

Table 14.1: Toolbox for the understanding of the epidemiology of chronic kidney disease

Disability adjusted life years (DALYs)	• The sum of years of potential life lost due to premature mortality and the years of productive life lost due to disability. • For CKD, it is calculated as the sum of the years of life lost (YLL) due to premature mortality in the population and the years lost due to disability (YLD) for people living with the CKD or its consequences.
Years of life lost (YLL)	• The years of life lost refers to the number of deaths multiplied by the standard life expectancy at the age at which death occurs.
Years lived with disability (YLDs)	• As a measure of the overall disease burden, this metric refers to the number of years that an individual lives with a functional impairment caused by a disease. • The formula for calculating YLD is the number of cases in a particular time period multiplied by the average duration of the disease, combined with a weight factor that represents the severity of the disease on a scale from 0 (perfect health) to 1 (dead).

CKD, chronic kidney disease; YLD, years lived with disability; YLL, Years of life lost

Table 14.2: Prevalence of chronic kidney disease in adults in China

Renal impairment			Albuminuria		CKD prevalence (95% CI)
Stage of CKD	**n**	**Prevalence (95% CI)**	**n**	**Prevalence (95% CI)**	
1	29,244	65.2 (64.4–66.1)	1,877	8.7 (8.–9.30)	5.7 (5.2–6.1)
2	16,775	33.0 (32.2–33.9)	1,385	10.3 (9.3–11.2)	3.4 (3.1–3.7)
3	1,106	1.6 (1.4–1.8)	221	21.1 (16.1–26.1)	1.6 (1.4–1.8)
4	59	0.1 (0.06–0.2)	25	34.3 (9.6–58.9)	0.1 (0.06–0.2)
5	20	0.03 (0.01–0.05)	9	56.6 (22.6–90.5)	0.03 (0.01–0.05)
Total	47,204	100	3,517	9.4 (8.9–10.0)	10.8 (10.2–11.3)

Data resource: Zhang L, et al. Lancet 2012; 379: 815–22.
CKD, Chronic kidney disease; albuminuria was defined as a urinary albumin-to-creatinine ratio > 30 mg/g creatinine; CKD was defined as an eGFR < 60 mL/min per 1.73 m² or albuminuria

the accompanying changes in lifestyle have varied considerably between rural and urban areas in China, especially during the 2010s.

Dialysis is a resource-intensive therapy, and there is a relationship between the provision of dialysis and the overall economic development of a locality. Over 90% of ESKD patients in Hong Kong received dialysis services in public hospitals. As of 2019, roughly 4,600 (70%) and 2,100 (~30%) patients in Hong Kong were receiving PD and HD respectively. In China, the prevalence of dialysis patients had risen seven-fold during the period from 1999 to 2012, while the incidence of dialysis patients remained unchanged over the same period (~15 pmp). In the 2015 annual data report of the China Kidney Disease Network (CK-NET), the estimated prevalence of HD and PD was around 400 pmp and 40 pmp, respectively. Much diversity has been observed in the distribution of dialysis patients in different geographic areas, with significantly higher incidence and prevalence in major cities such as Beijing and Shanghai. Socio-economic development and improvement of the national medical insurance system have increased the coverage of dialysis therapy. By the end of 2012, up to 98% of rural residents were covered by the New Rural Co-operative Medical Care System. This contributes partly to the increased prevalence of dialysis in China, especially in urban areas. However, regional disparities in medical resource accessibility to RRT still exist in China. For all prevalent dialysis patients, HD is the major modality (~90%). While it was estimated that over 70,000 Chinese ESRD patients were on continuous ambulatory peritoneal dialysis in 2016, the utilization rate of automated PD was only 1.4% in China.

Table 14.3: Methodology or scenario with implications on false estimation of prevalence of CKD

	Measurement and study methodology	Implications on estimation inaccuracy
Falsely high estimation of CKD prevalence	• Single time-point creatinine measurement (instead of repeated measurements) or one-off investigation of proteinuria	• 'One-off' testing does not take into account the definition of CKD (requiring a three-month duration of abnormal glomerular filtration rate or markers of kidney damage). • Misclassification of patients with acute kidney injury overestimates the true prevalence of CKD, mostly with an over-inflated prevalence of stage 3 CKD. • A false positive for proteinuria, often encountered in mild proteinuria (dipstick +), could have misclassified normal people as having stage 1 or 2 CKD.
	• Survey population with higher proportion of elderly people	• Age distribution of the community affects the prevalence of CKD based on the eGFR equation currently in use. • Besides the rise of true CKD prevalence with age, there could have been an overestimation of CKD prevalence when the same threshold of defining kidney function is applied to elderly individuals with so-called renal senescence, namely, a normal 'physiologic decrease' in eGFR.
Falsely low estimation of CKD prevalence	• Study population with young or middle-aged adults with unclassifiable CKD	• The use of a 'cut-off' eGFR < 60 ml/min/1.73 m^2 might have missed certain patients who have a low eGFR for their age.
	• Population with high prevalence of altered muscle mass, such as elderly people with sarcopenia	• Serum creatinine-based equation for eGFR gives rise to overestimation of true kidney function in patient subgroups with reduced muscle mass.

CKD, chronic kidney disease; eGFR, estimated glomerular filtration rate

In 2017, 697 million cases of all-stage CKD were recorded worldwide, bringing the global prevalence to 9.1%. Between 1990 and 2017, the global age-standardized prevalence of CKD has remained stable with a 1–2% change, although the all-age prevalence had markedly increased by almost 30%. These observations highlight the effect of ageing and population growth on the prevalence estimates. One should appreciate that an accurate estimation of the global incidence and prevalence of CKD is difficult for several reasons. Besides worldwide variation of the disease, these data often referred to cohort studies or large-scale population-based screening programmes from higher-income countries. Indeed, many countries do not have high-quality nationally representative data, and the true incidence and prevalence are particularly difficult to examine in low-income countries where disease awareness is low even among high-risk patient groups. Compounding this issue is the heterogeneous case definitions or study methods. For instance, diagnosis based on laboratory data versus the International Classification of Diseases and Injuries (ICD) codes would differ substantially.

The impact of the study methodology on the accuracy of CKD prevalence estimation is summarized in Table 14.3. A common approach of most published studies is to define CKD on the basis of an arbitrary single measurement, without incorporating the chronicity criterion. Conceptually, CKD should be diagnosed only when there is persistence of the damage or decreased function for at least three months. A single measurement of a young adult with transiently abnormal serum creatinine concentration after a severe bout of diarrhoea, for example, could overestimate the prevalence of CKD. The investigation of proteinuria to a one-off event or the use of haematuria as part of the screening may also affect the estimation of CKD prevalence. Indeed, previous studies have demonstrated that the introduction of screening for haematuria will increase the prevalence of CKD. Tools for estimating CKD, therefore, should be specified when comparing the prevalence across studies and regions.

Estimation of glomerular filtration rate (GFR) using different formulae also contributes to variations in CKD stages or prevalence. At best, the proportion of values of eGFR that lie within 30% of measured (or true) GFR is 75–85%. In other words, up to 25% of people could have been staged incorrectly with their estimates being more than 30% above or below the measured GFR. The accuracy or reliability of estimation equations is further reduced when there is reduced muscle mass, as occurs in general malnourishment, limb amputation, or muscle disease.

Etiology of Chronic Kidney Disease: Local, Regional, and Global Perspectives

In Hong Kong, the leading causes of ESKD in incident patients are diabetic kidney disease (DKD) (53%), followed by glomerulonephritis (GN) (18%), and hypertensive nephropathy (HTN) (13%). The major causes of ESKD in prevalent patients are GN (33%), DKD (31%), unknown cause (15%), and HTN (10%). According to the CK-NET 2015 annual report, the leading causes of CKD in China included DKD (27.0%), HTN (20.8%), obstructive nephropathy (ON, 15.6%), and GN (15.1%). DKD has overtaken GN as a cause of CKD in both the general population and the hospitalized urban population in China, and such transition in aetiology is preceded by decades of increasing prevalence of DM in China. The spectrum of CKD aetiology also differs between urban and rural areas. Over half of the patients in the urban areas have DKD (32.73%) or HTN (22.98%), while in rural residents the leading causes are ON (21.41%), GN (18.53%), and DKD (17.36%). Geographic variations of aetiology are also observed, with a relatively high percentage of DKD in northern China but a high percentage of ON in southern China. Globally, the causes of CKD vary with geographical region, with DKD and HTN being the predominant causes in most localities.

Estimating Disease Burden in Chronic Kidney Disease

The years lived with disability (YLDs), mortality, years of life lost (YLLs), and DALYs are important tools for estimating disease burden in CKD (Table 14.1). DALYs are, in fact, a composite of YLLs and YLDs. These figures are currently best captured by the Global Burden of Disease, Injuries, and Risk Factors Study, commonly known as GBD. The study allows a broad collection of data sources and statistical modelling approaches. Arguably, the study provides the hitherto best metrics although their data representativeness index (which is a measure of the

percentage of locations with data for a given time period) remained less than 30%.

To allow comparison of diseases, attributable mortality is often modelled by diagnostic codes, namely ICD codes. In terms of global mortality, CKD was estimated to result in 1.2 million deaths in 2017 and contribute to an additional 1.4 million deaths from cardiovascular disease. Based on such estimates from the GBD study, CKD was ranked the 12th leading cause of death, higher than tuberculosis or HIV. To better reflect the CKD burden, DALYs is perhaps a better metric that captures both death and disability. In 2017, CKD resulted in 35.8 million DALYs. To look at DALYs from the perspective of public health, the DALYs rate for impaired kidney function was higher than that for drug use, unsafe sanitation, low physical activity, and second-hand smoke. Although the aged-standardized CKD DALYs rates have remained stable from 2007 to 2017, the all-age DALYs rate has increased by 21.7%, a change largely driven by population growth and ageing. In terms of the age-standardized CKD DALYs, type 2 DM was the only cause of CKD associated with a significant rise of 9.5% from 1990 to 2017. A significant increasing trend of DM being the primary diagnosis of incident dialysis patients was also observed in Hong Kong, whereas there as a steady decrease of GN causing ESKD since 1995. In other words, the aggregate epidemiologic data from the CBD study strongly suggest an increase in the burden associated with DM (as compared to that of glomerulonephritis, for instance). Identification of 'hot spots' among and within countries deserves a push for the stratification of efforts, allocation of resources, as well as global health policy decisions.

Along with the rapid growth of the economy and gradual changes in lifestyle, China is facing an ever-increasing burden of CKD. CKD is associated with high morbidity and increased healthcare utilization. Both the medical expenditure and the length of stay of inpatients with CKD are important indicators for healthcare resource utilization. In the CK-NET 2015 annual data report, the total medical expenditure of inpatients with CKD was over 23 billion RMB, accounting for 6.3% of the overall costs in the dataset, while the number of inpatients with CKD accounted for 4.8% of the overall hospitalized population. Hospitalized patients with CKD were also associated with higher medical costs, increased mortality rates, and longer lengths of stay compared with those without CKD.

Conclusion

CKD has become a significant health issue in China, including Hong Kong, and worldwide. The rapid increase in the prevalence of risk factors including DM, HT, and obesity will cause a greater burden of CKD in the future and is likely to have substantial socio-economic and public health consequences at local, regional and, global levels. It is important to apply the appropriate tools in assessing the disease burden in CKD and be cognizant of the pitfalls, as an accurate estimation of the CKD burden is vital to public health policy planning.

15

Chronic Kidney Disease: Clinical Manifestations and Management

Benjamin So, Desmond Yap, and Sing Leung Lui

Introduction

Chronic kidney disease (CKD) is associated with various systemic complications and increased patient mortality. This chapter provides an overview of the causes and natural history of CKD and also highlights the pathophysiology and management of some common and important CKD complications.

Definitions of Chronic Kidney Disease

The Kidney Disease: Improving Global Outcomes (KDIGO) guidelines define CKD as abnormalities of kidney structure or function, present for over three months, with implications for health. CKD is distinguished from acute kidney injury (AKI) primarily by its chronicity. CKD often has different aetiologies, requires different interventions, and is associated with a distinct set of short- and long-term clinical outcomes.

Evidence of kidney damage can be subtle, especially at early stages. For the purposes of diagnosis of CKD, such evidence can manifest as either:

- abnormalities in various markers of kidney damage, such as but not limited to: albuminuria, microscopic haematuria and other abnormalities in the urinary sediment, structural anomalies on imaging (such as evidence of polycystic kidneys), aberrant findings on histology, or evidence of electrolyte or acid–base disorders suggestive of renal tubular disorders;
- persistently decreased glomerular filtration rate (GFR) to less than 60 mL/min/1.73 m^2.

The kidney has a myriad of functions including excretory, endocrine, and metabolic functions. Though measurement of the GFR primarily reflects excretory function, a decline in other kidney functions often parallels the decrease in GFR. Systemic complications of CKD, as well as all-cause mortality and other adverse clinical outcomes, also increase progressively with deteriorating GFR. Accordingly, CKD is classified into five stages based on the estimated GFR (eGFR) (Table 15.1).

Table 15.1: Classification of chronic kidney disease

Stage	GFR (mL/min/1.73 m^2)	Description
1	≥ 90	Kidney damage with normal or ↑GFR
2	60–89	Kidney damage with mild ↓GFR
3a	45–59	Moderate ↓GFR
3b	30–44	
4	15–29	Severe ↓GFR
5	<15 (or requiring dialysis)	Kidney failure

GFR, glomerular filtration rate

Causes of Chronic Kidney Disease

While CKD is associated with a distinct constellation of clinical sequelae, it is not sufficient as a diagnosis in and of itself. Identification of the underlying cause is important for both prognostication and management of CKD. In developed countries, the leading causes of CKD in adults nowadays are diabetes mellitus (DM) and hypertension (HT) (see also

Chapter 14). While this is also the case in Hong Kong, there is also a significant disease burden of chronic glomerulonephritis (GN), such as IgA nephropathy, in East Asia. CKD due to systemic autoimmune diseases (e.g. systemic lupus erythematosus), obstructive uropathy, and cystic kidney disease are also important aetiologies of CKD. In children, unlike in the adult population, congenital anomalies such as renal dysplasia or agenesis, and urological abnormalities such as vesicoureteric reflux are the major causes of CKD (see Chapter 13).

Evaluation of Chronic Kidney Disease

A high index of suspicion is required to identify patients with CKD, especially at earlier stages when renal abnormalities are often clinically silent. There is no evidence to suggest that screening for CKD in otherwise healthy populations alters outcomes meaningfully, but targeted screening for groups at high risk appears to be more worthwhile. In this context, patients with conditions such as DM, HT, rheumatological disease, urological problems, or those requiring chronic use of potentially nephrotoxic drugs such as calcineurin inhibitor (CNI) or non-steroidal anti-inflammatory drugs may benefit from regular screening for the development of CKD.

The current guidelines recommend that CKD be classified according to the cause, GFR, and albuminuria category (CGA). This serves as a useful schema for the evaluation of CKD. When a patient is found to have a low calculated GFR, it is important to follow up by observing the evolution of renal function over time to establish chronicity, and to identify a likely cause. Comprehensive evaluation of history, physical examination, blood tests, examination of the urinary sediment, and radiologic imaging can reveal the cause in many cases of CKD, with renal biopsies reserved for selected cases for definitive diagnosis or prognostication. Objective markers of kidney damage, especially albuminuria, should be assiduously sought for, as this not only affects diagnosis and management but also has prognostic significance.

Natural History and Evolution of Chronic Kidney Disease

CKD tends to be progressive over time, irrespective of the underlying cause. Certain kidney diseases such as diabetic nephropathy, may show a more accelerated disease course during the later stages of CKD and progress rapidly to end-stage kidney disease (ESKD). Glomerulosclerosis, tubular atrophy, and tubulointerstitial fibrosis inevitably ensue in patients with established CKD. These pathological changes are due to a series of secondary maladaptive changes in intra-renal haemodynamics, as well as inflammatory and metabolic factors. Complications of CKD, which will be elaborated in subsequent sections, develop in tandem with this process.

As nephrons become scarred or senescent with acute or chronic injury, the remaining nephrons compensate by increasing blood flow and glomerular hyperfiltration to maintain the same GFR. The elevated intraglomerular pressure increases wall stress and endothelial injury, causing chronic glomerular damage with time. This triggers a complex neurohormonal response, including activation of the renin-angiotensin-aldosterone system (RAAS) and various profibrotic pathways, which contribute to progressive tubulointerstitial fibrosis (see also Chapter 7). Modification of several of these pathways have been shown to attenuate renal injury and fibrosis in animal models, but aside from RAAS blockers, few treatments have been effective in human subjects.

Complications of Chronic Kidney Disease

Complications of CKD can develop in different organ systems as renal function declines. However, significant symptoms generally do not occur until GFR falls to below 15 mL/min/1.73 m^2, when patients begin to develop clinically overt features of the uraemic syndrome. Many patients present for the first time in late-stage disease, when the time window for intervention has elapsed and complications have already become established.

Cardiovascular complications

Cardiovascular disease is the leading cause of death at all stages of CKD. Individuals diagnosed with CKD have a ten- to twentyfold increased risk for cardiovascular death compared to age- and sex-matched controls. CKD is also associated with increased risk for adverse outcomes for patients diagnosed with different cardiovascular conditions, including acute coronary syndrome, valvular disorders, and congestive heart failure. Many patients with CKD may have comorbid conditions such as DM and HT, which further aggravates the risk of cardiovascular disease.

Hypertension and fluid overload

The single most common cardiovascular diagnosis in CKD is HT. HT is both a cause and effect in CKD. Uncontrolled essential or secondary HT can lead to both albuminuria and reduction in GFR with time. Conversely, up to 85% of patients with CKD, regardless of the underlying cause, may have HT. The pathogenesis of HT in CKD is multifactorial; sodium and water retention, and aberrations in neurohormonal pathways all play significant roles in the disease process (see also Chapter 10). Of note, the RAAS and sympathetic nervous systems are often active in CKD and serve as logical targets for blood pressure control. The corollary is that the numerous systemic complications of HT, including stroke and coronary artery disease, are also more prevalent in the CKD population. The patient with CKD is less able to cope with an acute sodium load and is prone to developing fluid overload. However, in the absence of other disorders, such as heart failure, liver cirrhosis, or nephrotic syndrome, significant oedema is uncommon until the patient reaches stage 4 or 5 CKD. In advanced CKD, gross fluid overload can result in peripheral and pulmonary oedema, pleural effusions, and occasionally ascites.

Arterial diseases

Coronary artery disease, cerebrovascular disease, and peripheral vascular disease are all more prevalent in the CKD population. Arterial disease develops via atherosclerosis as well as arteriosclerosis. The former is characterized by deposition of lipid-laden plaques in the arterial intima, especially in the carotid bifurcation, coronary arteries, renal arteries, femoral arteries, and infrarenal aorta, causing progressive arterial occlusion. The latter, arteriosclerosis, is predominantly driven by medial degeneration with distortion of the elastic lamellae and secondary fibrosis, calcification, and hypertrophy of the media and intima, especially in the aorta and central arteries.

The process of atherosclerosis is enhanced in CKD, accelerating exponentially with decreasing GFR. Part of this is attributable to the significant burden of concomitant cardiovascular risk factors including DM, HT, and dyslipidaemia in patients with CKD. Additionally, altered bone mineral metabolism in CKD further compounds the progression of atherosclerosis as well as arteriosclerosis. Arteriosclerosis tends to be far more common in advanced CKD than in the general population and portends a more sinister prognosis than the 'normal' arteriosclerosis that occurs with ageing.

Diseases of the myocardium

Left ventricular hypertrophy (LVH) is frequently present in CKD patients. Contributing factors of LVH in CKD patients include chronic volume overload, anaemia, systemic HT, aortic valve calcification, and activation of multiple neurohormonal and fibrotic pathways. LVH leads to diastolic dysfunction and is aggravated by coexisting ischaemic and valvular heart disease. These pathophysiological changes collectively cause a syndrome known as uraemic cardiomyopathy, which is associated with pulmonary oedema and cardiac arrhythmias. Patients with CKD often tolerate treatments for heart failure more poorly, show a higher propensity for cardiac decompensation, and require renal replacement therapy (RRT) at an earlier stage due to prominent fluid overload symptoms.

Diseases of the heart valves and pericardium

Calcification of the aortic valve and mitral valve parallels the process of vascular calcification throughout the whole body. Pericarditis with pericardial effusion occurs in a small percentage of patients with ESKD, often when RRT is not initiated in a timely manner. Pericardiocentesis yields a sterile, exudative pericardial fluid with lymphocytic infiltrate. Many patients may be relatively asymptomatic until they present with clinical manifestations of cardiac tamponade. Concomitant bleeding tendency may lead to life-threatening haemopericardium in these patients.

Arrhythmias

Atrial fibrillation (AF) affects up to 20% of pre-dialysis CKD patients. Incident AF is associated with an accelerated decline in renal function due to clinically silent renal thromboembolism. Anticoagulation for AF may be complicated with an increased risk of haemorrhage in patients with impaired renal function. Sudden cardiac death is common in the CKD population, especially in the dialysis population. The incidence of sudden cardiac death within the first year of initiating haemodialysis (HD) is around 5–7%. Loop recorder studies show that most episodes are due to bradyarrhythmias and asystole rather than ventricular tachyarrhythmias. As most arrhythmias in patients with advanced CKD tend not to be shockable rhythms, the installation of implanted cardioverter/defibrillators in this high-risk population remains controversial.

Haematologic complications

Anaemia

Anaemia is common in CKD, affecting 20–40% of patients with stage 3 CKD and over 70% of stage 5 patients. Multiple factors contribute to anaemia in CKD patients. Conditions that result in reduced oxygen delivery to peripheral tissues (e.g. anaemia or chronic hypoxaemia) promote stabilization of hypoxia-inducible factor (HIF), which in turn enhances the production of erythropoietin (EPO). The kidney is normally responsible for the production of 90% of EPO in the body. Therefore, decreased EPO production is the key mechanism for renal anaemia and the frequency and severity of anaemia correlate with the reduction in nephron mass. Iron deficiency is another important cause of anaemia in patients with CKD. It is estimated that up to 50% of patients with stage 3 to 5 CKD have iron deficiency, based on the gold standard of bone marrow examination. Iron deficiency in CKD may be either absolute or relative. Absolute iron deficiency occurs in the setting of chronic blood loss (e.g. gastrointestinal bleeding, or blood loss during HD), while relative (functional) iron deficiency is usually due to a supply-demand mismatch in iron stores. Functional iron deficiency is often triggered by the use of erythropoietin-stimulating agents (ESA), as the available store of iron cannot be mobilized fast enough to cope with the accelerated rate of red blood cell production. Furthermore, elevated hepcidin (a crucial regulator of iron homeostasis) in CKD patients can also lead to functional iron deficiency, and thus renal anaemia and resistance to ESA. Vitamin B12 and folic acid deficiencies can occur in ESKD patients as a result of malnutrition and excessive removal by dialysis. Secondary/tertiary hyperparathyroidism exerts negative effects on EPO production and integrity of red blood cells, and in severe cases may cause secondary myelofibrosis and ESA resistance. Microcytic hypochromic anaemia due to aluminium overload is less commonly seen nowadays due to more restricted use of aluminium-containing phosphate binders.

Bleeding tendency

Increased risk of haemorrhage is observed in CKD patients, especially in those with more severe renal impairment. While patients with severe uraemia often have prolonged bleeding time, the results of other quantitative haematological parameters (e.g. platelet count and coagulation profiles) are generally unremarkable. The increased bleeding tendency in uraemic patients is thought to be related to platelet dysfunction as result of dysfunctional glycoprotein IIb/IIIa (a platelet membrane glycoprotein that normally interacts with von Willebrand factor and fibrinogen), leading to impaired platelet aggregation and adhesion. A low haematocrit may also contribute to bleeding tendency in CKD.

Electrolyte and acid–base disturbances

Given the pivotal role of the kidney in the regulation of electrolyte and acid–base status in the body (see Chapter 1), it logically follows that electrolyte and acid–base disturbances ensue in patients with CKD and ESKD. Salient electrolyte and acid–base abnormalities in CKD and ESKD patients include hyperkalaemia, metabolic acidosis, hypocalcaemia, and hyperphosphataemia.

The incidence of hyperkalaemia increases with reducing GFR, owing to impaired regulation by the distal nephron and concomitant metabolic acidosis. Other precipitating factors for hyperkalaemia in CKD patients include the use of RAAS blockers, potassium-sparing diuretics, and CNI. Hyperkalaemia due to hyporeninaemic hypoaldosteronism (type 4 renal tubular acidosis) is common among DM patients, even at earlier stages of CKD.

Metabolic acidosis is also frequently observed in CKD patients as they have compromised capacity for bicarbonate conservation and generation through ammoniagenesis. In earlier stages of CKD, this is compensated for by buffer systems in the extracellular fluid, tissues, and bone. Acidaemia usually develops in later stages of CKD when these systems become overwhelmed progressively. The anion gap may remain normal in CKD until late stages, when anions such as phosphate, sulphate, urate, and hippurate accumulate. Metabolic acidosis can promote protein catabolism and muscle breakdown, and may accelerate CKD progression by induction of tubulointerstitial fibrosis.

Mineral and bone disorder

Changes in bone mineral metabolism in CKD

As GFR declines, regulation of calcium and phosphorus becomes increasingly disturbed as a result of a complex interplay between the various factors that affect bone mineral homeostasis (Figure 15.1). These hormonal factors include vitamin D compounds (such as vitamin D2 and D3, and their 25-hydroxylated

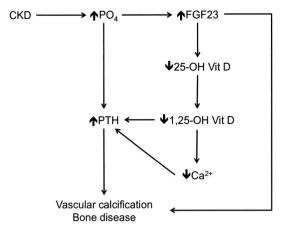

CKD ⟶ ↑PO₄ ⟶ ↑FGF23

↓25-OH Vit D

↑PTH ← ↓1,25-OH Vit D

↓Ca²⁺

Vascular calcification
Bone disease

Figure 15.1: A schematic diagram showing the pathogenesis of chronic kidney disease-mineral bone disease (CKD-MBD)

and 1,25-hydroxylated compounds), parathyroid hormone (PTH) and fibroblast growth factor 23 (FGF23) (see also Chapter 1).

The kidney's ability to excrete a phosphate load decreases as renal function deteriorates, resulting in phosphate retention. Hyperphosphataemia is a key driving event leading to elevated PTH and FGF23 levels. Increased FGF23 diminishes 1α-hydroxylation of 25-hydroxyvitamin D (calcidiol) to 1,25-hydroxy-vitamin D in renal tubules, resulting in reduced intestinal calcium absorption and hypocalcaemia which further promotes PTH secretion. Secondary hyperparathyroidism in CKD is characterized by excessive PTH production and hyperplasia of parathyroid glands in response to hypocalcaemia. As it is a compensatory mechanism to hypocalcaemia and hyperphosphataemia, it does not usually result in hypercalcaemia. With persistent severe secondary hyperparathyroidism, the parathyroid glands may become autonomous (i.e. tertiary hyperparathyroidism) and patients often show both hypercalcaemia and hyperphosphataemia. The skeletal and systemic manifestations of altered mineral metabolism in CKD were previously generalized as 'renal osteodystrophy', but the term 'chronic kidney disease–mineral and bone disorder' (CKD-MBD) is now preferred. 'Renal osteodystrophy' now largely refers to the skeletal pathologies diagnosed from a bone biopsy.

Bone disease in chronic kidney disease

In general, a diagnosis of CKD-MBD is made starting from later stages of CKD, from at least stage 3

onwards, when the clinical behaviour and fracture risk of patients begin to diverge from the healthy general population. The skeletal abnormalities in CKD patients can show distinct or mixed pathologies (mixed uraemic osteodystrophy), which have potential implications for management. Bone biopsy is the gold standard for diagnosing skeletal disease in CKD, but is rarely done in practice due to its invasiveness. Instead, the type of bone disease in CKD patients can often be inferred from various laboratory parameters, including alkaline phosphatase, PTH, vitamin D, and aluminium levels. Some specific tests such as deferoxamine (DFO) test may aid the diagnosis of aluminium-related bone diseases in CKD patients.

Classification of bone histology in renal osteodystrophy now follows a 'turnover, mineralization, volume' (TMV) system as defined by the National Kidney Foundation. Mechanistically, bone turnover refers to the rate of bone remodelling due to osteoclast-mediated bone resorption and osteoblast-mediated bone formation, with the generation of an osteoid, which is an extracellular matrix that needs to be further mineralized. Mineralization is the process by which calcium phosphate crystals are deposited into the matrix; this is governed by osteoblasts but can be limited by other factors like vitamin D deficiency or skeletal resistance to PTH. Finally, bone volume represents the end-result of bone resorption, formation, and mineralization. Impaired bone volume is associated with increased bone fragility and susceptibility for fractures.

Osteitis fibrosa cystica is one of the most classical forms of renal osteodystrophy. This is usually attributable to the skeletal effects of elevated PTH, and is characterized by high bone turnover, with increased osteoclastic activity and excess bone resorption, as well as increased osteoblastic activity leading to more rapid formation of osteoid. A bone biopsy may show marrow fibrosis, woven osteoid with disordered collagen fibres, and increased osteoclasts and osteoblasts. Clinically, patients may suffer from an escalated risk of bone fracture and tendon rupture, as well as anaemia due to secondary myelofibrosis.

Adynamic bone disease (ABD) may occur in CKD patients and is characterized by low bone turnover together with abnormal mineralization. Osteoclast and osteoblast activity are both depressed, and there is also a consequent defect in mineralization. The amount of osteoid is not increased, as osteoblastic activity is low. The most common cause of ABD is excessive suppression of PTH, often related to the use of high doses of vitamin D analogues and calcimimetics. Other important causes of ABD include

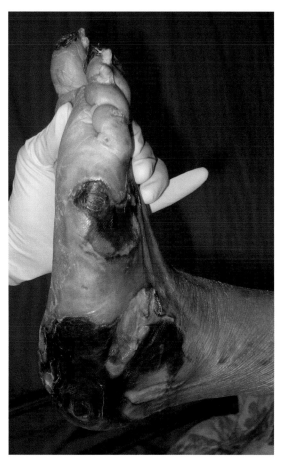

Figure 15.2: Calciphylaxis, which typically presents with a characteristic painful ischaemic ulcer with necrosis

calcification. Current guidelines suggest screening for vascular calcification in patients on dialysis, such as lateral abdominal X-rays to look for calcifications of the abdominal aorta and echocardiogram to identify valvular calcifications.

Calciphylaxis is a form of calcific uraemic arteriolopathy that involves medial calcification of small arteries (including cutaneous arteries). Patients suffering from calciphylaxis typically present with a characteristic painful ischaemic ulcer with necrosis (Figure 15.2). Such necrotic lesions can become foci for bacterial superinfection and are also associated with ischaemic lesions in other organs. As such, calciphylaxis portends a very poor prognosis and is associated with high short-term mortality.

Malnutrition and protein-energy wasting

Appetite and most parameters of nutritional status (such as serum albumin) remain largely preserved until patients reach stage 3b or above CKD. As GFR declines, a series of changes lead to loss of fat and lean muscle mass in many patients, a process denoted as protein-energy wasting syndrome (PEWS). This is different from malnutrition, a condition that is often attributed solely to inadequate dietary intake; while malnutrition also occurs in some patients with CKD, the term PEWS better captures the overall clinical picture, as patients demonstrate wasting, with abnormalities that cannot be corrected simply by increasing the diet.

Many factors contribute to the development of PEWS, including reduced appetite secondary to aberrant hypothalamic regulation of appetite and altered levels of appetite-regulating hormones, gastroparesis, and sometimes even inappropriate dietary advice from healthcare professionals. Hypermetabolism, particularly that due to chronic inflammation, plays an instrumental role in causing PEWS in patients with advanced CKD. CKD patients with intercurrent sepsis, severe cardiovascular disease, and poorly controlled DM frequently show exaggerated protein catabolism and consequent muscle breakdown. Dialysis itself also promotes catabolism; for instance, intermittent HD can trigger the release of various proinflammatory mediators. Disturbances in systemic neurohormonal pathways also play an important role in aggravating PEWS. In this context, insulin resistance blunts the anabolic effects of insulin on skeletal muscle, thereby favouring muscle breakdown. Uraemia, metabolic acidosis, elevated levels of angiotensin II, glucocorticoids, and proinflammatory cytokines can interact with

post-parathyroidectomy and aluminium accumulation. Clinically, these patients may have non-specific bone pain and a very high risk of fracture. They are also prone to hypercalcaemia as the bone fails to act as an effective buffer for calcium.

Osteomalacia is characterized by a mineralization defect with an increased amount of unmineralized osteoid. Historically, most cases of osteomalacia complicating advanced CKD were related to aluminium toxicity. Vitamin D deficiency may also contribute to this clinical entity.

Vascular calcification and other extra-skeletal manifestations

Calcification can affect any organ in the body, with vascular calcification being of particular concern. The pathogenesis of vascular calcification in CKD is complex, but *in vitro* data suggests that vascular smooth muscle cells are induced to differentiate into an osteoblast-like phenotype leading to progressive neurohormonal pathways, resulting in enhanced muscle protein breakdown. Hormonal perturbations such as hyperprolactinaemia with hypogonadism and growth hormone resistance are common in CKD patients, and these endocrine disturbances can retard growth and normal pubertal development in the paediatric CKD population.

Clinically, the presence of PEWS can be inferred from various clinical and laboratory criteria. These include low albumin and cholesterol levels, low body mass index (BMI), unintentional weight loss, reduced fat mass, low lean muscle mass (measured by anthropometric means or inferred from a reduced rate of creatinine appearance in blood tests), and reduced dietary protein intake. A high index of suspicion is required to pick up less overt cases of PEWS, as the syndrome has been tied with adverse outcomes including excess mortality.

Management of Chronic Kidney Disease

Principles of management in chronic kidney disease

The management of CKD can be clinically challenging and should take into consideration the underlying renal disease, severity of CKD and associated complications, other medical comorbidities, and psychosocial issues (Table 15.2). As a general renoprotective measure, all patients with CKD should receive RAAS-blocking agents unless there is an absolute contraindication. Treatments specific to the underlying renal disease should be instituted to limit further attrition of nephrons. For instance, glycaemic control needs to be optimized in patients with DM nephropathy and sodium-glucose cotransporter 2 (SGLT2) inhibitors must be commenced to help reduce adverse renal outcomes. Patients with immune-mediated GN should receive adequate maintenance immunosuppression to prevent disease relapse and consequent renal parenchymal damage. It is important to avoid further renal insults such as hypoperfusion, nephrotoxic agents (e.g. drugs or iodine contrast), and urinary obstruction in CKD patients. Caution should be exercised during drug prescription in CKD individuals, which include the avoidance of nephrotoxic medications and appropriate dosage modification according to the degree of renal impairment. The indication of contrast studies should be carefully reviewed, and if possible, avoided in CKD patients. In CKD patients who require iodine contrast studies, one ought to ensure adequate hydration and the minimum amount of contrast

should be administered. Magnetic resonance imaging with gadolinium contrast can often be a viable alternative to iodine-based contrast. While rare but serious nephrogenic systemic fibrosis has previously been reported with the administration of gadolinium contrast in patients with advanced CKD, the newer gadolinium compounds used nowadays are not associated with such side effect. The focus of care in CKD patients gradually shifts towards the management of CKD complications as renal function declines, which will be discussed in the following sections. Patients approaching ESKD should be prepared for RRT or referred to RPC services in a timely manner.

Management of hypertension and fluid overload

Good hypertensive control is crucial for retardation of renal disease progression and reduction of cardiovascular complications in CKD patients. The optimal treatment targets for HT in CKD remains poorly defined. Historically, many guidelines have referenced a target of 130/80 mmHg for patients with DM or proteinuric kidney disease. RAAS blockers including ACE inhibitors and angiotensin II receptor blockers (ARBs) are considered first-line antihypertensives for most patients with CKD. This is corroborated by trials in certain kidney diseases such as diabetic kidney disease, as well as basic science data that show activation of the RAAS system in CKD. RAAS blockers are also superior to other antihypertensives in reducing proteinuria, a surrogate marker of kidney damage. Very often, CKD patients may require multiple antihypertensive agents to achieve optimal blood pressure control. Fluid overload in CKD should be managed with a combination of a low-sodium diet (ideally, less than 2g of sodium per day) and judicious use of diuretics. High doses of loop diuretics (sometimes in combination with thiazides) may be required in patients with advanced CKD.

Management of electrolyte and acid–base disturbances

Acute severe hyperkalaemia can be life-threatening and thus require urgent medical attention (see also Chapter 4). CKD patients tend to tolerate chronic hyperkalaemia and aggressive treatment may not always be necessary. Management of chronic hyperkalaemia in CKD patients includes dietary restriction of potassium, dosage modification/discontinuation

Table 15.2: A general approach of management for chronic kidney disease

1. Disease-specific treatments for underlying causes of CKD

Examples:
- DKD: Optimization of glycaemic control, RAAS blockade, SGLT2 inhibitors
- Lupus nephritis, ANCA-associated GN, anti-GBM disease: immunosuppressive treatments
- IgAN: RAAS blockade; immunosuppression in selected patients

2. General reno-protective measures for CKD
- Optimization of blood pressure and proteinuria control (RAAS blockers)
- Early identification and treatment of hypoperfusion (e.g. dehydration, septic shock)
- Avoidance and prevention of iodine-contrast nephropathy
- Avoidance of nephrotoxic medications and appropriate dosage modification
- Early detection and treatment of urinary obstruction

3. Management of systemic complications of CKD
- Management of hypertension and fluid overload (RAAS blockers, diuretics)
- Management of electrolyte and acid–base disturbances
- Management of CKD-MBD (e.g. phosphate binders, vitamin D analogues, calcimimetics)
- Management of renal anaemia (e.g. ESA, iron therapy)
- Management of bleeding tendency in patients requiring major surgery or invasive procedures
- Renal nutrition and management of PEWS
- Vaccination as appropriate (e.g. HBV, influenza, pneumococcus, herpes zoster)

4. Preparation for ESKD
- Renal counselling (introduction of different modalities of RRT; assessment of hand–eye coordination, cognitive function, family support and home environment)
- Planning and creation of dialysis access (e.g. PD catheter, AVF, AVG)
- Explore potential live kidney donors

Anti-GBM, anti-glomerular basement membrane; ANCA, anti-nuclear cytoplasmic antibody; AVF, arteriovenous fistula; AVG, arteriovenous graft; CKD, chronic kidney disease; DKD, diabetic kidney disease; ESA, erythropoiesis-stimulating agent; ESKD, end-stage kidney disease; GN, glomerulonephritis; HBV, hepatitis B virus; IgAN, IgA nephropathy; MBD, mineral bone disease; PD, peritoneal dialysis; PEWS, protein–energy wasting syndrome; RAAS, renin angiotensin aldosterone system; RRT, renal replacement therapy; SGLT2, sodium glucose transporter 2

of RAAS blockers, correction of metabolic acidosis, loop or thiazide diuretics (especially in the presence of fluid overload), and the use of potassium-binding resins. Side effects of long-term prescription of binding resins include colonic necrosis and perforation. Novel potassium-binding resins such as patiromer acetate and sodium zirconium cyclosilicate appear to be efficacious and safe for chronic hyperkalaemia.

Mild to moderate metabolic acidosis can be corrected by administration of oral sodium bicarbonate, but patients with severe metabolic acidosis generally require intravenous sodium bicarbonate. Rapid correction of metabolic acidosis by sodium bicarbonate may be complicated by fluid overload, hypernatraemia, and rarely paradoxical CNS acidosis. Refractory or recurrent hyperkalaemia and severe metabolic acidosis are indications for initiation of dialysis. The management of hypocalcaemia and hyperphosphataemia will be elaborated on in the following section.

Management of mineral and bone disorder

Management of hypocalcaemia

Mild hypocalcaemia in CKD is often of little clinical consequence and may not warrant aggressive treatment. For patients with severe hypocalcaemia (e.g. adjusted calcium < 2.0 mmol/L), intravenous calcium gluconate/chloride may be indicated in the acute setting, especially in the presence of a related arrhythmia or neuromuscular instability. Concomitant severe hypocalcaemia must be normalized before one attempt to correct metabolic acidosis in CKD patients. For patients with chronic hypocalcaemia, oral treatments should be initiated to prevent excessive stimulation of PTH and other complications of hypocalcaemia. The amount of calcium supplementation should be limited as long-term excessive calcium loading is associated with increased vascular calcification. CKD patients with relative vitamin D deficiency should also receive active vitamin D, calcitriol, or other vitamin D analogues. In patients already receiving HD or peritoneal dialysis (PD), chronic hypocalcaemia can also be corrected accordingly by adjusting the calcium content in the respective dialysates.

Management of hyperphosphataemia

While restricting intake of phosphorus-rich foods is important for the management of hyperphosphataemia, this is often impractical because phosphorus is present in high quantities in most protein-rich foods and overzealous dietary discretion can put patients at risk of malnutrition. In this context, phosphate binders are often required in CKD patients. Calcium-based compounds are the most commonly prescribed phosphate binders, and have the advantages of established efficacy, safety, and low cost. Other common phosphate binders include sevelamer, aluminium-containing compounds, and lanthanum carbonate (Table 15.3). Although adequate dialysis can improve phosphate control, most ESKD patients still require phosphate binders to achieve the target phosphate levels.

Management of renal osteodystrophy and hyperparathyroidism

Management of patients with high turnover bone disease should focus on the treatment of hyperparathyroidism. Treatment of hyperparathyroidism not only ameliorates bone disease but also reduce cardiovascular sequela. Activated vitamin D (calcitriol) or vitamin D analogues such as alfacalcidol and paricalcitol can bind directly to vitamin D receptors in the parathyroid gland to suppress PTH secretion. Supra-physiological doses of calcitriol or vitamin D analogues are often required for cases with severe hyperparathyroidism. Calcimimetics (e.g. cinacalcet and etelcalcetide) bind to the calcium-sensing receptor (CaSR) and act to downregulate PTH secretion. Calcimimetics are particularly useful in patients with severe hyperparathyroidism and hypercalcaemia as these drugs can decrease both calcium and phosphate levels. Parathyroidectomy is the definitive treatment for severe hyperparathyroidism, especially in patients who are refractory to medical therapy. Re-implantation of one parathyroid gland in the forearm or thigh is frequently performed to prevent ABD. Hungry bone syndrome may occur in the early post-operative period after parathyroidectomy, in which blood calcium levels can drop precipitously due to shifting into the bones with the abrupt reduction in PTH levels.

For patients with ABD, the treatment approach is to stimulate PTH secretion or remove factors that overtly suppress PTH or precipitate ABD. Such approaches include the use of low-calcium dialysate

Table 15.3: Common phosphate binders and their advantages and disadvantages

Drug	Advantages	Disadvantages/side effects
Aluminium-containing compounds		
Aluminium hydroxide	• Low cost • Highly effective	• Anaemia • Osteomalacia • Encephalopathy ('dialysis dementia')
Calcium-containing compounds		
Calcium carbonate/acetate	• Low cost • Established efficacy and safety	• Vascular calcification • Constipation
Sevelamer		
Sevelamer carbonate	• May improve lipid profile • Does not cause metabolic acidosis	• Constipation/intestinal obstruction • More expensive than calcium- or aluminium-based compounds • Less efficacious than calcium- or aluminium-based compounds
Sevelamer hydrochloride	• May improve lipid profile	• Theoretical risk of metabolic acidosis
Lanthanum carbonate	• Highly effective	• Gastrointestinal upset • High treatment cost
Magnesium-based compounds	• Less clinical experience	• Diarrhoea
Ferric citrate	• May act as iron supplement, especially in those with iron deficiency	• Constipation • Iron overload

to stimulate PTH production in ESKD patients, discontinuation of vitamin D analogues/calcimimetics or aluminium-containing medications, and DFO chelation therapy in patients with aluminium toxicity. For patients with osteomalacia, the treatment objective is to manage the underlying causes such as aluminium accumulation or vitamin D deficiency.

Management of anaemia

Correction of anaemia in CKD patients can alleviate anaemic symptoms and mitigate cardiovascular complications. Nonetheless, previous studies have also demonstrated that overcorrection of haemoglobin levels in CKD patients is associated with a higher risk of death, and of cardiac and cerebrovascular events. In CKD patients with anaemia, iron deficiency should be excluded and repleted. Oral iron supplements can be used to treat iron deficiency, but constipation is a common side effect, leading to poor compliance. Intravenous iron should be considered in patients with low transferrin receptor saturation, but this treatment is associated with a risk of anaphylactoid reaction and precipitation of ferrophilic bacterial infection. The use of erythropoiesis-stimulating agents (ESA) is an established therapy for renal anaemia and can significantly reduce the need for blood transfusion and its related complications. Nowadays, most patients receive long-acting ESA (e.g. darbepoetin or continuous erythropoietin receptor activators). Common side effects include elevation of blood pressure (particularly diastolic blood pressure), increased risk of stroke, and, rarely, pure red cell aplasia due to anti-EPO antibodies. Oral hypoxia-inducible factor prolyl hydroxylase inhibitors (HIF-PHI) are novel treatments for renal anaemia and the current data suggests that these agents show efficacy comparable to ESA. Oral HIF-PHI are generally well-tolerated and one important advantage over ESA is the avoidance of injection.

Management of bleeding tendency in patients requiring major surgery or invasive procedures

Bleeding diathesis needs to be corrected in CKD patients who require major surgery or invasive procedures. The bleeding tendency caused by severe uraemia can be improved by dialysis. Desmopressin (DDAVP) increases the release of factor VIII: von Willebrand factor multimers from the vascular endothelium and thus improves platelet dysfunction. DDAVP is generally safe but potential side effects include hyponatraemia, reduced urine volume, and precipitation of thrombotic events (especially in patients with a history of severe arterial or venous thrombosis). Other therapeutic options for uraemic bleeding tendency include transfusion of cryoprecipitate and conjugated oestrogens.

Renal nutrition and management of protein-energy wasting syndrome

Excessive nutrition in patients with CKD can lead to sodium and volume overload, accumulation of phosphate and uraemic toxins, glomerular hyperfiltration, and increased intraglomerular pressure, which perpetuates renal damage. Some previous studies have advocated low protein diets (0.6–0.8 g/kg/day of protein, or even lower) or ketoacid-amino acid supplements to retard CKD progression. While there is some limited evidence suggesting the role of dietary modifications in preventing the progression of CKD, the small benefits of dietary restrictions must be balanced against the significant risks of undernutrition. Patients receiving intermittent HD and PD have distinct nutritional requirements. PD patients tend to require more protein but less caloric intake, whereas patients on intermittent HD need more stringent restrictions on salts (especially sodium and potassium) and fluids. In patients with PEWS, preservation and restoration of muscle mass must take precedence as the most important treatment goal. Concurrent comorbidities that contribute to catabolism, including systemic inflammation, metabolic acidosis, and insulin resistance need to be addressed. Nutritional supplementation should then be instituted, with the oral/enteral route more preferred to parenteral nutrition. In HD patients with poor response to oral nutritional supplements, intradialytic parenteral nutrition may be considered. Amino-acid-containing PD solutions may also be a viable option to improve nutrition in PD patients.

Historically, poor appetite has been viewed as a part of the uraemic syndrome, and initiation or intensification of dialysis has been proposed as part of the treatment for this condition. There is a ceiling effect; beyond conventionally accepted minimum requirements for 'dialysis adequacy', additional dosing of dialysis does not improve nutritional status. There has also been some success in the use of exogenous hormones such as anabolic steroids or megestrol acetate to treat PEWS. These interventions need to be used in tandem with intensive physical training and nutritional supplementation to be truly effective.

Preparation for renal replacement therapy

Clinicians should prepare patients well for RRT as they approach stage 5 CKD. The decision regarding whether a patient should receive RRT, as well as the timing and modality, is influenced by medical, socio-economic, and psychological factors. 'Renal counselling' is usually arranged for the patient and their family prior to their decision to undergo RRT. During the counselling, a specialist renal nurse and/or nephrologist will introduce to the patient and their family the various options of RRT and assess their suitability for each modality of dialysis.

Patients who have committed to chronic dialysis should be referred early to surgeons for the creation of dialysis access (e.g. Tenckhoff catheter or arteriovenous fistulas). Any potential live kidney donor should be explored, so as to facilitate pre-emptive or early transplantation after the commencement of dialysis. Patients who are deemed unsuitable for dialysis or kidney transplantation should be referred early to renal palliative care services (see Chapter 22). The timing of initiation of chronic dialysis should take into consideration medical indications, the trajectory of renal function decline, and psychosocial factors. In general, dialysis should be commenced in patients who develop uraemic symptoms (e.g. nausea, loss of appetite) or complications (e.g. encephalopathy or pericardial diseases), fluid overload, refractory hyperkalaemia, and severe metabolic acidosis. Clinicians should be cognizant that many of the symptoms in advanced uraemia may be non-specific, and timely initiation of dialysis in these instances can potentially alleviate the symptoms and prevent severe uraemic complications.

16

Peritoneal Dialysis: Principles and Practice

Terence Yip, Ping Nam Wong, Wai Ling Chu, and Cheuk Chun Szeto

Introduction

Peritoneal dialysis (PD) is one of the modalities of renal replacement therapy (RRT). It replaces some of the functions performed by the healthy kidneys in patients suffering from end-stage renal disease (ESRD). PD removes solutes and water accumulated in the body into the dialysis solution (dialysate) infused into the peritoneal cavity. The acid–base and electrolyte status are also corrected and maintained during the process of PD.

Solute Transport

The average surface area of the peritoneal membrane is around 1.7–2.1 m² in adults. During PD, it is mainly the parietal peritoneum that participates in peritoneal transport. The peritoneal membrane functions as a semi-permeable membrane, which is composed of three layers: the mesothelium, the interstitium, and the capillary endothelium. The capillary endothelium is the most important barrier between the dialysate and the capillary blood. According to the three-pore model of solute transport, the capillary endothelium contains three different-sized pores (large, small, and ultra-small), restricting solute transport. The ultra-small pore, also called aquaporin-1, is permeable only to water.

Solute transport across the peritoneum occurs via diffusion and convection. Diffusion varies directly with the magnitude of the concentration gradient, and inversely with the size of the solute. Convection or solvent drag refers to solute transport that occurs with water transport, a process mediated by the frictional forces between water and solute. The transport of small solutes (e.g., urea, potassium, creatinine) across the peritoneum primarily occurs by diffusion. The rate of diffusion depends upon the concentration gradient, the peritoneal surface area, and peritoneal permeability. Peritoneal transport of large molecules (e.g., vitamin B12, beta-2-microglobulin) occurs at a much slower rate. Both peritoneal permeability and the surface area of the peritoneal membrane influence the transfer of large solutes. The transport of these solutes out of the peritoneal cavity primarily occurs via the subdiaphragmatic and peritoneal lymphatics. This process is independent of molecular size.

The weekly Kt/V_{urea} is commonly used to measure solute clearance by PD. The daily peritoneal urea clearance (Kt) is the product of the total 24-hour peritoneal drain volume and the ratio of the urea concentration in the pooled drained dialysate to that in the plasma (D/P urea). The volume of distribution of urea (V_{urea}) approximately equals that of body water (60% of ideal body weight in kg in men; 55% of ideal body weight in kg in women). Total solute clearance equals the peritoneal Kt/V_{urea} plus the 24-hour urea clearance by the kidney (residual renal function). Residual renal function is predictive of survival in PD patients.

Water Removal

Water moves between the peritoneal capillary blood and peritoneal dialysate fluid via aquaporin-1 water channels and small pores. Net water removal (ultrafiltration or UF) equals water removed by osmosis minus water absorbed into the body. Glucose is the most commonly used osmotic agent in peritoneal dialysate. Glucose is an effective osmotic agent with a predictable UF profile. It has a high osmotic driving force at relatively low concentrations, and a large UF volume per unit mass absorbed.

The net transcapillary UF rate is maximal at the beginning of the dialysate exchange when the glucose concentration gradient is maximum. The concentration gradient then decreases by a combination of glucose absorption and dilution by the ultrafiltrate. The UF volume peaks at around two to three hours after an exchange of dialysate. The rate of lymphatic absorption is independent of osmosis and is more or less constant, at around 50–100 ml/hour. When the transcapillary UF rate falls below that of lymphatic absorption, negative UF will occur. PD solutions are available with variable amounts of glucose (1.5%, 2.5% and 4.25%). UF typically increases with higher concentrations of peritoneal dialysate glucose.

Peritoneal Equilibration Test

The peritoneal equilibration test (PET) is commonly used in clinical practice to assess transperitoneal transfer. In this test, 2 litres of 2.5% dextrose dialysate is instilled into the peritoneal cavity. After an equilibration time of four hours, the dialysate-to-plasma concentration ratio (D/P) of creatinine and the dialysate glucose-to-baseline dialysate glucose concentration ratio (D/D0) are measured. There is a reverse correlation between D/P creatinine and D/D0 glucose. Peritoneal transport characteristics are defined according to D/P creatinine at four hours: > 0.81 is high; > 0.65–0.81 is high-average; > 0.5–0.65 is low-average; and < 0.5 is low transporters (Figure 16.1). Patients with high peritoneal equilibration rates (high transporters) have lower UF during a four-hour dwell. In these patients, peak UF occurs early during an exchange due to rapid dissipation of osmotic gradient with continuous lymphatic fluid reabsorption. These patients, therefore, tend to have adequate peritoneal Kt/V_{urea} but are prone to fluid overload due to negative UF. In patients with low equilibration rates, peak UF occurs late in the exchange. UF continues over four hours of dwell. Low transporters remove fluid easily but may have difficulty in removing solute. Peritoneal Kt/Vurea may be low. Patients with solute equilibration rates between these two extremes have intermediate patterns (high-average and low-average transporters). The PET can assist in the management of patients with poor UF and guide dialysis prescription.

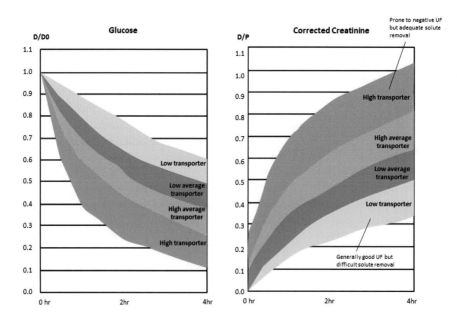

Figure 16.1: Peritoneal transport status according to peritoneal equilibration test (PET) results (adapted from Twardowski ZJ et al. Peritoneal equilibration test. Perit Dial Bull 1987; 7: 138–147)
D, dialysate concentration at 4 hours; D0, dialysis concentration at baseline; P, plasma concentration
High transporter: D/PCr above 0.81
High-average transporter: D/P Cr 0.65–0.81
Low-average transporter: D/PCr 0.5–0.65
Low transporter: D/PCr Cr 0.34–0.5

Constituents and Bag Design of Peritoneal Dialysis Solution

The typical constituents of PD solution are shown in Table 16.1. Glucose, present in different concentrations, is commonly used as the osmotic agent to achieve UF in PD. Icodextrin (a large glucose polymer with an osmolarity similar to that of plasma) can be used as an alternative osmotic agent in PD solutions. Icodextrin-based solutions pursue UF in PD patients using colloid osmosis. The absorption of icodextrin by the peritoneum is very limited as it only takes place by convection via the lymphatics. Icodextrin produces more UF during the long dwell than conventional glucose-based solutions, which is especially helpful to high transporters who require long dwell cycles. PD solutions also contain lactate which will be converted into bicarbonate by the liver after absorption to correct acidosis. The absence of potassium in PD solution facilitates the removal of potassium from the blood, and PD solutions with different calcium contents can be used in patients with different medical conditions. For instance, PD solutions with lower calcium concentrations are available for patients with high blood calcium level due to secondary hyperparathyroidism.

Bicarbonate-containing PD solutions are now available in the form of a two-bag system. Bicarbonate cannot be used as the buffer in the single-bag system because it reacts with the calcium in the dialysate and forms calcium carbonate precipitates. Before the dialysis exchange procedure in the two-bag system, the patient breaks a frangible

connection that separates the two compartments. The PD solution is then ready for use after mixing.

Peritoneal Access

The success of PD as RRT depends upon a safe, functional, and durable catheter access to the peritoneal cavity provided in a timely fashion. The most widely used catheter for PD patients is the Tenckhoff catheter. This catheter is made of silicone rubber and has two cuffs made of Dacron. The Dacron cuff permits profuse collagen tissue ingrowth between the fibres, providing strong bondage between the cuff and the surrounding tissue. The Dacron cuffs minimize dialysate leakage and act as barriers against the entry of bacteria into the peritoneum.

The PD catheter is functionally recognized as having three segments:

1. The intraperitoneal segment with multiple side holes
2. The intramural segment consisting of two Dacron cuffs
3. The outer segment positioned outside the skin for easy connection for dialysate delivery

The technique for catheter implantation varies from centre to centre and is greatly influenced by local surgical practices. The four main PD catheter implantation approaches are:

1. Percutaneous needle-guidewire technique
2. Open surgical dissection
3. Peritoneoscopic procedure
4. Surgical laparoscopy

Dialysis Procedure and Types of Peritoneal Dialysis

During PD, dialysate is infused into the peritoneal cavity through a PD catheter. After a variable dwell period, the dialysate is drained. The main types of PD regimens are shown in Figure 16.2.

Continuous peritoneal dialysis regimens

The term 'continuous' means PD treatment is given 24 hours a day, seven days a week, with no interruption.

Continuous ambulatory peritoneal dialysis

Continuous ambulatory peritoneal dialysis (CAPD) is the most commonly adopted regimen. The procedure can be performed manually in any place that is

Table 16.1: Constituents of conventional peritoneal dialysis solution

Common constituents	Common values in PD dialysate
Sodium	132 mmol/L
Chloride	96 mmol/L
Potassium	0 mmol/L
Calcium	1.25 or 1.75 mmol/L
Magnesium	0.25 mmol/L
Lactate	40 mmol/L
Dextrose*	Usually different concentrates available (1.5%, 2.5%, 4.25%)
pH	5.3

*Some PD dialysate may contain icodextrin (7.5%) or amino acids (1.1%) instead of dextrose
PD, peritoneal dialysis

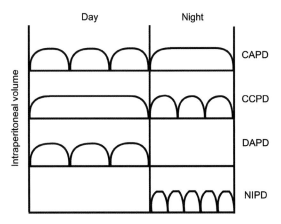

Figure 16.2: Schematic diagram showing the different regimens of peritoneal dialysis
CAPD, continuous ambulatory peritoneal dialysis; CCPD, continuous cyclical peritoneal dialysis; DAPD, daytime ambulatory peritoneal dialysis; NIPD, nocturnal intermittent peritoneal dialysis

clean and well lit. In standard CAPD, 2-litre volume is used per exchange and patients usually perform three to four exchanges every day. Drainage of the previous bag of dialysate is immediately followed by the instillation of a new bag. The overnight exchange time is usually eight to ten hours. The amount of fluid absorbed during this long overnight exchange can be significant, especially in high transporters. In that case, the use of higher glucose concentration dialysate or icodextrin-based dialysate should be considered.

Continuous cyclic peritoneal dialysis

In continuous cyclic peritoneal dialysis (CCPD), a PD machine (cycler) is used to perform exchanges at night while the patient is sleeping. The usual volume is 2–2.5 litres per exchange, three to five exchanges over eight to ten hours at night. After the instillation of the last bag in the morning, the cycler is disconnected from the patient. The dialysate dwells for 14–16 hours and is drained at the beginning of the next nightly CCPD treatment. The amount of fluid absorbed during this long day-dwell can be significant.

Intermittent peritoneal dialysis regimens

The term 'intermittent' means periodic treatment interspersed with periods with no treatment. Intermittent regimens are suitable for patients with significant residual renal function.

Daytime ambulatory peritoneal dialysis

Dialysis treatment is given during the day for 12–16 hours when the patient is ambulatory. Dialysate is drained before going to bed. This regimen avoids fluid absorption during the long overnight dwell. The regimen is suitable for patients who are high transporters with significant residual renal function.

Nocturnal intermittent peritoneal dialysis

Dialysis treatment is given with the help of a cycler every night while the patient sleeps, lasting for eight to ten hours. Dialysate is drained after the last cycle in the morning. The peritoneal cavity is left empty during the daytime. This offers better dialysis acceptability for workers and school students because of the reduced intra-abdominal pressures during the daytime.

Intermittent peritoneal dialysis

Dialysis treatment is given over 20–24 hours with the help of a cycler, twice a week. Between treatments, the peritoneal cavity is kept empty. This regimen serves as a temporary measure before home dialysis training. Intermittent peritoneal dialysis (IPD) is also useful for the management of patients with acute kidney injury who are unsuitable for haemodialysis (HD) or haemofiltration, or CAPD patients with inguinal hernias or retroperitoneal leakage, or those in severe fluid overload.

Automated peritoneal dialysis

Nocturnal intermittent peritoneal dialysis (NIPD) and CCPD are collectively called automated PD (APD). The benefits of APD over CAPD include fewer connections, reduced fill volumes, and exchange procedure-free during the daytime. APD therefore has lifestyle advantages when compared with CAPD. APD is especially suitable for schoolchildren, patients in full-time employment where daytime CAPD exchanges can be a disruption, and elderly people requiring caregivers to perform the exchange procedures. Recently, some new cyclers have chips to record information on each treatment such as treatment time, number, and volume of each cycle. Dialysis units can download these data to review the details of the dialysis treatment process. This is also useful to monitor patients' compliance with treatment. The latest automated PD system is integrated with a web-based connectivity platform. Healthcare providers can have improved access to monitor their patients' home PD treatment and adjust PD prescriptions remotely as necessary. These cyclers may enhance adherence with proper connection procedures and very likely, make the training of the patient easier.

Complications of Peritoneal Dialysis

Peritonitis

Peritonitis is a serious complication of PD. It may lead to structural and functional damages of the peritoneal membrane, resulting in membrane failure. Peritonitis is a major cause of technique failure. Micro-organisms may enter the peritoneal cavity by the following routes:

1. Intra-catheter, e.g., after contamination during the exchange procedure
2. Peri-catheter, especially in the presence of exit-site infection and tunnel infection
3. Transmural, through the gut wall
4. Haematogenous
5. Ascending from the female genital tract

Patients with peritonitis usually present with cloudy PD effluent, with or without abdominal pain. On physical examination, abdominal tenderness is usually generalized. Localized pain or tenderness should raise the suspicion of underlying surgical pathologies, e.g., appendicitis, cholecystitis. The exit site and catheter tunnel should be examined for signs of infection.

When peritonitis is suspected, PD effluent should be sent for cell count with differential, Gram stain, and culture by using the blood culture bottle. Recommended by the International Society for Peritoneal Dialysis (ISPD), peritonitis can be diagnosed when two out of the following three criteria are present:

1. Abdominal pain or cloudy effluent
2. Dialysis effluent white cell count > 100/μL (after a dwell time of at least two hours), with > 50% polymorphonuclear cells
3. Positive dialysis effluent culture

After obtaining microbiological specimens, one to two rapid exchanges are often performed for pain relief. Analgesics may also be required. Empirical antibiotics therapy should then be initiated as soon as possible. Empirical antibiotics regimens should cover both gram-positive and gram-negative organisms. Gram-positive organisms are usually covered by a first-generation cephalosporin or vancomycin; gram-negative organisms by an aminoglycoside or a third-generation cephalosporin. Intraperitoneal (IP) is the preferred route of administration of antibiotics unless the patient shows features of systemic sepsis. IP dosing results in higher IP drug levels. Moreover, it avoids venepuncture and can be administered by the patient at home after training. Subsequent antibiotic regimens will be adjusted according to the culture results. IP antibiotics can be given as continuous or intermittent dosing. In intermittent dosing, the antibiotic-containing dialysis solution must be allowed to dwell for at least six hours to allow adequate absorption. The ISPD recommended dosages of antibiotics for the treatment of PD-related peritonitis are summarized in Table 16.2.

Patients with cloudy effluent may benefit from the addition of IP heparin to prevent occlusion of the catheter by fibrin. Peritoneal permeability to water and glucose typically increases during peritonitis, resulting in a reduction in UF and fluid overload. Temporary use of hypertonic or icodextrin-containing dialysate may be needed to achieve adequate fluid removal. Protein loss during peritonitis is also increased, and malnutrition often occurs during and after peritonitis.

The duration of antibiotic treatment is usually 14–21 days, depending on the culture results and clinical response. Patients who show poor clinical response to IP antibiotics should have their PD-catheters removed and be put on temporary HD. Re-insertion of a new PD catheter may be attempted after peritonitis resolution. After severe episodes of peritonitis, around 50% of patients could return to PD.

Patients with peritonitis due to multiple enteric organisms should be evaluated for underlying intra-abdominal pathologies when there is no prompt clinical response. They should be treated with IP antibiotics that cover anaerobes (e.g., metronidazole), in conjunction with antibiotics that cover aerobic enteric organisms. Most patients with tuberculous peritonitis can be managed with antituberculous treatments without the need for catheter removal. The initial antimicrobial regimen generally comprises rifampicin, isoniazid, pyrazinamide, and a quinolone. In general, pyrazinamide and the quinolone could be stopped after two months, while rifampicin and isoniazid should be continued for a total of 12–18 months. Pyridoxine (50–100 mg per day) should be given to avoid isoniazid-induced neurotoxicity. For fungal peritonitis, the PD catheter should be removed as soon as possible, and an appropriate antifungal agent should be given for at least two weeks.

Table 16.2: Recommended dosing of some common intraperitoneal antimicrobials for the treatment of PD-related peritonitis

	Intermittent regimen (1 exchange/day)	Continuous regimen (all exchanges)
Penicillins		
Penicillin G	No data	LD 50,000 units/L, MD 25,000 units/L
Cloxacillin	No data	LD 500 mg/L, MD 125 mg/L
Ampicillin	No data	LD 500 mg/L, MD 125 mg/L
Ampicillin/Sulbactam	2 g/1 g every 12 hrs	LD 750–1000 mg/L, MD 100 mg/L
Piperacillin/Tazobactam	No data	LD 4 g/0.5 g, MD 1 g/0.125 g
Aminoglycosides		
Amikacin	2 mg/kg/bag	LD 25 mg/L, MD 12 mg/L
Gentamicin	0.6 mg/kg/bag	LD 8 mg/L, MD 4 mg/L
Tobramycin	0.6 mg/kg/bag	LD 3 mg/kg, MD 0.3 mg/kg
Cephalosporins and carbapenems		
Cefazolin	15–20 mg/kg/bag	LD 500 mg/L, MD 125 mg/L
Cefepime	1000 mg/bag	LD 250–500 mg/L, MD 100–125 mg/L
Ceftazidime	1000–1500 mg/bag	LD 500 mg/L, MD 125 mg/L
Imipenem	No data	LD 500 mg/L, MD 200 mg/L
Meropenem	1 g daily*	LD 500 mg/L, MD 200mg/L
Quinolones		
Ciprofloxacin	No data	LD 50 mg/L, MD 25 mg/L
Ofloxacin	No data	LD 200 mg, MD 25 mg/L
Others		
Vancomycin	15–30 mg/kg every 5–7 days	LD 30 mg/kg, MD 1.5 mg/kg/bag
Clindamycin	No data	LD 600 mg/bag, MD 150 mg/L
Daptomycin	No data	LD 100 mg/L, MD 20 mg/L
Teicoplanin	15 mg/kg every 5 days	LD 400 mg/bag, MD 20 mg/bag
Antifungals		
Fluconazole	IP 200 mg every 24–48 hrs	No data
Voriconazole	IP 2.5 mg/kg daily	No data

LD, loading dose; MD, maintenance dose; IP, intraperitoneal; APD, automated peritoneal dialysis; PD, peritoneal dialysis
*Supplemental doses may be needed for APD patients
(Modified from ISPD Peritonitis Recommendations 2016: https://journals.sagepub.com/doi/pdf/10.3747/pdi.2016.00078)

The following strategies may help prevent PD-related peritonitis:

1. Systemic prophylactic antibiotics for catheter insertion
2. The use of 'flush before fill' disconnect PD system
3. Meticulous PD training for patients and carers
4. Application of prophylactic antibiotic cream or ointment to the catheter exit site
5. Prompt treatment of exit-site and tunnel infection
6. Antibiotics prophylaxis prior to colonoscopy and invasive gynaecological procedures
7. Anti-fungal prophylaxis when patients receive antibiotics courses to prevent fungal peritonitis
8. Prophylactic antibiotics after wet contamination

Exit-site and tunnel infections

Exit-site infections (ESIs) and tunnel infections are the major predisposing factors for PD-related peritonitis. ESI is defined as the presence of purulent discharge, without or without erythema of the skin at the catheter-epidermal interface. A positive culture with a normal-appearing exit site is indicative of colonization rather than infection. The spectrum of severity of ESI can range from increased crust formation, to erythema around the exit site, to purulent discharge, to abscess formation. Tunnel infection is defined as the presence of clinical inflammation or ultrasonographic evidence of collection along the catheter tunnel. A tunnel infection may present as erythema, oedema, induration, or tenderness over the subcutaneous pathway but is often clinically occult. Clinical examination involves gross inspection of the exit site, palpation of the tunnel tract, and expression of discharge from the exit site. The discharge should be sent for Gram smear and culture.

ESI and tunnel infections may be caused by a variety of micro-organisms. The most common and serious ESI pathogens are *Staphylococcus aureus* and *Pseudomonas aeruginosa*. Other micro-organisms such as *coagulase negative staphylococcal* species, *Streptococcal* species, *Burkholderia* species, atypical mycobacteria, and fungi can also be involved.

Patients with ESI should be treated with effective antibiotics for at least two weeks. ESI caused by *Pseudomonas* species and tunnel infection should be treated for at least three weeks. Catheter removal should be considered when ESI fails to respond to a three-week course of effective antibiotics. Other interventions that may be considered for persistent ESI include cuff-shaving, un-roofing with or without *en bloc* resection of the skin and tissue around the external cuff, partial catheter re-implantation, catheter diversion with exit-site renewal, and simultaneous removal and re-insertion of the PD catheter. The following strategies may help prevent ESI:

1. A prophylactic antibiotic administered immediately before catheter insertion
2. Keeping the exit site dry post-operatively until it is well healed
3. Good hand hygiene practice during routine handling of the PD catheter and its exit site
4. Daily cleansing of the exit site with antiseptic agents and topical application of an antibiotic cream or ointment
5. Eradication of nasal carriage of *Staphylococcus aureus* by topical mupirocin

Inadequate ultrafiltration

Inadequate UF may lead to hypervolaemia in PD patients. It is a significant cause of technique failure for PD. Inadequate UF may be caused by catheter flow dysfunction or by peritoneal membrane failure. The most common cause of catheter flow dysfunction is constipation. The distended rectosigmoid colon may block the catheter side holes or displace the catheter tip into a position of poor drainage function. Extrinsic bladder compression on the catheter due to urinary retention may also cause catheter flow dysfunction. Mechanical kinking of the catheter tubing or an intra-luminal fibrin clot is usually accompanied by two-way obstruction. Flow failure can also be due to either catheter-tip migration or obstruction by adherent intraperitoneal tissues, such as the omentum. Both conditions may have the radiologic appearance of a catheter tip displaced from the pelvis, while the latter can also occur with the normal pelvic position. Inadequate UF can also be caused by peritoneal membrane failure. In this context, UF failure is defined as the failure to achieve at least 400 ml of net UF during a four-hour dwell using 4.25% glucose dialysate. There are three types of UF failure:

1. Type 1: There is very rapid membrane solute transport, resulting in rapid equilibration and dissipation of the osmotic gradient. Type 1 is the most common type of UF failure and maybe transient during an episode of peritonitis.

2. Type 2: There is a decrease in aquaporin function, resulting in an isolated decrease in water transport. Solute transport is not affected.
3. Type 3: There is a loss of effective peritoneal membrane surface area due to sclerosis or adhesion. Both solute and water transports are decreased.

Type 1 UF failure patients with volume overload are treated with short dwells and the use of icodextrin for long dwells. In addition, they may benefit from being switched to APD where the cycler performs short-dwell exchanges during the sleeping period. Type 2 UF failure patients with volume overload may benefit from resting the peritoneum, to allow aquaporin function to be regained. Patients may benefit from being switched to temporary HD. Type 3 UF failure patients are more difficult to treat, and frequently necessitate the use of high glucose concentration dialysate and icodextrin. These patients often need to change to HD or combined PD and HD therapy to achieve adequate fluid and solute removal. Occasionally, inadequate UF may be caused by an increase in the rate of lymphatic absorption of fluid in the peritoneal cavity. The peritoneal membrane function is intact in this case.

Encapsulating peritoneal sclerosis

Encapsulating peritoneal sclerosis (EPS) is a rare complication of PD that is characterized by inflammation and fibrosis of the peritoneum, leading to the encasement of bowel loops. The two major risk factors for EPS are the duration of time on PD (generally more than five years), and severe recurrent peritonitis. The use of high glucose concentration or bio-incompatible dialysate may also be predisposing factors. EPS is a slowly progressive disorder. The early symptoms are non-specific which include nausea, anorexia, diarrhoea, and intermittent abdominal pain. Late symptoms resulting from the encapsulation of the bowel include severe abdominal pain, constipation, and vomiting. A computed tomography scan may reveal peritoneal calcification, bowel thickening, bowel tethering, and dilatation. There is no radiographic feature that is diagnostic in patients with EPS, however. Nutritional support, often by parenteral nutrition, is crucial in managing patients with EPS. Treatment with tamoxifen and corticosteroids may be beneficial, and surgical interventions may be considered in patients refractory to medical treatment at specialized centres. Mortality associated with

EPS remains very high. Minimizing dialysate glucose exposure, the use of neutral-pH, low-glucose degradation product dialysate, and preventing PD-related peritonitis may help prevent the development of EPS.

Complications due to increased intraperitoneal pressure

The empty peritoneal cavity has an intra-abdominal pressure of 0.5–2.2 cmH$_2$O. IP pressure rises in direct proportion to the amount of fluid infused into the peritoneal cavity, and is higher when ambulatory than when supine. Further elevations in intra-abdominal pressure can be induced by straining due to constipation, weight-lifting, and coughing. Complications that arise from increased IP pressure in PD patients include:

1. Hernia formation
2. Acute hydrothorax due to pleuroperitoneal communication
3. Gastroesophageal reflux disease

Hernia formation

An abdominal hernia is not an uncommon problem in patients treated with PD. The sites of anatomic weakness that predispose to hernia formation include the inguinal canals, umbilicus, patent processus vaginalis, exit site, and site of a prior surgical incision. Symptoms associated with an abdominal hernia in PD patients include painless swelling at different sites, discomfort or disfigurement, and problems related to a complication from the hernia (e.g. intestinal obstruction, incarceration, strangulation, peritonitis). Leakage of peritoneal fluid into adjacent body structures can lead to either an abdominal wall or genital oedema. It is therefore important to assess for pre-existing hernias and to repair them before the commencement of PD. Combined hernia repair and PD catheter placement, in experienced hands, is also an option. Patients who develop a hernia after the initiation of PD should undergo elective repair. The use of a mesh prosthesis appears to decrease the risk of hernia recurrence. After the repair surgery, IPD may be resumed within a few days with gradual reinstitution of the former PD regimen in the subsequent two to four weeks. For dialysate leakage in patients without an associated hernia, temporary IPD may be tried. Short-term transfer to HD may be needed if the leakage persists during IPD.

Acute hydrothorax due to pleuroperitoneal communication

The development of pleural effusion in patients on PD may be due to fluid overload, heart failure, or a local pleural process. In patients with acute hydrothorax without other signs of heart failure or peripheral oedema should prompt a search for pleuroperitoneal communication. Acute hydrothorax due to pleuroperitoneal communication is an uncommon but well-recognized complication of PD. The pathogenesis of pleuroperitoneal communication remains unclear. Leakage via diaphragmatic lymphatics, the thoracic duct, or through congenital or acquired defects or blebs with a one-way valve mechanism in the diaphragm have all been implicated. The fact that anatomic defects are more commonly situated in the right hemidiaphragm may account for the preponderance of right-sided hydrothorax. Regardless of the underlying abnormality, the physiologic negative intrapleural pressure and the positive intraperitoneal pressure in PD act in concert to promote the transfer of dialysate from the abdominal to the pleural cavity, if a physiologic weak point exists.

Presenting symptoms and signs of pleuroperitoneal communication include dyspnoea and inadequate UF. The patient may be asymptomatic with the recognition of fluid in the pleural space as an incidental finding. The right side is more commonly affected than the left side, with unilateral right-sided effusions found in 50–90% of cases. The diagnostic approach includes chemical analysis of pleural fluid, methylene blue discolouration of the dialysate followed by thoracocentesis, imaging modalities that demonstrate the transfer of radio-opaque or radioactive media across the diaphragm, and direct visualization under thoracoscopic surgery. In the analysis of fluid chemistry, the basic principle is to demonstrate a similarity between the fluid composition in the two body cavities. High glucose and low protein content in the pleural fluid are suggestive of pleuroperitoneal communication.

The treatment of acute hydrothorax due to pleuroperitoneal communication depends on the acuity and severity of the patient's symptoms and the need to continue with PD as the treatment modality. Acute thoracocentesis to remove pleural fluid may be required. Small communication may be resolved by switching the patients to temporary IPD or HD. Chemical pleurodesis may be offered to patients with recurrent pleural effusion. Video-assisted thoracoscopic pleurodesis or repair may also be an option for patients who failed conservative management.

Gastroesophageal reflux disease

Gastroesophageal reflux disease (GERD) is common among PD patients. The presenting symptoms include nausea, vomiting, heartburn, acid regurgitation, fullness, and epigastric discomfort. In addition to general measures and pharmacological treatment, the management of GERD in PD patients involves minimizing IP fluid volume. Since achieving adequate dialysis in PD patients depends largely on the exchange volume, this strategy requires careful tailoring of the PD prescription to avoid inadequate solute clearance.

Systemic effects due to glucose absorption

PD patients absorb around 100–300 g of glucose per day, or about 30–100 kg per year, depending upon their prescription and transporter type. Excessive IP glucose absorption leads to obesity, dyslipidaemia, hyperglycaemia, hyperinsulinaemia, and insulin resistance. Hypertonic glucose may also have the effect of increasing blood pressure, heart rate, and stroke volume. These metabolic and haemodynamic effects of excessive glucose absorption contribute to the high morbidity and mortality of PD patients.

Detrimental effects of glucose on peritoneal membrane function

During the manufacturing of glucose-containing PD solution, glucose degradation products (GDPs) are the inevitable by-products of the heat sterilization process. An ambient acidic pH will reduce the formation of GDPs in dialysate, and for this reason, the pH of unused peritoneal dialysate is low. Another challenge with formulating peritoneal dialysate for storage is that bicarbonate cannot be used as the buffer, because it reacts with the calcium in the dialysate and forms calcium carbonate precipitates. Therefore, lactate is used in lieu of bicarbonate and is converted into bicarbonate in vivo. The presence of GDPs, the low pH, high lactate, and the absence of bicarbonate make conventional PD fluid not 'biocompatible'. These non-physiologic components in the dialysate damage the peritoneum and ultimately lead to the development of peritoneal failure.

The use of GDP-sparing biocompatible dialysate may help preserve peritoneal function. A bag of biocompatible PD fluid is divided into two subcompartments. One compartment contains glucose and electrolytes. This subcompartment has a very low pH, which slows the formation of GDPs. The other compartment contains bicarbonate. Because calcium is stored in the glucose-containing compartment, there is no calcium-bicarbonate interaction during storage. Before the dialysis exchange procedure, the patient breaks a frangible connection that separates the two compartments, and when the components are mixed, the final pH is close to physiologic. Fluids with neutral pH and low GDP have been shown to preserve residual renal function and urine volume, particularly when used for more than 12 months. Glucose-sparing by the use of icodextrin-based or amino acid–based solutions may also help preserve peritoneal membrane function. In addition, the use of the amino acid–based solution may improve nutritional parameters in PD patients.

Protein-energy wasting

Protein-energy wasting (PEW) (malnutrition) is highly prevalent in PD patients and is an important predictor of morbidity and mortality (see also Chapter 15). The diagnosis of PEW is based on biochemical measures, anthropometric parameters (body mass and muscle mass), and dietary intake. The following factors contribute to the development of PEW in PD patients:

1. Inadequate dialysis
2. Protein and amino-acid loss in the peritoneal dialysate
3. Protein loss in urine
4. Suppressed appetite due to increased IP pressure and excessive glucose absorption

To prevent malnutrition, optimal dietary protein intake is important. The recommended protein requirement in PD patients is 1.2–1.3 g of protein/kg/day. Constant monitoring of nutritional status, early detection, and the institution of therapeutic strategies for the prevention and treatment of PEW are important in the management of PD patients.

17

Haemodialysis and Haemodiafiltration: Principles and Practice

Maggie Ming Yee Mok, Hon Lok Tang, Chiu Cheuk Wong, Samuel Ka Shun Fung, and May Ki Lam

Introduction

Long-term intermittent haemodialysis (HD) therapy for the treatment of end-stage renal disease (ESRD) began in 1960 after the development of the Teflon arteriovenous shunt by Belding Scribner and colleagues at the University of Washington in Seattle, years after the first practical artificial kidney was developed by Willem Kolff in the Netherlands in 1942. Funding was an initial problem. With the establishment of Medicare insurance coverage in the 1970s, and the growing population with ESRD, the demand for and growth of HD increased in the United States. In Hong Kong, the chronic HD service was first established in 1969 and the treatment became widely available from the 1980s onwards.

Principles of Haemodialysis

HD is a treatment that aims to remove accumulated metabolic waste products and to correct blood electrolyte and acid–base composition by means of an exchange between the patient's blood and dialysate fluid across a semi-permeable membrane. The transport of solute involves two main mechanisms: diffusion and convection. Diffusion refers to the transport of substances down a concentration gradient, and substances with larger molecular size generally show slower diffusion rates. Convection transport involves an ultrafiltration (UF) drag, which is a force driven by osmotic, oncotic, or hydrostatic pressures. It is independent of molecular weight and size, as long as the solute is able to pass through the pores of the dialysis membrane. The rate of UF is determined by the pressure difference across the membrane between the blood and the dialysate compartment, known as the transmembrane pressure. In HD, the transport of most solute is mainly diffusive. Removal of larger and poorly diffusible solutes can be achieved by haemofiltration, which involves a high volume of UF coupled with the infusion of a replacement fluid to enhance their removal by convection. Haemodiafiltration (HDF) is a hybrid modality that combines HD and haemofiltration.

Components of the Haemodialysis Apparatus

Vascular access

Vascular access can be classified as temporary or permanent. Temporary accesses are venous catheters used for acute HD therapy. They can be cuffed or uncuffed, and are inserted at the internal jugular, subclavian, or femoral vein using the Seldinger technique, under ultrasonographic guidance. The right internal jugular vein is the most preferred site. The tip of the catheter should be ideally placed at the mid-right atrium for a cuffed catheter and superior vena cava for an uncuffed catheter. Non-cuffed catheters should not be used for more than a few weeks due to a high risk of infection. Permanent accesses refer to arteriovenous fistula (AVF) or arteriovenous graft (AVG). Albeit with worse outcomes, sometimes cuffed catheters may be used as permanent access for patients whom arteriovenous access cannot be created, such as those with small vessels (e.g. elderly, women), severe peripheral vascular disease, morbid obesity or severe heart failure who are unable to sustain adequate blood pressure and access flow.

Arteriovenous accesses are created by 'arterialization' of the vein (by connecting an artery directly to an adjacent vein in AVF or by bridging the two with native saphenous vein or synthetic material polytetrafluoroethylene in AVG). AVF generally requires two to six months to mature but they have excellent long-term patency and low infection rates. AVGs mature in around four weeks, but they carry higher thrombosis and infection rates than AVF.

Water treatment

Municipal water must be purified before it can be used to prepare dialysis solution as it contains a lot of organic and inorganic contaminants, bacteria, and endotoxins. Water is first pre-treated by a water softener and adsorption of chloramines by activated carbon, followed by a reverse osmosis process for further purification. Purified water in dialysis units has to be monitored regularly for bacterial and endotoxin levels to ensure it meets qualified microbiological standards.

Dialysis solution

Subsequent dialysis solution is formed by mixing a bicarbonate and an acid concentrate with the purified water. The correct proportioning of the final dialysis solution is monitored by conductivity testing before passing through the dialyser. The usual composition of dialysis solutions is shown in Table 17.1.

Table 17.1: Usual composition of dialysate in haemodialysis

Composition	Concentration (mmol/L)
Sodium	*130–150
Potassium	*2
Calcium	*1.25/1.5/1.75
Magnesium	0.25–0.5
Chloride	104.5
Bicarbonate	*30–40
Acetate	2–4
Glucose	0–11
pH	7.1–7.3

*Commonly adjusted to tailor for individual patient needs

Haemodialyser

Modern dialysers have a hollow-fibre design in which fibres are bundled inside a cylindrical shell. These hollow fibres comprise semi-permeable membranes where blood constituents pass through to the dialysis solution. Blood passes through these hollow fibres whereas the dialysate flows outside in a counter-current direction. Parallel-plate designs where blood and dialysis solution pass through alternate membrane sheet spaces have become obsolete nowadays.

Dialyser membranes are designed to mimic the permeability characteristics of the glomerular basement membrane. There are three types of dialyser membrane. The traditional cellulose membrane is made from processed cottons and contains many free hydroxyl groups at its surface, which leads to complement activation (bio-incompatibility). Modified cellulose membranes have most of the free hydroxyl group substituted by other moieties such as acetate. Modern dialysers are mostly made of synthetic membranes with no hydroxyl group such as polysulfone, polyacrylonitrile, polycarbonate, polyamide, polymethyl-methacrylate, and thus exhibit markedly improved biocompatibility. The hydroxyl group in the cellulose membrane triggers complement activation causing a drop in both neutrophil and platelet count within the first 30 minutes of dialysis. Activation of white cells leads to the release of cytokines such as interleukin-1 and tumour necrosis factor, thereby inducing the production of β2-microglobulin (β2-M) to cause dialysis-related amyloidosis. The exposure to bio-incompatible dialysis membranes, together with dialysate contaminants during HD, places patients in a state of chronic inflammation, with deleterious effect on the susceptibility to infection, protein catabolism, and malnutrition.

Solute transport within a dialyser is determined by blood flow and dialysate flow distribution, membrane characteristics and blood membrane interaction. The efficiency of a dialyser (K_oA) is defined by urea clearance. Dialysers of $K_oA < 450$ ml/min are considered to have low efficiency and $K_oA > 700$ ml/min are considered highly efficient. The flux of a dialyser refers to the clearance of β2-microglobulin which is a middle molecule of 11.8 kDa. In the Haemodialysis (HEMO) study, β2-microglobulin clearance of at least 20 ml/min was regarded as high-flux and < 10 ml/min was defined as low-flux. The size and shapes of pores within the membrane are designed to achieve different clearance goals. However, the permeability of dialysers has to be balanced against the leakage of useful polypeptides and albumin. So far, the mortality benefits with the use of high-flux dialysers have only been shown in a subgroup of patients who have been on HD for more than 3.7 years in the HEMO study, which implies that the detrimental effects of middle-sized uremic molecules take time to emerge. High cut-off (HCO) and medium cut-off (MCO) dialysers will be discussed later in this chapter.

Anticoagulation

Haemodialysis involves blood flow to an extracorporeal circuit. Anticoagulation is required to prevent blood clot formation along the blood tubings and the dialyser. Dialyser clogging could result in loss of the dialyser and tubings, accompanied by around 100–150 ml of blood trapped in the clotted dialyser and blood lines. Heparin is the most commonly used anticoagulant, either in the form of unfractionated heparin or low molecular weight heparin (LMWH). Unfractionated heparin is given by a single bolus followed by continuous infusion or by a single bolus and a mid-dose or repeated boluses. The whole blood partial thromboplastin time or activated clotting time (ACT) are commonly used to titrate heparin doses. The target is to keep ACT about 150–180% of the baseline value. LMWH has a longer half-life and can be given as a single bolus at the beginning of HD treatment (e.g. Enoxaparin at 100 anti-factor Xa IU/kg as a bolus dose and Tinzaparin at 2,000–4,500 anti-factor Xa IU). Routine monitoring of clotting profiles in patients using LMWH is generally not required. Besides ease of administration, LMWH is preferred to heparin as it is associated with better lipid profiles, less hyperkalaemia, and a lower risk of heparin-induced osteoporosis.

In patients with bleeding diathesis, heparin doses may have to be reduced or totally avoided. Heparin induced thrombocytopenia (HIT) is a complication of heparin therapy which manifests in two clinical forms. Type I HIT shows a time- and dose-dependent thrombocytopenia which is mild and transient, and the platelet count usually recovers without any change in heparin dose. Type II HIT is an immune-mediated thrombocytopenia caused by IgG antibodies formed against the multimolecular complex of heparin and platelet factor 4. This occurs more commonly with conventional heparin than LMWH. Type II HIT typically results in a 40–50% decline in platelets 5–10 days after heparin exposure and may result in paradoxical thrombosis requiring systemic anticoagulation. The diagnosis is confirmed by the presence of heparin-PF4 antibody (platelet aggregation assay/ELISA) and the serotonin release assay. Further heparin exposure should be avoided. LMWH should also not be used due to the cross-reactivity of heparin-PF4 antibodies.

When heparin needs to be avoided, the patency of the HD circuit may be maintained by continuous or periodic saline rinsing. Other measures include increasing the blood flow rate, avoiding blood product or lipid administration via the inlet blood line, and the use of dialysers with heparin coating. Regional citrate anticoagulation is another measure for this purpose. Citrate binds with plasma calcium to inhibit coagulation, and thus administration of sodium citrate to the arterial limb of the blood circuit together with calcium-free dialysate can achieve regional anticoagulation. Calcium has to be re-infused at the venous limb and ionized calcium levels need to be closely monitored to ensure normalization of plasma calcium before blood is returned to the patient. Plasma bicarbonate levels also need to be monitored as the metabolism of sodium citrate generates bicarbonate. Citric acid can be used as a replacement for acetate in the dialysate. This citrate dialysate results in reduced clotting compared with heparin-free dialysis. A small reduction in serum-ionized calcium occurs, but no clinically relevant hypocalcaemia has been observed. Regional anticoagulation with vasodilator prostanoids (e.g. prostacyclin, epoprostenol, prostaglandins E1 and F1) reduces platelet activation in the extracorporeal circuit, but may lead to hypotension. Other anticoagulation strategies include the use of direct thrombin inhibitors (e.g. argatroban, lepirudin) and heparinoids which consist of non-heparin glycosaminoglycan heparan sulfate (e.g. danaparoid, fondoparinux), but these alternatives should be used with caution in patients with type II HIT as cross-reactivity has been reported.

Other components in the haemodialysis circuit

In the blood circuit, a roller blood pump drives blood through the circuit. The arterial pressure is measured by a pressure gauge before the blood pump. There is another venous pressure monitor after blood passes through the dialyzer. Before the dialysed blood is returned to the patient, there is a venous air trap and detector to prevent air embolism.

The dialysis solution circuit involves the water purification system (as above) and the concentrate proportioning system mixing concentrated electrolyte solution/powder with the purified water to form the desired dialysis solution, which is then heated. There are both temperature and conductivity sensors and alarms. A proportioning system moves the dialysate to the dialyser and then a second pump moves it out of the dialyser into a drain. The amount of UF is determined by the difference in pumping rates between the two and is monitored by UF control. In the dialysis outflow, blood leak detectors sense blood when there is a leak developing through the dialyser membrane.

Haemodialysis Adequacy and Urea Kinetic Modelling

The dose of dialysis delivered to a patient can be measured by urea kinetic modelling, the calculation of which is based on the blood-side kinetics or the dialysate-side kinetics.

Blood-side urea kinetic modelling

Urea reduction ratio

This is an extraction ratio that reflects the fraction of solutes (urea) removed from blood in a single pass through the dialyser. The urea reduction ratio (URR) is determined as

$$(C_{in} - C_{out})/C_{in}$$

where C_{in} is the solute (urea) concentration in the blood entering the dialyser and C_{out} is the concentration in the blood exiting the dialyser. The extraction ratio is dependent on the blood and dialysate flow rates, the dialyser membrane properties, and the characteristics of the solute itself (e.g. molecular size, protein binding).

Clearance (Kt/V)

The removal of solute could also be assessed by the concept of clearance, which is the volume from which the solute is removed during a specific period. It is expressed as Kt/V, where K is the plasma urea clearance, t is the dialysis session length in minutes, and V is the urea distribution volume in litres (i.e. total body water). K is determined by the blood flow rate, dialysate flow rate, and the efficiency of the dialyser. A high-efficiency dialyser has a thin membrane with a large surface area and wide pores to maximize contact between the blood and dialysate. Kt/V is calculated by determining the slope of the logarithmic decline of blood urea level. This is because the blood urea level entering the dialyser is not constant but

falls continuously during the dialysis process. In this context, urea in the body declines exponentially, thus removal of urea is the most efficient at the beginning of HD but falls as blood is gradually cleared of urea. The relationship between Kt/V and URR is expressed as:

$$Kt/V = \ln(1\text{-URR})$$

Taking into account both the small amount of urea generated during dialysis and the urea removed by convection, the equation is modified (Daugirdas, 1995) as below:

$$spKt/V = -\ln(R\text{-}0.008 \times t) + (4\text{-}3.5 \times R) \times UF/W$$

where sp stands for 'single pool', R is defined as $C_{out(urea)} / C_{in(urea)}$ (i.e. R = 1 − URR), t is the dialysis time in hours, UF is the ultrafiltration volume in litres, and W is the post-dialysis weight.

This single-pool urea kinetic model assumes that urea is distributed in the body in a single-pool of volume. In real life, urea is sequestrated in other tissues during dialysis, mainly muscles, where there is a low ratio of blood flow to remove urea leading to urea sequestration. After completion of dialysis, there is urea rebound as urea from these sequestrated tissues redistributes back to the vascular pool. Therefore, spKt/V overestimates the true Kt/V due to the falsely low post-dialysis urea level. The post-dialysis rebound is largely completed by 30–60 minutes. Post-dialysis urea taken at this time is used to calculate the equilibrated Kt/V (eKt/V), which is roughly 0.2 unit lower than spKt/V.

Dialysate-side urea kinetic modelling: Solute removal index

The solute removal index (SRI) is based on the urea removed in the spent dialysate. It is defined as the percentage of body urea nitrogen content removed during an HD treatment.

$$SRI\ (\%) = (R\text{-}G \times t) / (C \times V) \times 100$$

where R is the total urea nitrogen removed from the body during HD in g; G is the urea generation rate in g/min; t is the HD session length in minutes; (G × t) is the amount of urea nitrogen generated during HD; C is the pre-dialysis urea in g/L; V is the pre-dialysis urea distribution volume in L; and (C × V) will be the pre-dialysis urea nitrogen content in the body in g.

Since the calculation of SRI does not involve post-dialysis blood urea, it is not affected by post-dialysis urea rebound. R can be measured by collecting spent dialysate using Ing's partial dialysate collection method, in which a T-tube system is used to collect a representative sample of the total spent dialysate.

Haemodialysis Prescription

Based on results from several large clinical trials such as the National Cooperative Dialysis Study and HEMO study, the current guidelines recommend a minimum HD requirement of spKt/V of 1.2 per session in a thrice-weekly schedule of HD (in patients with residual native kidney clearance Kru < 2 ml/min). Dialysate flow rate is usually set to twice the blood flow rate to enhance urea clearance. Other modifiable parameters to achieve the spKt/V target include increasing dialysis time, frequency, using dialysers with a larger surface area, and the use of anticoagulation to minimize fibre bundle clotting in the dialyser.

A common chronic intermittent HD prescription is usually scheduled 2–3 sessions per week and 4–5 hours per session (Table 17.2). Blood flow rates are usually set at 200–300 ml/min and the dialysate flow rate at 13 ml/hour/kg. A UF goal is set to achieve the desired weight loss to reach a patient's target ideal or 'dry weight', but should preferably be not more than 500 ml/hour. It must be remembered that maintenance dialysis provides only a fraction of the normal renal function. Even if the dialysers are as efficient as the native kidneys in clearing waste products across the entire molecular size range, HD for 10 to 12 hours a week provides only 12/(24x7), i.e. < 7% of normal renal function.

One should appreciate that the minimum spKt/V target of 1.2 per session for a thrice-weekly HD schedule (i.e. 3.6 per week) cannot be directly compared to the minimum Kt/V target of 1.7 for patients on peritoneal dialysis. This is because the urea clearance is intermittent in HD, whereas it is continuous in peritoneal dialysis. When comparing the different frequency and intensity of HD across different dialysis modalities, one can use the weekly standardized Kt/V (std Kt/V) derived by Gotch, which incorporates the generation rate and clearance of urea and corrects for the intermittent decline in urea after each HD therapy.

Acute Complications of Haemodialysis

Hypotension

Hypotension is the most common complication of HD. As fluid is removed from the intravascular compartment, hypotension may occur if the UF rate exceeds the refill rate from the interstitium. Haemodialysis is a catabolic process that generates heat and the heated dialysate transfers thermal energy to the blood leading to vasodilation. Blood pressure and cardiac output are normally maintained by an increase in heart rate and contractility. However, these mechanisms may be blunted in the presence of autonomic dysfunction, background cardiovascular diseases, and the use of multiple antihypertensive medications, all of which are prevalent in the HD population.

The acute management of hypotension during HD include stopping UF, reducing the blood flow rate and the dialysate flow rate, putting the patient in the Trendelenburg position, and replacing the intravascular volume with intravenous fluid or albumin. The dry weight of the patient and the UF rate need to be re-adjusted if there is no clinical fluid overload. In patients with large weight gain in between HD sessions, hypotension may occur before reaching one's dry weight if fluid redistribution from the interstitium to the intravascular space is not fast enough. In such cases, it is necessary to increase the frequency and duration of HD to allow more gentle

Table 17.2: Common regimens of various haemodialysis strategies

	Conventional	Short daily	Long intermittent	Long frequent	Nx stage	Common home haemodialysis regimen in Hong Kong
Sessions/week	3	≥ 5	3–4	≥ 5	≥ 5	3.5
Time/session (hrs)	4	2.5–3.5	≥ 5.5	≥ 5.5	2.5–3.5	6–8
Blood flow rate (ml/min)	200–400	400	200–400	200–300	400	200–250
Dialysate flow rate (ml/min)	500		500–800	300–500	300–500	130	300

removal of excess fluids. Anti-hypertensive medications are generally withheld four hours before HD. Cool temperature dialysis can be used to prevent intradialytic hypotension (IDH), but the dialysate temperature should not be lowered to < 35°C. The sodium level of dialysate can also be modelled to prevent IDH. The sodium concentration can be adjusted to a fixed higher level to prevent the decline in plasma osmolality and thus osmotic fluid loss from the interstitium and cells. Dialysate sodium concentration can also be set up to 150–160 mmol/L at the start of HD, and then continuously, exponentially, or step-wise decreased to around 140 mmol/L at the end of the dialysis (called 'sodium profiling'). However, the association of increased inter-dialytic weight gain and hypertension with this modality precludes its routine use. Food intake is generally avoided before and during HD in patients who are prone to develop hypotension. Factors resulting in tissue ischemia such as anaemia should also be corrected. α1-adrenergic agonist (e.g. midodrine) and fludrocortisone can be tried if the problem persists. A blood volume-controlled feedback system is a function in new generation HD machines to prevent IDH. The machine adjusts the UF rate and dialysate sodium level throughout the dialysis session to achieve a more physiological blood volume reduction along a predefined trajectory. This modality can be used in patients with refractory IDH.

Muscle cramps

This frequently occurs when UF is too rapid or excessive or when a low sodium dialysate is used, which leads to vasoconstriction and thus muscle hypoperfusion. Symptoms can be improved by avoiding large intradialytic weight gains, slowing the UF rate, and administering a bolus of normal saline and hypertonic solution (e.g. saline, glucose, mannitol) to raise plasma osmolarity and expand the intravascular volume. Drug treatments with diazepam may alleviate symptoms and quinine sulphate, L-carnitine, and vitamin E may help to prevent cramps. Electrolyte disturbances such as low pre-dialysis levels of potassium, calcium, and magnesium should also be corrected.

Nausea, vomiting, and headache

Most of these symptoms are related to hypotension, but they could be early symptoms of dialysis disequilibrium syndrome and dialyser reactions (below).

Dialysis disequilibrium syndrome

Dialysis disequilibrium syndrome occurs when acute patients with high blood urea levels are dialysed too aggressively. This is due to the rapid fall in plasma osmolality by the removal of solute during HD, which subsequently leads to water shifting from plasma into the brain tissue causing cerebral oedema. Milder symptoms include nausea, vomiting, headache, and restlessness. Seizure and coma may occur in severe cases. The target reduction in plasma urea level should be limited to about 40% at the initial acute HD treatment setting. Intravenous mannitol can be administered during dialysis to prevent this syndrome.

Dialyser reactions

These are broadly categorized into two types. Type A (anaphylactic type) dialyser reaction manifests as those of anaphylaxis. Dyspnoea, a sense of impending doom, a feeling of warmth throughout the body, urticaria, and abdominal cramps are common presenting symptoms. Cardiac arrest and death could occur in severe cases. Symptoms usually occur in the first few minutes up to 30 minutes after the start of dialysis. This is usually attributed to allergic reactions towards ethylene oxide used for the sterilization of dialysers and blood lines, especially when it has not been adequately rinsed off. Disinfection of dialyser and blood line by alternative methods such as steam or gamma radiation have to be considered in such cases.

AN69 membrane, a copolymer of polyacrylonitrile and sodium methallyl sulfonate, can also cause anaphylactoid reactions when used in patients who are taking angiotensin-converting enzyme inhibitors (ACEI). This is related to the negatively charged methallyl sulfonate binding to the Hageman factor (factor XII) of the intrinsic pathway of coagulation, followed by the conversion of kininogen to bradykinin. The concomitant use of ACEI inhibits the degradation of bradykinin, leading to the accumulation of bradykinins. The effect on bradykinins is less pronounced with angiotensin receptor blockers. Rare reactions to polysulfone, polyethersulfone, or polyacrylonitrile membranes made with other copolymers may also occur. Anaphylactoid reaction can also occur when the dialysis solution is contaminated by bacteria or endotoxin or with the use of contaminated reuse dialysers. These reactions generally occur within minutes of HD and are associated with fever and chills. It is important to stop the HD procedure immediately when anaphylaxis occurs without returning blood already in the circuit back to the patient. Other steps in usual management for anaphylaxis should also be promptly initiated.

Type B dialyser reactions are non-specific. They are generally less severe and manifest commonly as chest and back pain during the early phase of the HD session. This is usually attributed to membrane bio-incompatibility. Management is supportive and symptoms usually disappear after the first hour. Other causes of chest and back pain should be excluded.

Hypoglycaemia

Patients with ESRD have abnormal carbohydrate metabolism, prolonged insulin half-life, and reduced peripheral insulin resistance. Thus, diabetic patients on insulin are especially prone to hypoglycaemia and glucose-containing dialysate may help to avoid this complication.

Arrhythmia

Arrhythmia is common during HD due to the rapid fluctuation in haemodynamics and electrolyte concentrations (e.g. potassium). The presence of left ventricular hypertrophy, coronary artery and pericardial disease, valvular calcifications and calcific deposits in the conduction system, and autonomic dysfunction in ESRD patients may further compound the issue. A step-wise lowering approach of the potassium level in the dialysate is less arrhythmogenic than a constant dialysate potassium level. The use of higher calcium dialysate may alleviate arrhythmia and intradialytic hypotension, but is associated with an increased risk of tissue calcification.

Haemolysis

Patients usually present with chest tightness, back pain, and shortness of breath. This occurs when there are problems with the dialysis solution such as overheating, dialysate hypotonicity due to insufficient concentrate-to-water ratio, and contamination by formaldehyde, bleach, chloramine, fluoride, nitrates (from the water supply), and copper and zinc (from water pipelines). Mechanical stress to red blood cells may also arise from kinking of blood lines and poorly constructed blood tubing, and this can result in severe hyperkalaemia if not detected early. Haemodialysis should be stopped without returning the haemolysed blood in the circuit to the patient.

Air embolism

The entry of air into the HD circuit commonly occurs via the arterial needle, the pre-pump arterial tubing segment, or an inadvertently opened end of a central venous catheter. This is usually prevented by the presence of air leak detectors and pressure alarms. When air embolism accidents occur, the venous blood line should be clamped and the blood pump stopped. Resuscitation measures should be commenced and the patient should lie in the recumbent position on the left side with the chest and head tilted downwards.

Long-Term Complications of Haemodialysis

Dialysis-related amyloidosis

Dialysis-related amyloidosis is a disorder characterized by the accumulation and tissue deposition of β2-M amyloid in bones, joints, soft tissue, and viscera of patients with ESRD. β2-M, as mentioned earlier, is a middle-sized solute (MW 11.8 KDa) which is normally cleared by the kidneys. Even with the use of high-flux haemodialyser and convective therapy, its clearance by HD still lags far behind its production. β2-M may also be modified by an advanced glycation end-product which increased its affinity to collagen and renders it more difficult to be cleared. In HD, the use of bio-incompatible dialyser membranes and the presence of endotoxins in dialysate stimulate reactive inflammation and intradialytic generation of β2-M. HD therapy also leads to a faster loss of residual renal function, which, however minimal, still contributes significantly to the clearance and catabolism of β2-M.

The incidence of dialysis-related amyloidosis increases with dialysis vintage. Common presentations include carpal tunnel syndrome, shoulder pain related to scapulohumeral periarthritis and rotator cuff infiltration by amyloid, flexor tenosynovitis of the hands, and neck pain due to destructive spondyloarthropathy. Occasionally there may be involvement of the gastrointestinal tract leading to bleeding. The gold standard of diagnosis is by Congo red and immunohistochemical staining of biopsy specimens, although the diagnosis can be established by the typical clinical features and characteristic radiological findings in most cases. Ultrasound examination of the shoulder and hip joints may show synovial thickening due to amyloid infiltration. X-ray, computed tomography and magnetic resonance imaging show rapidly enlarging bony cysts. Management is mainly symptomatic although the application of HDF may enhance the clearance of β2-M. Kidney transplantation is the only definitive treatment.

Aluminium toxicity

In the past, aluminium toxicity in HD patients was caused by the use of aluminium sulphate in water treatment. This is now rarely seen due to the improvement in water purification methods and the reduction in the use of aluminium-containing phosphate binders. The neurological manifestations in affected patients include apraxia, myoclonic jerks, seizures, progressive dementia, and encephalopathy. The accumulation of aluminium can also disturb the mobilization of iron, resulting in microcytic anaemia and resistance to erythropoietin therapy. Aluminium accumulation in the bones could interfere with parathyroid function and bone turnover, which often presents as severe bone pain and multiple fractures. Typically, serum calcium rises dramatically after vitamin D administration due to inhibition of bone turnover. The bony lesions are either adynamic or unmineralized (osteomalacia). The mainstays of management are discontinuation of aluminium-containing medications and chelation with desferrioxamine (DFO). Aluminium is highly protein-bound and poorly eliminated during HD. DFO combines with aluminium to form a dialysable complex aluminoxamine, which is more readily removable by HD and peritoneal dialysis. A low starting dose should be used to prevent encephalopathy due to redistribution of mobilized aluminium into the brain.

Renal osteodystrophy

Renal osteodystrophy is a common and important complication in HD patients (see also Chapter 15).

Other Modalities of Haemodialysis

Hemodiafiltration

HDF combines the process of HD and haemofiltration to remove solutes by diffusion and convection. UF by convection carries toxins through membrane pores by fluid movement and is independent of molecular size (as long as the toxin molecule can pass through the membrane pores). Infusion of a significant amount of fluid is required to replace the ultrafiltrate and should be accurately controlled to prevent fluid imbalance. Substitution fluid can be replaced before or after the dialyser, or both (pre-dilution, post-dilution, or mixed). In the pre-dilution mode, since the solute concentration in blood entering the dialyser is reduced, a higher infusion rate is required to achieve the same clearance. More stringent microbiological standards in dialysate water treatment are required as the substitution fluid directly enters the blood circuit during replacement. Dialysers for HDF also require a better hydraulic permeability to facilitate convective clearance. The relative survival benefit of HDF therapy compared to HD has been shown to be a function of the convection volume, requiring up to >23 L or 26 L/1.73 m^2 per treatment (post-dilution). HDF provides better clearance of small and middle molecules such as β2-M and other uremic toxins including some proinflammatory mediators, leptin, and advanced glycation end-products. HDF may be a potential treatment for patients with high levels of β2-M and dialysis-related amyloidosis. HDF may sometimes confer superior hemodynamic stability than HD due to replacement fluid infusion and the removal of vasodilatory mediators. On-line HDF is a method of HDF using on-line prepared substitution fluid for replacement of ultrafiltration. This method enables a large volume of convention.

Intensive haemodialysis

Any HD therapy which has either a longer duration or higher frequency compared with standard HD regimen (three times per week, four hours per session) is considered as intensive HD. It can be performed in the daytime or at night, at HD facilities or at home (Table 17.2). Intensive HD is intended to enhance the clearance of middle molecules due to the higher frequency and duration, increased UF, and augmented clearance of protein-bound molecules (e.g. indoxyl sulfate, p-cresyl sulphate). To date, data from observational studies have demonstrated that intensive HD is associated with better survival than conventional HD. The lower rates of blood and dialysate flow and UF in each treatment allows for more stable intradialytic haemodynamics and less intradialytic discomfort such as cramps. The longer overall treatment time also enables more total fluid removal to improve long-term fluid and blood pressure control, thus reducing the development of left ventricular hypertrophy and cardiovascular diseases. Intensive HD can be performed in form of nocturnal home HD to facilitate employment and daytime activities. Various studies have demonstrated beneficial effects of nocturnal home HD in terms of anaemia control, serum phosphate and calcium phosphate product reduction, blood pressure control, dialysis adequacy, and quality of life. The greater removal of fluid and phosphate also allows a more liberal diet. Other indications for intensive HD therapy are inadequate control of uraemia, obstructive sleep apnoea, and pregnancy. New and smaller machines such as NxStage are in place which is portable and easy to set-up. The dialysate is prepared in a bag by a build-in dialysate preparation system and circumvents the need for an external water purification system.

High cut-off haemodialysis and expanded haemodialysis

HCO dialysers are employed clinically to clear large molecular weight serum free light chains (e.g. κ-FLC: 22.5 kDa; λ-FLC 45 kDa) in multiple myeloma cast nephropathy patients who require HD treatment. Together with appropriate chemotherapy, HD therapy with high cut-off dialysers shows better removal of serum-free light chains than conventional high-flux dialysers. Superflux dialysers remove molecules with mass up to 60 kDa, and is used mainly in the intensive care setting to remove cytokines typical for severe sepsis and inflammatory mediators. The dialyser membrane is hydrophobic and has an affinity to adsorb proteins to increase the clearance of protein-bound solutes, but is associated with greater loss of albumin, useful drugs, and other nutrients.

Middle molecules have a wide range of molecular weights from 500 Da to 60 kDa. The clearance of middle molecules with molecular weight > 15 kDa (large middle molecules) is low with high-flux membranes. The development of a new generation of dialysis membranes, the medium cut-off (MCO) membranes, has allowed the removal of these large middle molecules up to approximately 50 kDa. The dialysis using this MCO membrane is known as expanded haemodialysis (HDx). Unlike HCO membranes, the MCO membranes have significantly less albumin loss due to the tighter distribution of pores. In dialysis patients, these molecules have been shown to be involved in the development of atherosclerotic cardiovascular disease, e.g. IL-6 (24.5 kDa), IL-18 (24 kDa); cardiac hypertrophy, e.g. FGF23 (32 kDa); secondary immunodeficiency, e.g. Ig light chains (κ 22.5 kDa, λ 45 kDa), retinol-binding protein 4 (21.2 kDa); and chronic inflammation, e.g. IL-6, IL-1β (17.5 kDa), and TNF-α (17 kDa). A recent randomized controlled trial has shown improvement of quality-of-life outcomes and uraemic pruritus in patients dialysed with MCO dialyser compared with high-flux dialyser.

Haemoperfusion and continuous renal replacement therapy

The other important modalities of HD, continuous renal replacement therapy and haemoperfusion, will be discussed in chapters 19 and 20 respectively.

18

Kidney Transplantation: Principles and Practice

*Maggie Ma, Simon C. Y. Cheung, Cindy Choy, Gavin Chan, Janette Kwok,
and Tak Mao Chan*

Introduction

Successful kidney transplantation offers better survival and quality of life than dialysis in patients with end-stage kidney disease (ESKD). This chapter will provide an overview of transplant immunology, evaluation of renal transplant recipients and donors, use of immunosuppression, and the complications and management of kidney transplantation.

Immunology of Organ Transplantation

The immune system primarily serves to defend against infections related to various pathogens. In the context of organ transplantation, immune responses can lead to rejection of the transplanted organ. Despite the use of various effective immunosuppressive therapies, acute and chronic rejection remain major causes of kidney allograft loss. Human leukocyte antigens (HLA), expressed on the surface of the donor cells, are the principal molecules that trigger or mediate an immune response during organ transplant rejection.

Human leukocyte antigen system

The human leucocyte antigen (HLA), which corresponds to the major histocompatibility complex (MHC) in human, is located on chromosome 6p21.3. It plays a pivotal role in enabling the immune system to distinguish between 'self' and 'non-self'. The classical HLA Class I antigens include HLA-A, HLA-B, and HLA-C while classical HLA Class II includes HLA-DR, HLA-DQ, and HLA-DP. HLAs are largely responsible for adaptive immunity and govern the rejection of allogeneic transplantation. HLA Class I proteins are expressed in most cell types and they are heterodimers that consist of α and β2-microglobulin chains (Figure 18.1). They load intracellular antigens (self or foreign antigens, e.g. viral peptides) in the endoplasmic reticulum and subsequently translocate to the cell surface. HLA Class II proteins are mainly expressed on professional antigen-presenting cells (APC) such as B cells and dendritic cells. They are also heterodimers that consist of α and β chains and are responsible for presenting extracellular antigens (Figure 18.1).

Allo-recognition

Allo-recognition is the process by which T lymphocytes recognize the foreign antigens on the transplanted organ. T cells recognize the presented antigens via T-cell receptors. T-cell allo-recognition can be direct or indirect. The former recognizes the unprocessed allogeneic HLA molecule presented by *donor* APC, while the latter recognizes the processed allo-peptide presented by *recipient* APC in the context of self (recipient) HLA (Figure 18.2). CD8+ cytotoxic T cells recognize the antigens presented by HLA Class I and exert cytotoxicity to the cells. On the contrary, CD4+ helper T cells recognize antigens presented by HLA Class II and provide help to B cells to produce antibodies.

T-lymphocyte activation

Activation of T lymphocytes is the prelude to rejection, and involves three important signalling

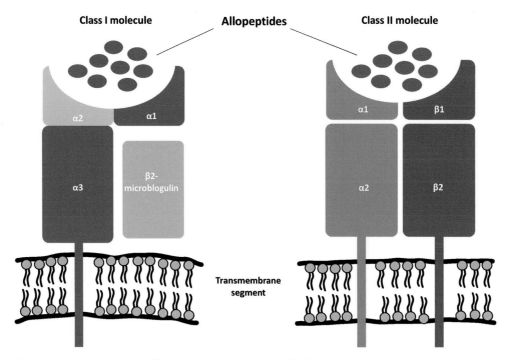

Figure 18.1: Structure of class I and II human leucocyte antigen (HLA) molecules

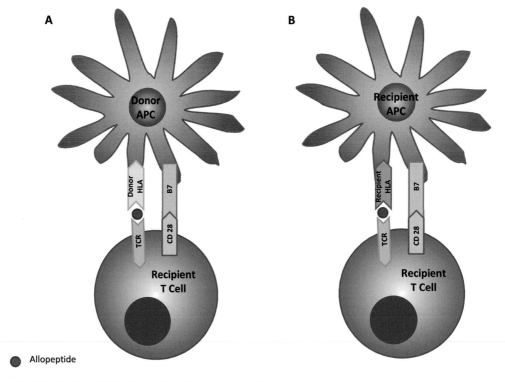

Figure 18.2: (A) direct and (B) indirect alloantigen presentation
APC, antigen-presenting cell; HLA, human leukocyte antigen; TCR, T-cell receptor

pathways. The binding of allo-peptide/HLA molecules on APC to the TRC/CD3 complex on T-cell surfaces constitutes the first signal. This is followed by the synthesis of the second messengers, which leads to an increase in intracellular calcium level and activation of calcium-dependent phosphatase which is crucial to cytokine gene induction. Calcineurin is a calcium-calmodulin complex-dependent phosphatase that plays a key role in T-cell activation. The second signal is the non-antigen specific costimulatory signal of engagement of the B7 on APCs with the CD28 on T cells. These signals lead to the induction of cytokine genes, most notably the production of IL-2 and increased expression of IL-2 receptors. The binding of these cytokines to their respective receptors provides the third signal, leading to the progression of T-cell activation, cell proliferation, and clonal expansion.

Role of B lymphocytes

Activated CD4+ T helper cells interact with B cells to trigger humoral immune responses, i.e. production of specific antibodies targeting exposed antigens. It is increasingly recognized that alloantibodies can be major effectors of both acute and chronic immune-mediated injury in the graft kidney. Alloantibodies are mostly directed against HLAs but can also target other kinds of antigens (e.g. endothelial or epithelial antigens).

Evaluation of Kidney Transplant Recipients and Donors

Kidney transplant recipients

Early kidney transplantation is associated with favourable patient survival and allograft outcomes. ESKD patients can undergo 'pre-emptive' kidney transplantation before initiation of maintenance dialysis if a donor is available. Various medical comorbidities can increase peri-operative risks or jeopardize patient or allograft survival after kidney transplantation, and some may even preclude patients from renal transplantation (Table 18.1).

Kidney donors: Deceased and live donors

Deceased donors can be classified as heart-beating donors who meet the criteria of brain death (donation after brain death, DBD) or as non-heart beating donors (donation after cardiac death, DCD).

Table 18.1: Contraindications to kidney transplantation

- Active infection
- Active malignancy
- Any other medical illness with short life expectancy
- Poorly controlled psychosis
- Medical non-compliance or active substance abuse

Certification of brain death should be performed by a neurologist or intensivist not associated with the transplant team. Organ shortage has led to the increasing use of marginal donors (expanded criteria donors, ECDs) to maximize the opportunities for transplantation. It is important to ensure that all deceased donors have reasonable kidney function and without any uncontrolled sepsis. Utmost precautions should be taken to avoid transmission of infections such as hepatitis B virus (HBV), hepatitis C virus (HCV), or human immunodeficiency virus (HIV) from the donor to the recipient. Nowadays, it is feasible to transplant a kidney from an HBsAg-positive donor to a recipient who is HBsAg-positive or HBsAg-negative but with protective levels of anti-HBs antibody. Prior to the advent of effective antiviral therapies, kidneys from HCV-positive donors were allocated to HCV-positive recipients. The arrival of highly effective direct-acting antiviral agents (DAA) has changed the management of HCV infection, and treatment of HCV in patients with CKD can be done before or after kidney transplantation. Also, there is accumulating data to show that with antiviral treatment it is safe and feasible to transplant kidneys from HCV-positive donors to HCV-negative recipients. There is also emerging data supporting kidney transplantation in selected CKD patients who have HIV infections.

Live kidney donation is a unique medical situation, in which the patient (donor) receives no direct medical benefit from an operation that is associated with risks. Therefore, proper counselling and informed consent are obligatory, with the donor fully aware of the potential short- and long-term implications of donor nephrectomy. The process has to be free from coercion. Involvement of unrelated donors or non-first-degree relatives usually requires approval from the local human organ transplant board. The medical evaluation of live donor also needs to ensure that:

1. The potential donor is in good health and fit for surgery.

2. The potential donor has normal kidney function and is at low risk of kidney disease or medical complications in the future.
3. The immunological barrier of incompatible pairs can be overcome (see next section).

Compatibility and immunological evaluation

Human leucocyte antigen compatibility

Histocompatibility testing is the standard practice to evaluate HLA compatibility between transplant candidates and potential donors for the assessment of immunological risks in solid organ, tissue, or stem cells transplantations. The current histocompatibility test consists of three major elements: HLA typing of both donor and recipient, identification of anti-HLA antibodies in the recipient to determine their HLA sensitization, and cross-matching between the donor and the recipient.

HLA typing

HLA typing refers to the determination of the HLA antigens/alleles of an individual. The routine techniques have evolved from serological typing using complement-dependent cytotoxicity (CDC) assay to molecular typing methods (e.g. sequence-specific oligonucleotide, sequence-specific primer, sequence-based typing, or next-generation sequencing) (Table 18.2). An example of HLA typing and mismatches calculation is illustrated in Figure 18.3.

Identification of anti-HLA antibodies

Sensitization of allogeneic HLA can result from prior transplantation, pregnancy, transfusion of blood products, and infections which may induce antibodies against the exposed HLA antigens. An anti-HLA antibody with specificity against the donor HLA is called a donor-specific antibody (DSA). Kidney transplant recipients with pre-formed DSA before transplant are at high risk of hyperacute rejection. Panel Reactive Activity (PRA) is a measure of the degree of sensitization. Traditionally, the patient's serum is tested against a panel of donor lymphocytes and PRA is expressed as the percentage of positive cross-matches over the total number of donors tested. PRA predicts the likelihood of finding a cross-match incompatible donor in the local organ donor pool and correlates with the immunological risk. Nowadays, anti-HLA antibodies of IgG subclass can be detected by solid-phase assays using luminex technology. Single antigen beads are coated with recombinant HLA antigens that allow a sensitive tool to identify the specificities and measure the semi-quantitative levels of anti-HLA antibodies. The anti-HLA antibody detected can be listed as 'unacceptable antigen'. In recent years, the concept of calculated PRA (cPRA) has been introduced and is defined as the percentage of donors expected to have HLA antigens that are unacceptable for a candidate. In some countries, cPRA is incorporated in the kidney allocation system and extra scores will be granted to highly sensitized individuals to enhance their access to potentially compatible donors.

Table 18.2: A comparison between serological and molecular HLA typing

	Serological typing	Molecular typing
Methodology	• HLA typing using complement mediated cell lysis when mixing well-defined anti-HLA antibodies (antisera) with lymphocytes of the individual to be typed	• DNA-based typing
Advantages	• Quick and inexpensive to perform	• More accurate and allows typing at higher resolution (allelic level) • Highly efficient technique with only a small amount of sample needed • Does not require viable lymphocytes • Inexhaustible supply of reagents
Disadvantages	• Only defines broad antigen family • Potential cross reactivity of antisera • Some antisera are no longer available	• Techniques used are complex

DNA, deoxyribonucleic acid; HLA, human leukocyte antigens

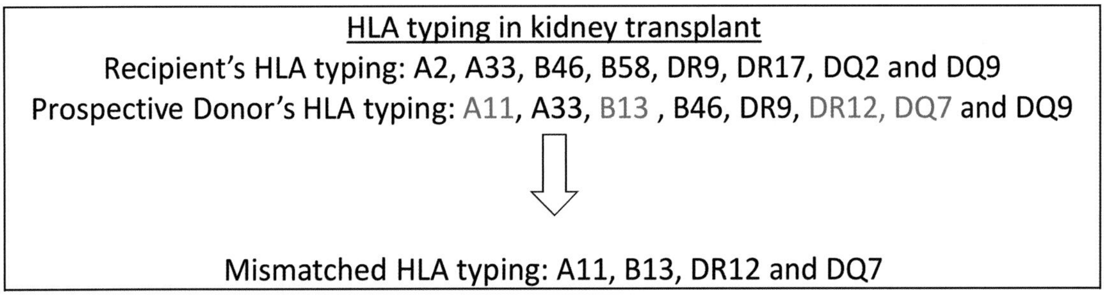

HLA typing in kidney transplant
Recipient's HLA typing: A2, A33, B46, B58, DR9, DR17, DQ2 and DQ9
Prospective Donor's HLA typing: A11, A33, B13 , B46, DR9, DR12, DQ7 and DQ9

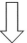

Mismatched HLA typing: A11, B13, DR12 and DQ7

Figure 18.3: An example of human leukocyte antigen (HLA) typing in kidney transplant. Mismatched antigen(s) refer to the HLA antigen(s) that is/are found in the prospective donor but not in the recipient.

Table 18.3: Interpretation of histocompatibility test results

Scenario	Solid phase antibody results	XM results	Risk of Rejection
Absent of DSA	Negative	Negative	Low
Anti-HLA antibodies positive but not against donor's HLA typing	Positive	Negative	Low
On anti-CD20 treatment	Negative	B-cell FCXM negative (after pronase treatment)	Low
Presence of DSA	Positive	Positive	High
Presence of non-HLA antibodies and absent of DSA	Positive/Negative	Positive	Uncertain

DSA, donor-specific antibody; FCXM, flow cytometric cross-match; HLA, human leukocyte antigen; XM, cross-match

HLA cross-match

Physical cross-match is performed to demonstrate the response of DSA using the live donor's cells and the recipient's serum. A conventional CDC cross-match assay detects the presence of cytotoxic DSA which is a contraindication for transplantation. Flow cytometric cross-match assay is highly sensitive to detect low levels of DSA bound to the donor's T cells and B cells. Rejection risk assessment based on the combination of anti-HLA antibodies identification and cross-match results is shown in Table 18.3.

Blood group compatibility

Transplantation in subjects with incompatible blood groups is generally avoided due to the risk of hyperacute rejection mediated by pre-formed anti-A or anti-B antibodies against the blood group antigens. Nevertheless, blood group incompatible kidney transplantation is technically possible nowadays with desensitization prior to transplantation and can achieve comparable patient and graft survival to blood group compatible transplants. Blood group incompatible renal transplantation can also confer a survival benefit in ESKD patients who do not have compatible live donors as they might otherwise face long waiting times for deceased donor kidneys.

Strategies to overcome incompatibility

Paired kidney exchange programme

Kidney paired donation refers to the matching of a potential kidney transplant recipient who has a willing but incompatible donor to another incompatible pair (Figure 18.4). Such an approach gives both recipients the chance to receive a compatible kidney. However, potential recipients who have blood group O or broad sensitization may have difficulty in finding a matched kidney.

Desensitization

This process involves the removal of antibodies against blood group antigens or HLA by plasmapheresis or immunoadsorption to achieve safe target titres, and depletion of B lymphocytes with anti-CD20

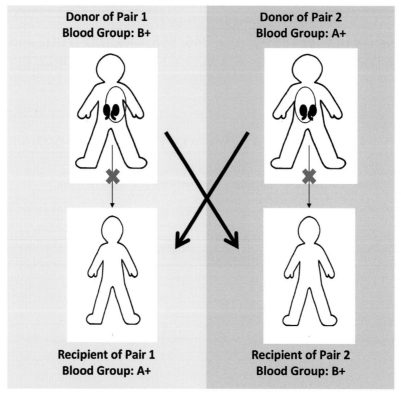

Figure 18.4: Paired kidney exchange. There are two pairs of kidney donors and recipients who have incompatible blood groups (Pair 1 and Pair 2). The recipient of Pair 1 receives the kidney allograft from the donor of Pair 2, who is ABO blood group-compatible, and vice versa.

treatment or splenectomy prior to transplantation. Desensitization presents a viable strategy for 'difficult-to-match' patients, but patients who have high initial antibody titres and high rebound titres early after transplant are at increased risk of rejection.

Immunosuppression in Kidney Transplantation

The use of immunosuppressive treatments is the cornerstone for preventing allograft rejection. Induction therapy, given at the time of kidney transplantation, aims to deplete or modulate T-cell responses upon alloantigen presentation. The use of induction agents can help reduce acute rejection and facilitate decreased exposure of concomitant immunosuppressants such as CNI or corticosteroids. Maintenance immunosuppression for kidney transplant recipients consists of a combination of immunosuppressive medications with different targets of action. A triple immunosuppressive regimen comprising corticosteroids, calcineurin inhibitor (e.g. tacrolimus), and an antimetabolite (e.g. mycophenolate) is commonly used for preventing rejection in kidney transplant recipients. The three-signal model of allo-recognition and T-lymphocyte activation provides a useful framework for understanding the mechanisms of action of immunosuppressive agents used in kidney transplantation (Table 18.4).

IL-2 receptor antagonist

Basiliximab is a monoclonal antibody against CD25 (IL-2 receptor α chain) which inhibits T-cell activation by blocking IL-2 engagement. While IL-2 receptor antagonist (IL-2RA) significantly reduces the risk of acute rejection and allograft loss, it shows little impact on all-cause mortality, malignancy, or cytomegalovirus (CMV) infection in renal transplant recipients. IL-2RA is generally well-tolerated and health-economic analysis also suggests that it is cost-effective in kidney transplant patients. The Kidney Disease: Improving Global Outcomes (KDIGO) guidelines recommend IL-2RA be used as the first-line induction therapy for kidney transplantation.

Table 18.4: Commonly used immunosuppressive agents in kidney transplantation

Site of action	Relevant immunosuppressive medications	Phase of use
Signal 1: Binding of TCR/CD3 complex on T-cell surface to the peptide/HLA complex on APCs		
CD3	• Lymphocyte-depleting antibodies: monoclonal (e.g. OKT3) or polyclonal (e.g. ATG, thymoglobulin)	Induction
Calcineurin	• Corticosteroids	Induction and maintenance
	• CNI: CYA, TAC	Maintenance
Signal 2: Non-antigens specific costimulatory signal by engagement of B7 on APCs with CD28 on T cells		
Co-stimulatory signal	• CTLA-4 Ig: Belatacept	Maintenance
Signal 3: Stimulation of IL-2 (CD25) leads to mTOR activation and cell proliferation		
IL-2 receptor	• IL-2RA: basiliximab	Induction
mTOR	• mTOR inhibitors: sirolimus, everolimus	Maintenance
Nucleotide synthesis	• Anti-metabolites: AZA, MPA	Maintenance

APCs, antigen-presenting cells; ATG, anti-thymocyte globulin; AZA, azathioprine; CNI, calcineurin inhibitors; CTLA-4 Ig: cytotoxic T-lymphocyte-associated protein 4 immunoglobulin; CYA, cyclosporine A; HLA, human leukocyte antigen; IL-2RA, IL-2 receptor antagonist; mTOR, mammalian target of rapamycin; MPA, mycophenolic acid; TAC, tacrolimus; TCR, T-cell receptor

Lymphocyte-depleting antibodies

These animal-derived biological agents can be monoclonal (e.g. OKT3) or polyclonal (e.g. antithymocyte globulin, thymoglobulin). They recognize lymphocyte (especially T cells) surface markers, and upon binding to these targets lead to paralysis or depletion of T lymphocytes. Adverse effects include fever, chills, arthralgia and leucopenia, and rarely cytokine release syndrome in which patients can develop fever, diarrhoea, and even potentially life-threatening complications such as bronchospasm and pulmonary oedema. With the advent of potent immunosuppressive agents such as mycophenolate and tacrolimus, OKT3 is rarely used for induction therapy nowadays. Lymphocyte-depleting antibodies remain a useful treatment for steroid-refractory acute cellular rejection or recurrent acute cellular rejections. Owing to their profound immunosuppressive actions, these lymphocyte-depleting therapies are associated with an increased risk of opportunistic infections and post-transplant lymphoproliferative disorders (PTLD).

Corticosteroids

Corticosteroids exert diverse effects on various immune-reactive cell types and their cytokine expressions, and are generally included in most immunosuppressive regimens for kidney transplantation. Intravenous pulses of corticosteroids are given as an initial treatment at the time of kidney transplantation and also as the first-line therapy for acute allograft rejections. Important side effects of corticosteroids include Cushingoid facies, acne, infections, diabetes mellitus, hypertension, hyperlipidaemia, reduced bone density, and neuropsychiatric complications (e.g. depression or psychosis). Many of these adverse effects are dose-dependent and elderly transplant patients are particularly susceptible. For instance, an increased risk of steroid myopathy has been observed in elderly patients. Corticosteroids minimization or withdrawal approaches may be considered in selected patients who are at low immunological risk and receive induction therapy with a biologic agent, but these patients need to be carefully monitored for allograft rejection.

Calcineurin inhibitor

The outcomes of kidney transplantation have improved considerably after the first calcineurin inhibitor (CNI), cyclosporin A (CYA), was introduced in the mid-1980s. While CYA and tacrolimus (TAC) are both commonly used CNIs, they are structurally unrelated agents that form complexes with cyclophilin and FK-binding protein (FKBP) respectively. They both inhibit calcineurin and thus the expression of cytokines (e.g. IL-2, IL-4, interferon-gamma and tumour necrosis factor-alpha) that are important for T-cell activation. With accumulating evidence suggesting its lower risk of acute rejection and better allograft outcomes compared with CYA, TAC has become the first-line CNI in many transplant centres around the world and also a rescue therapy in patients who develop rejection despite a therapeutic level of CYA being maintained. Therapeutic drug monitoring of CNI exposure in kidney transplant recipients is essential for ensuring adequate immunosuppression while minimizing the risk of nephrotoxicity and other potential side effects. In this context, a 12-hour (C12) blood level is commonly used for therapeutic drug monitoring of CNI exposure. The 2-hour (C2) blood level can also be checked in patients who are on CYA.

The pharmacokinetics of CNI can be significantly influenced by various concomitant medical conditions and drug-drug interactions. Both CYA and TAC are metabolized by cytochrome P450 CYP3A enzymes in the liver. Therefore, close monitoring of drug concentrations and sometimes pre-emptive dosage adjustments are required in patients with hepatic dysfunction and those receiving medications that affect P450 CYP3A enzymatic activity. For instance, blood levels of CNI can be substantially elevated in patients receiving erythromycin, ketoconazole, or diltiazem, but can be precipitously reduced in those taking rifampicin or phenytoin. Careful therapeutic drug monitoring of CNI is also indicated when patients present with conditions that affect gastrointestinal transit or absorption (e.g. diarrhoea or vomiting).

CNI-associated nephrotoxicity is an important concern for its use in renal transplant recipients and can be categorized as acute or chronic CNI nephrotoxicity. Acute CNI nephrotoxicity is associated with increased intra-renal vasoconstriction and decreased glomerular filtration rate. Such nephrotoxicity is often related to high blood levels and is largely reversible upon reduction of drug dosage. Histological findings of acute CNI nephrotoxicity include isometric vacuolization of proximal tubular cells and peritubular capillary congestion, and giant mitochondria can sometimes be seen ultrastructurally (Figure 18.5A). Chronic CNI is characterized by arterial hyalinosis and striped fibrosis (Figures 18.5B and C), and is very often irreversible and shows a less direct relationship with blood concentrations. Thrombotic microangiopathy is an uncommon but distinct form of CNI-induced endothelial toxicity. It can be systemic or limited to the kidney, and usually resolves with discontinuation of CNI. CYA and TAC often show different patterns of non-renal side effects. For instance, patients receiving CYA experience more cosmetic side effects (e.g. hirsutism and gingival hyperplasia) while patients receiving TAC have an increased risk of developing post-transplant diabetes and hand tremors. The common and important side effects of CYA and TAC are summarized in Table 18.5.

Table 18.5: Common and important side effects of calcineurin inhibitors

- Hypertension
- Hyperuricaemia
- Hyperkalaemia
- Hyperlipidaemia (CYA)
- Glucose intolerance and diabetes mellitus (TAC)
- Gingival hyperplasia and hirsutism (CYA)
- Alopecia (TAC)
- Hand tremors (TAC)

CYA, cyclosporine A; TAC, tacrolimus

Mycophenolate acid

Mycophenolate mofetil (MMF) is a prodrug that is hydrolysed into the active drug mycophenolate acid (MPA). Lymphocytes depend exclusively on *de novo* purine synthesis because they lack the salvage pathway. MPA inhibits inosine monophosphate dehydrogenase, the enzyme that is critical for the *de novo* purine synthesis pathway, and thereby selectively suppresses lymphocyte proliferation. MMF is associated with a lower risk of rejection compared with azathioprine (AZA), and is generally quite well-tolerated. The major side effects of MMF are haematological abnormalities (e.g. anaemia and leucopenia) and gastrointestinal disturbances (e.g. abdominal pain and diarrhoea). Enteric-coated mycophenolate sodium is another preparation of MPA whose immunosuppressive efficacy is comparable to MMF, and it is associated with slightly improved gastrointestinal tolerability. MPA has teratogenic potential and therefore female kidney transplant recipients of childbearing age receiving MPA should be reminded to adopt effective contraceptive measures. The C12 MPA level in patients on twice-daily MMF dosing has been shown to be a useful surrogate for MPA exposure, with good clinical correlations in kidney transplant recipients.

Azathioprine

Azathioprine (AZA) is metabolized in the liver to 6-mercaptopurine, which interrupts purine synthesis and hence DNA replication in lymphocytes. Side effects of AZA include marrow suppression

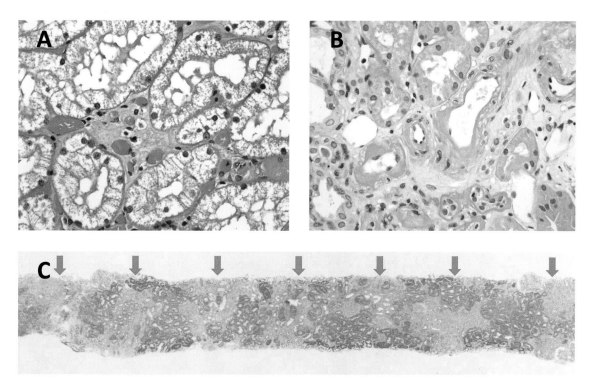

Figure 18.5: Calcineurin inhibitor toxicity. (A) The presence of isometric vacuolation in the tubular cells is commonly seen in acute phase of calcineurin inhibitor toxicity (H&E, ×400, Dr A. H. N. Tang). (B) Nodular hyaline deposition in the arterioles with extension into the tunica media is a characteristic finding of calcineurin inhibitor toxicity (PASD, ×400, Dr A. H. N. Tang). (C) Striped pattern fibrosis (arrows) is a characteristic feature of chronic calcineurin inhibitor toxicity, as shown in this low-power microscopic photo (Masson Trichrome, ×20, Dr A. H. N. Tang).

and hepatotoxicity. Thiopurine S-methyltransferase (TPMT) is an enzyme that is responsible for the metabolism of AZA, and hence patients with TPMT deficiency who receive AZA can develop life-threatening myelosuppression. Testing for TPMT deficiency with either genotyping or functional essays for this enzyme before initiation of AZA can help avoid this serious complication. AZA is eliminated both by the kidneys and liver through metabolic degradation by xanthine oxidase and thus the concomitant use of allopurinol can result in severe marrow suppression.

mTOR inhibitor

Sirolimus, also known as rapamycin, is a macrolide antibiotic that binds to FKBP. Unlike TAC, this complex acts on the mammalian target of rapamycin (mTOR) pathway (Signal Three), and thereby inhibits lymphocyte activation and proliferation. Everolimus is another mTOR inhibitor that is closely related to sirolimus chemically but with a shorter duration of action. mTOR inhibitor is an established treatment for the prevention of kidney transplant rejection, and can be used in combination with CNI or as a substitute for CNI in the early or late phases of transplantation. Owing to its antiproliferative and antitumour properties, mTOR inhibitors are often introduced in transplant recipients who have a history of malignancy. The commencement of mTOR inhibitors in patients with advanced allograft dysfunction or significant proteinuria, however, is not preferable. Therapeutic drug monitoring of sirolimus and everolimus are useful in dosage optimization. Common side effects of mTOR inhibitors include aphthous ulcers, dyslipidaemia (especially hypertriglyceridaemia), myelosuppression, lymphocele, and impaired wound healing. Non-infectious pneumonitis is also a rare complication.

Belatacept

Belatacept is a second-generation fusion protein composed of the Fc fragment of human IgG1 linked to the extracellular domain of CTLA-4, which selectively blocks the costimulatory signal that is essential for T-lymphocyte activation. Regular intravenous belatacept infusion can prevent rejection in kidney transplantation, and data from both *de novo* and conversion studies suggested that belatacept treatment was associated with superior kidney function and metabolic parameters compared with CNI-based regimens. Although belatacept has been approved by the FDA as a maintenance immunosuppressant in kidney transplantation since 2011, its routine use in kidney transplantation is limited by its high costs.

Kidney Transplantation: Operative and Early Post-Operative Management

Once the donor kidney is procured, it is important to have an appropriate organ preservation method to optimize the graft viability and quality under the condition of prolonged ischaemia. To date, the most commonly used graft kidney preservation method is static cold storage, i.e. to flush the graft kidney with a cold preservation solution (e.g. University of Wisconsin solution), and transport it in ice. Another organ preservation strategy is machine perfusion (MP). During MP, the graft kidney is connected to a perfusion device and the preservation solution is pumped continuously through the renal vasculature. MP can be further classified according to the temperature of the perfusate as hypothermic MP or normothermic MP. There is emerging evidence demonstrating the advantage of machine perfusion over static cold preservation in reducing delayed graft function and improve graft survival, particularly in DCD kidneys.

During kidney implantation, the renal allograft is placed in the iliac fossa. The graft renal artery is usually anastomosed end-to-side to the internal iliac artery while the graft renal vein is anastomosed end-to-side to the common iliac vein. The ureter is implanted into the bladder with the creation of a submucosal tunnel to prevent reflux.

Factors affecting renal allograft survival

The long-term survival of renal allografts is influenced by the following factors:

1. Donor factor: this indicates the quality of the donor kidney. Kidneys from live donors are associated with the best allograft survival, while renal allografts from ECD donors are associated with less favourable outcomes.
2. Recipient factor: fewer HLA mismatches are associated with better graft survival. Patients with high circulating levels of pre-formed antibodies against a wide panel of donors have a higher risk of rejection. Transplantation of kidney from children or small-built adults to recipients with large body size is associated with less favourable long-term allograft survival. Patients who have been dialysed for longer periods or have other comorbidities such as cardiovascular disease also have inferior outcomes.
3. Peri-operative factor: Ischaemic time refers to the time lapse between the cessation of circulation in the donor and the re-establishment of circulation in the recipient. The ischaemia and subsequent reperfusion cause injury to the graft kidney and are associated with delayed graft function in the immediate post-operative period.
4. Complications after transplantation: rejection, infection (e.g. BK polyomavirus), recurrence of disease in the graft kidney, and chronic allograft nephropathy adversely affect the renal allograft outcomes. These will be further elaborated in subsequent sections.

Complications of kidney transplantation

Surgical complications of kidney transplantation

Vascular complications

Graft renal artery thrombosis is a rare but serious complication. It can be caused by technical errors, thrombotic tendency, complicated anatomy (e.g. kidney with multiple vessels), or atherosclerotic arteries in donor or recipient. Clinical presentation varies from an acute reduction of urine output to complete anuria during the post-operative period. Graft renal vein thrombosis also occurs in the early post-operative period and can be caused by kinking of graft renal vein, stenosis of venous anastomosis, hypotension, hypercoagulable states, and acute rejection. A high index of suspicion is needed to identify these vascular complications and the diagnosis can be confirmed with Doppler ultrasound. Emergency thrombectomy is usually indicated but graft salvage is rarely successful. Transplant renal artery stenosis should be suspected if the renal allograft function is deteriorating without obvious reason, especially if the patient's blood pressure has become difficult to manage. Patients can first be screened with Doppler ultrasound, and suggestive cases can be confirmed by conventional or magnetic resonance angiography. Surgical revision of arterial anastomosis is preferred in the early post-operative period while balloon angioplasty can be attempted after one month post-transplantation.

Lymphocele

Lymphocele is a collection of lymphatic fluid that occurs adjacent to the kidney allograft after transplantation. Differential diagnoses of per-inephric collection after kidney transplantation include seroma, haematoma, and urinoma. Small, asymptomatic lymphocele is usually managed con-servatively. Image-guided percutaneous drainage will be required for a larger collection that causes obstruction/compression or partially occludes the transplant ureter or renal vein, and with associated renal allograft dysfunction or ipsilateral leg swelling. Fluid yielded from percutaneous drainage should be tested for chyle and creatinine, which can help distinguish the different types of perinephric collec-tions. Sclerotherapy or marsupialization should be considered in cases requiring repeated percutane-ous drainage.

Ureteric complication

Urine leakage can occur in the post-operative period while ureteric stenosis must always be excluded if a patient shows deterioration in renal allograft function.

Medical complications of kidney transplantation: Renal

Rejection

This should always be suspected in patients who show a rise in the serum creatinine level. The florid signs of fever, graft tenderness, and decreased urine output are often absent in the current era when most patients receive effective immunosuppressive treat-ments. Allograft biopsy remains the gold standard for diagnosis of graft rejection as clinical manifesta-tions can often be quite non-specific.

'Acute cellular rejection' is the consequence of an immune response after activation and proliferation of T cells. It occurs most commonly in the first few days to months after transplantation. Acute cellular rejec-tion is characterized by the presence of leucocyte (usually lymphocyte) infiltration of the interstitium and tubular epithelium (i.e. tubulitis) (Figures 18.6A and B), and sometimes accompanied by disruption of arterial intima (i.e. intimal arteritis, Figure 18.6C) on allograft biopsy. The mainstay of treatment for acute cellular rejection is pulse methylprednisolone.

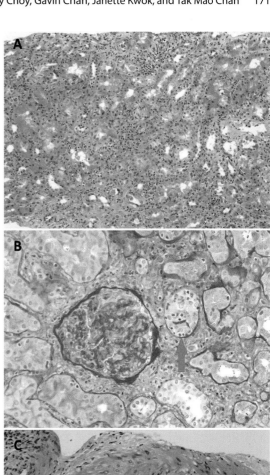

Figure 18.6: Acute cellular rejection. (A) There are scattered foci of interstitial inflammatory infiltrates comprising lymphocytes and plasma cells. Foci of tubu-litis are also noted (H&E, ×100, Dr G. S. W. Chan). (B) In addition to interstitial inflammation, tubulitis (arrow) is another characteristic feature of acute cellular rejec-tion (PASD, ×400, Dr G. S. W. Chan). (C) There is a small amount of lymphocytes in the intima of this arcuate artery, compatible with intimal arteritis. The presence of arteritis is not entirely specific to acute cellular rejec-tion, as it can also be seen in cases of antibody-medi-ated rejection (H&E, ×200, Dr G. S. W. Chan).

ATG or OKT3 may be used in patients who are refractory to pulse corticosteroids.

'Antibody-mediated rejection' (AMR) is caused by pathogenic antibodies that target donor HLA or ABO blood group antigens and, less commonly, a variety of non-HLA molecules. AMR can occur at any time after transplantation and its clinical presentation/prognosis can be quite variable (Table 18.6). Sensitized events that expose a patient to foreign HLAs such as prior transplantation, multiparity, and history of blood transfusion increase the risk of AMR. Diagnosis of AMR requires the presence of morphological evidence of tissue injury on allograft biopsy (Figures 18.7A to C), serological evidence of circulating antibodies to donor HLA or to other donor endothelial antigens, and immunopathologic evidence for antibody-mediated reactions (e.g. deposition of complement split product [C4d] in the peritubular capillaries, Figure 18.7D). Treatment of AMR includes plasmapheresis, intravenous immunoglobulin and anti-CD20 antibodies.

Chronic allograft nephropathy

Chronic allograft nephropathy (CAN) is a term used to describe progressive allograft dysfunction with histological evidence of interstitial fibrosis and tubular atrophy with non-specific cause identified. CAN remains one of the leading causes of graft loss in long-term kidney transplant recipients. Deteriorating renal function and proteinuria are the usual clinical presentations, although the condition can be subclinical and diagnosed only by allograft biopsy. The pathogenesis is multifactorial, and involves both immunological and non-immunological elements (Table 18.7).

Recurrent diseases in the graft kidney

Many forms of glomerulonephritis can recur in the graft kidney. The risk and timing of recurrence vary between different renal diseases. Focal segmental glomerulosclerosis (FSGS) may recur in the first few days to weeks after transplantation and can destroy the graft in a relatively short period of time. Recurrent FSGS may present as new-onset or aggravated proteinuria, often accompanied by worsening allograft function. Screening for urinary protein after kidney transplantation may allow early detection of FSGS recurrence, but allograft biopsy is generally required for definitive diagnosis. Recurrent membranous nephropathy occurs on average 10 months post-transplant and should be distinguished from de novo membranous GN, which usually occurs later and is the most common de novo glomerulopathy after transplantation. The incidence of recurrent IgA nephropathy can be up to 50–60% and its clinical presentations are similar to primary IgA nephropathy (e.g. microscopic haematuria, proteinuria, and slow decline in allograft function). Patients with ESKD due to lupus nephritis, anti-GBM disease, or ANCA-associated vasculitis should wait for the disease to become clinically quiescent before considering transplantation. In general, patients with crescentic forms of glomerulonephritis should not undergo transplantation within a year of the disease.

Table 18.6: The clinical characteristics and histological findings of the different types of antibody-mediated rejection

Types	Onset time	DSA involved	Histology	Clinical manifestations
Hyper-acute	• Within minutes to hours after transplantation	• Pre-existing DSA	• Vascular thrombosis and ischemic necrosis of graft kidney	• Infarction and even rupture of graft kidney, often leads to graft loss
Active	• Any time after transplantation	• Pre-existing or de novo DSA	• Microvascular inflammation (glomerulitis, peritubular capillaritis), intimal arteritis, acute tubular necrosis	• Rapid graft dysfunction
Chronic (active/ inactive)	• Months to years	• Mostly de novo DSA	• Transplant glomerulopathy, • PTC basement membrane multi-lamination • IFTA	• Slow but progressive loss of graft function, proteinuria, often difficult to control

DSA, donor-specific antibody; IFTA, interstitial fibrosis and tubular atrophy; PTC, peritubular capillary

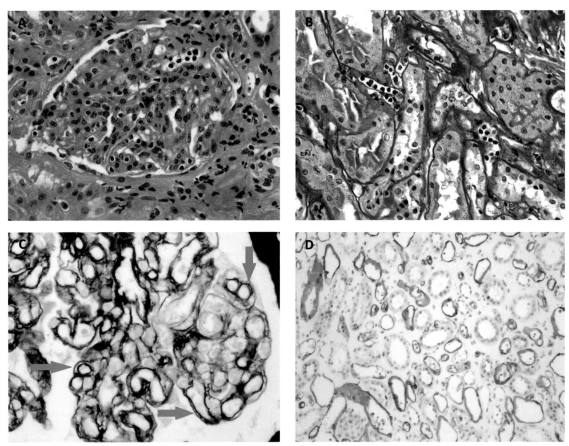

Figure 18.7: Antibody-mediated rejection. (A) Lymphocytes are present in multiple capillary loops in this glomerulus, a histologic feature known as glomerulitis (H&E, ×400, Dr G. S. W. Chan). (B) Lymphocytes are present in the peritubular capillaries, a histologic feature known as peritubular capillaritis. It is commonly seen in antibody-mediated rejection (PASD, ×400, Dr G. S. W. Chan). (C) Transplant glomerulopathy. Frequent double-contouring of GBM is identified in the glomerulus (arrow). This is commonly seen in chronic tissue injury of antibody-mediated rejection (PASM, ×400, Dr G. S. W. Chan). (D) Immunopathologic evidence of antibody-mediated rejection is confirmed by the presence of C4d immunostaining along the peritubular capillaries (Anti-C4d immunohistochemistry, ×200, Dr A. H. N. Tang).

Table 18.7: Immunological and non-immunological factors for chronic allograft nephropathy

Immunological
- HLA mismatches
- Sensitization
- Acute/chronic rejection

Non-immunological
- Donor factors (age, donor comorbidity)
- Ischemic reperfusion injury
- Infection
- CNI nephrotoxicity

CNI, calcineurin inhibitor; HLA, human leukocyte antigen

Other medical complications after kidney transplantation

Infection

Infection is an important cause of morbidity and mortality in kidney transplant recipients. The type and severity of the infection are influenced by patient and surgical factors, degree of immunosuppression, time after transplantation, local epidemiology of pathogens, and the use of antimicrobial prophylaxis. Bacterial infections involving the urinary and respiratory tracts as well as surgical wounds are common in the immediate post-operative period. Urinary tract infection is the most common bacterial infection requiring hospitalization in kidney transplant recipients. Complications of graft pyelonephritis such as abscess formation and emphysematous pyelonephritis generally require drainage and more prolonged courses of antimicrobial treatment.

CMV infection is the most common opportunistic infection in kidney transplant recipients. It can occur as a primary infection, reinfection, or reactivation of latent infection. Risk factors include donor seropositivity (especially if the recipient is seronegative) and the use of induction agents such as lymphocyte-depleting antibodies. CMV infection is defined as evidence of CMV replication regardless of symptoms, while CMV disease refers to CMV infection in the presence of clinical manifestations such as fever, malaise, leucopenia, thrombocytopenia, or evidence of tissue invasion (e.g. gastrointestinal tract ulcers, hepatitis, pneumonitis, and retinitis). The development of CMV infection has a negative impact on patient and renal graft survival. Measurement of viral load by polymerase chain reactions (PCRs) or CMV pp65 antigen levels are useful means for diagnosis and monitoring of CMV infection. CMV PCR is highly sensitive and a negative result virtually excludes CMV infection. The CMV pp65 antigenaemia level often correlates with disease manifestations and can be used to monitor treatment response. Histologic confirmation may be required for diagnosis, especially for those with gastrointestinal disease. Oral valgancicovir can be used to treat patients with mild CMV infections, but intravenous ganciclovir is generally required for patients with high viral loads or tissue invasions. Intravenous foscarnet can be given as rescue therapy in patients with ganciclovir resistance. Oral valganciclovir prophylaxis is indicated in patients with a high risk of CMV disease/reactivation (e.g. transplantation from a seropositive donor to a seronegative recipient, or recipients receiving lymphocyte-depleting antibodies).

BK polyomavirus (BKV) belongs to the polyoma family of viruses that are associated with the development of nephropathy in kidney transplant recipients. In most patients, BKV nephropathy manifests as renal allograft dysfunction, while some also develop ureteric obstruction from stenosis or stricture. Detection of BKV DNA in plasma is a sensitive method for identifying BKV infection, and BKV nephropathy can be confirmed by histology (Figure 18.8 A to C). Histological findings of BKV nephropathy, however, may sometimes closely resemble that of acute rejection. Identification of virus-infected cells and a positive immunohistochemical staining for SV40 can help to distinguish BKV nephropathy from rejection. There is no proven antiviral therapy

for BKV, and the mainstay of treatment is the judicious reduction of overall immunosuppression.

Chronic HBV infection is associated with excess patient mortality in kidney transplant recipients. HBV reactivation after kidney transplantation can result in serious complications such as fulminant hepatitis or fibrosing cholestatic hepatitis. HBsAg-positive kidney transplant recipients are also at increased risk of long-term complications such as cirrhosis or hepatocellular carcinoma (HCC). Wait-listed patients should receive HBV vaccination prior to kidney transplantation. The HBV status of the recipient and donor should be carefully assessed before transplantation for risk stratification. Antiviral therapy has significantly improved the short- and long-term clinical outcomes of HBsAg-positive kidney transplant recipients, and therefore should be initiated for kidney transplant recipients who are at risk for de novo HBV infection or HBV reactivation. In this context, entecavir is the treatment of choice because of its potent antiviral activity, low rates of resistance, and favourable safety profile. Tenofovir-based antivirals are associated with some nephrotoxic potential and so are often reserved for cases with lamivudine-resistance. The newer agent tenfovir alafenamide has an improved safety profile and is better tolerated in kidney transplant recipients. Serial HBV DNA levels should be monitored to assess for treatment response and development of viral resistance. HBsAg-positive kidney transplant recipients should undergo surveillance for HCC through regular alpha-fetoprotein (AFP) and liver ultrasonography.

HCV is associated with the development of glomerulonephritis, post-transplant diabetes mellitus (PTDM), and accelerated liver cirrhosis after kidney transplantation. Kidney transplant recipients with HCV infections usually show inferior patient and allograft survival compared with those who are not infected with HCV. In the past, pegylated interferon and ribavirin were the standard treatments for HCV infection. However, interferon is associated with an increased risk of allograft dysfunction and rejection while ribavirin is generally contraindicated in renal failure due to the risk of haemolytic anaemia. The introduction of safe and highly effective DAA-based interferon-free regimens has changed the landscape of HCV treatment in kidney transplant recipients. Timing of treatment (before or after transplantation) is tailored to the individual patient and the choice of DAA regimen in kidney transplant recipients depends on the HCV genotype, presence or absence of decompensated cirrhosis, and the renal allograft function. Measurement of HCV RNA can help monitor

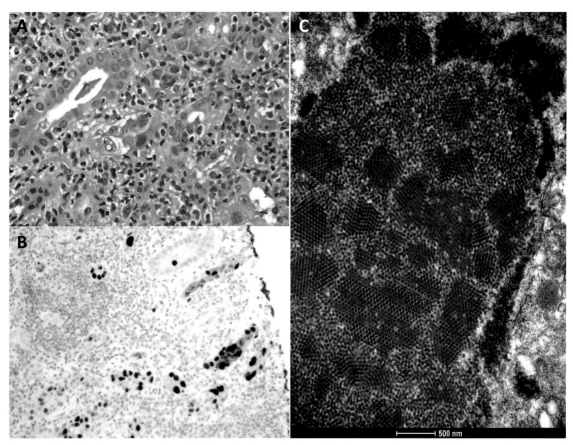

Figure 18.8: BK virus nephropathy. (A) The tubular epithelial cells display viral cytopathic changes characterized by nuclear enlargement, chromatin margination, and ground-glass nuclei (H&E, ×400, Dr A. H. N. Tang). (B) The presence of polyoma virus infection is confirmed by immunohistochemical staining for SV40, which is positive in the tubular epithelial cells (Anti-SV40 immunohistochemistry, ×400, Dr A. H. N. Tang). (C) Electron microscopy shows the presence of intranuclear viral particles in tubular epithelial cells (transmission electron microscopy, ×20000, Dr G. S. W. Chan).

treatment response and document viral eradication after completion of DAA therapy. Regular AFP and ultrasound surveillance for HCC should also be performed in kidney transplant recipients with HCV infections.

Pneumocystis jiroveci (previously known as *pneumocystis carinii*) is a potentially life-threatening infection in kidney transplant recipients, especially in the first six months after transplantation. Common clinical presentations of *pneumocystis jiroveci* pneumonia (PJP) include fever and dyspnoea. Chest radiography can be normal or show diffuse bilateral interstitial infiltrates. Cotrimoxazole (for 6–12 months) is the preferred prophylactic agent, while inhaled pentamidine can be used for patients who are intolerant or allergic to cotrimoxazole. Diagnosis depends on the identification of the organism in sputum, bronchoalveolar lavage, or transbronchial

biopsy samples. Optimal treatments of PJP include high-dose cotrimoxazole or intravenous pentamidine. The glucose-6 phosphate dehydrogenase status should be determined before commencing cotrimoxazole to avoid severe haemolysis.

Mycobacterium tuberculosis (TB) remains one of the major post-transplant infections and disseminated disease or extra-pulmonary involvements are not uncommon. Detection of *M. tuberculosis* in culture from clinical specimens, demonstration of caseating granuloma in a histologic examination, detection of *M. tuberculosis* DNA using PCR, and chest radiography are the diagnostic tests of choice. Interferon-gamma release assays may give false negative results in kidney transplant recipients. Rifampicin treatment leads to a precipitous fall of CNI and mTOR-inhibitor blood levels. Therefore, the dose of these immunosuppressive medications should be increased at the time of starting rifampicin and their blood levels must be closely monitored. Kidney transplant recipients suffering from TB infections may require prolonged treatment, very often for up to one year or more.

Fungal infections can occur in many different forms in kidney transplant recipients. Oral candidiasis is common and can be prevented with oral nystatin. Invasive fungal infections can also occur in kidney transplant patients, commonly in patients receiving potent immunosuppressive treatments or after antirejection therapy. *Candida* and *Cryptococcus* species are the most frequently isolated yeasts, while most frequent filamentous fungi (moulds) isolated are *Aspergillus* species. Choice of antifungal agents should take into consideration the expected pathogen, site of infection, renal toxicity, and potential for drug interactions. Amphotericin B is highly effective for most medically important fungal species (e.g. *Candida*, *Aspergillus*, and *Cryptococcus species*), but its substantial nephrotoxicity remains an important concern in kidney transplant patients. Liposomal amphotericin B, with relatively fewer renal side effects, is an efficacious but expensive alternative in kidney transplant recipients. Azole derivatives (e.g. fluconazole, voriconazole) are also active against many medically important fungal species, but these agents inhibit CYP450 enzymatic activity and thus significantly increase CNI drug levels. Echinocandins (e.g. micafungin, caspofungin, and anidulafungin) are not associated with nephrotoxicity and have relatively few drug interactions with immunosuppressive agents, and thus are gaining popularity as a treatment for invasive fungal infections in renal transplant patients.

Cancer

Cancer emerges as a major cause of death among patients suffering from ESKD, especially after kidney transplantation. There has been a two- to threefold increase in the overall incidence of neoplasm in kidney transplant recipients when compared with age- and gender-matched general population but the magnitude of cancer risk varies by cancer site. The elevated risk of neoplasm is a composite of the known risk factors for cancer in the general population, cumulative exposure to immunosuppressive treatments, and infections by oncogenic viruses. Certain malignancies, such as renal cell carcinoma and urinary tract cancers, are related to the duration of ESKD. Oncogenic viruses are associated with post-transplant malignancies, and important examples include Epstein–Barr virus (Hodgkin's or

non-Hodgkin's lymphoma and nasopharyngeal carcinoma), human papillomavirus (cancers of the cervix, anus, penis, vulva, vagina, and oropharyngeal cancer), human herpes virus 8 (Kaposi's sarcoma), HBV, and HCV (hepatocellular carcinoma). PTLD represents a heterogeneous group of lymphoid and plasmacytic proliferative diseases, occurring as a result of immunosuppressive therapy, and is one of the most common cancers in kidney transplant recipients. The use of lymphocyte-depleting antibodies has been found to be associated with a higher risk of PTLD/lymphoma, although the overall risk of cancer appears to be related to the cumulative exposure of immunosuppressive medications rather than individual components of the drug regimen. The mainstay of treatment for post-transplant cancers, especially those related to immunosuppressed status (e.g. non-Hodgkin's lymphoma and Kaposi's sarcoma), is the judicious reduction of immunosuppression. Cancer surveillance facilitates early detection of tumours and may potentially improve the clinical outcomes of kidney transplant recipients, and screening guidelines adopted in the general population have been used as the reference.

Cardiovascular disease

Kidney transplant recipients remain at higher risk of cardiovascular disease (CVD)-related mortality and morbidity compared to the general population. CVD is also the leading cause of death in kidney transplant recipients with a functioning allograft, and important risk factors include:

1. Hypertension: In addition to pre-existing hypertension, transplant-related factors such as kidney allograft dysfunction, vascular pathology, and immunosuppressive drugs such as steroids and CNI all contribute to the pathogenesis of *de novo* hypertension after kidney transplantation.
2. Post-transplantation diabetes mellitus (PTDM): The development of PTDM and worsening of pre-existing diabetes is a major cardiovascular risk factor after kidney transplantation. Corticosteroids, CNI and mTOR inhibitors are all associated with an increased propensity for PTDM. In this context, TAC shows a higher risk of PTDM than CYA and mTOR inhibitors.
3. Dyslipidaemia: Dyslipidaemia is common after kidney transplantation, which can be aggravated by obesity, PTDM, proteinuria, and certain immunosuppressive medications (e.g. corticosteroids and mTOR inhibitors).

Mineral and bone disorders

With a longstanding history of chronic kidney disease, kidney transplant recipients are still vulnerable to persistent hyperparathyroidism and mineral and bone disorder (MBD). Contributing factors of MBD in kidney transplant recipients include pre-existing renal osteodystrophy, transplantation-related therapies, and chronic allograft dysfunction. Other important bone disorders that affect kidney transplant recipients include osteoporosis and osteonecrosis (avascular necrosis). Osteoporosis increases the risk of fractures in renal transplant patients and is mainly related to the long-term use of glucocorticoids, but may also reflect changes associated with prior renal osteodystrophy. A DEXA scan helps predict fracture risk in kidney transplant recipients. Kidney transplant recipients should receive the lowest possible dose of maintenance corticosteroids to reduce the risk of osteoporosis while preventing rejection. Patients with normal serum calcium should receive calcium and vitamin D supplements, and those with osteoporosis and no evidence of low-turnover bone disease can be managed with antiresorptive therapies such as bisphosphonates. Denosumab is an alternative option in patients with osteoporosis and low GFR.

Erythrocytosis

Post-transplant erythrocytosis (PTE) is defined as a haemoglobin concentration >17 g/dL and/or haematocrit >51% that occurs after kidney transplantation, persists for more than six months, and occurs in the absence of another underlying cause. It can occur in up to 8–15% of kidney transplant recipients. Kidney transplant recipients with PTE may develop thromboembolic events that involve both veins and arteries (e.g. stroke, deep vein thrombosis, or pulmonary embolism). Treatment with renin-angiotensin blocking agents may be beneficial.

19

Drugs, Toxins, and the Kidneys

Becky Ma, Davina Lie, Shing Yeung, Siu Fai Cheung, Patrick Siu Chung Leung, Sik Hon Tsui, and Desmond Yap

Introduction

The prescription of drugs is an important but often challenging issue in clinical practice. On the one hand, patients with renal insufficiency show impaired handling of drugs and therefore are at increased risk of the adverse effects of medications. On the other hand, some pharmacological agents have nephrotoxic potential and often constitute an important cause of iatrogenic acute and/or chronic renal impairment. This chapter highlights the principles and pitfalls of prescription in renal failure, the effect of drugs on the kidneys as well as the approach in renal toxicology and extracorporeal removal of these toxic compounds.

Drug Prescription and the Kidneys

Pharmacokinetics of drugs in renal failure

The pharmacokinetics of a drug is influenced by absorption, distribution, metabolism, and elimination (Figure 19.1). Alterations in these pharmacokinetic processes have been observed in patients with renal failure, rendering them more susceptible to the adverse effects of medications. In this context, gastrointestinal absorption of drugs is diminished in nephrotic patients with gut oedema or severely uraemic patients with repeated vomiting. Drug absorption in patients with chronic kidney disease (CKD) is also affected by the frequent use of concomitant medications that interfere with gastric absorption. For example, in CKD patients receiving phosphate binders can interfere with the absorption of aspirin, digoxin, and quinolones.

Furthermore, first-pass hepatic metabolism is also impaired in patients with significant azotaemia, resulting in increased bioavailability of certain drugs. Patients with CKD or nephrotic syndrome also show abnormalities in drug distribution, often related to hypoalbuminaemia and changes in total body water. Drugs that are highly protein-bound (e.g. warfarin and penicillin) are especially affected by hypoalbuminaemia, as decreased protein-binding of these agents increases the free fraction of drugs, thereby enhancing pharmacological or untoward effects. Fluid retention in CKD patients can increase the volume of distribution (Vd) of medications, resulting in lower plasma concentration of drugs.

The kidneys are a major site of drug elimination, and involves various processes including glomerular filtration, drug metabolism as well as tubular secretion and reabsorption. Water-soluble drugs are directly excreted through the kidneys, while lipophilic drugs often need to be metabolized into hydrophilic molecules before they can be excreted. Normally, the kidneys take part in oxidative, reductive, hydrolytic reactions (collectively known as phase I reactions), and conjugative reactions (phase II reactions). Once filtered, drugs are reabsorbed from the renal tubular lumen back to the bloodstream by passive diffusion, the extent depending on the lipophilic properties, urine flow and the state of ionization. Active renal tubular secretion is important for drugs that are highly protein-bound. Patients with reduced glomerular filtration rates (GFRs) show impaired glomerular filtration and metabolism of medications, leading to excessive accumulation of drugs and their metabolites.

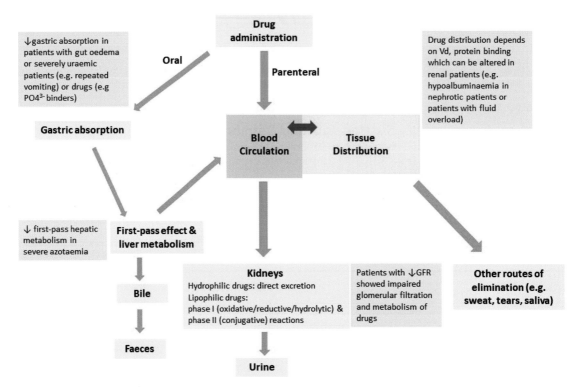

Figure 19.1: Schematic diagram showing the pharmacokinetic processes of drug handling and the processes that are affected in patients with renal impairment
GFR, glomerular filtration rate; Vd, volume of distribution

Principles of drug prescription in patients with renal impairment

Careful drug prescription is of paramount importance in patients with renal impairment. The clinical indications should be carefully reviewed and possible alternatives considered if one plans to use potentially nephrotoxic medications. Drugs with known nephrotoxic potential are best avoided in patients with CKD or during acute kidney injury (AKI). Drugs that depend substantially on renal clearance require dosage modification in patients with renal insufficiency. Renal adjustment of dosage generally can be achieved by reducing individual doses or the frequency of administration, depending on the characteristics of the drug. In clinical practice, physicians follow drug modification guidelines that are based on measurements of GFR. Examples of commonly used drugs in clinical practice and their dosage modifications and precautions in renal failure patients are listed in Table 19.1. Therapeutic monitoring of blood concentrations of some drugs (e.g. vancomycin, aminoglycosides) can help ensure treatment efficacy and minimize side effects. Dosage modification in

patients with renal impairment should also take into consideration the body size and composition, drug bioavailability, protein-and-tissue binding properties, drug-drug interactions, and pharmacogenomics variations.

Dialytic clearance of drugs

The elimination of drugs presents a significant challenge in patients receiving dialysis. The dialytic clearance of medications is determined by both drug properties (e.g. molecular size, extent of protein binding, Vd, and water solubility) and the delivery of dialysis (e.g. mode of dialysis, regimen, and membrane characteristics). In this context, the clearance of pharmacological agents in haemodialysis (HD) is dependent on the pore size of the dialyser as well as the blood and dialysate flow rates. Medications with lower molecular weights and protein-binding tend to be more readily removed by HD, and therefore supplementary doses are often required after an HD session. For patients receiving peritoneal dialysis (PD), elimination of drugs is generally poor, although medications with small

Table 19.1: Dosage adjustment and precautions for prescription of some commonly used drugs in patients with renal impairment

Drugs	Adjustments and precautions in renal impairment
Anti-arrhythmic agents	
• Amiodarone	• No dosage adjustment required
• Digoxin	• Dosage reduction depends on CrCl; consider alternative therapy in case of acute renal failure
Anti-coagulants	
• LMWH (e.g. enoxaparin, tinzaparin)	• Dosage reduction depends on CrCl
• Novel oral anticoagulants (NOACs)	• Apixaban: least dependent on renal excretion among different NOACs; avoid use in CrCl < 25 mL/min • Dabigatran, edoxaban, rivaroxaban: avoid use in CrCl < 30 mL/min
• Unfractionated heparin	• No dosage adjustment required; adjust dosage according to aPTT or anti-factor Xa activity
• Warfarin	• No dosage adjustment required • Patients with severe renal impairment have increased bleeding risk; INR should be monitored closely
Anticonvulsants	
• Gabapentin, levetiracetam, pregabalin	• Dosage reduction depends on CrCl
• Carbamazepine	• Increased risk of toxicity in moderate to severe kidney dysfunction • Consider measuring serum carbamazepine epoxide levels
• Phenytoin	• Monitoring of free (unbound) concentration is recommended
Antihistamines	
• Chlorpheniramine	• No renal adjustment required
• 2nd generation antihistamines (e.g. loratadine, cetirizine)	• Increase dosing interval with declining CrCl
• Metoclopramide	• Dosage reduction depends on CrCl
Antihypertensives	
• ACEIs (e.g. lisinopril, perindopril, ramipril, enalapril, captopril)	• Dosage reduction depends on CrCl
• ARBs (e.g. losartan, valsartan, irbesartan, candesartan)	• No dosage adjustment required
• Beta-blockers	• Avoid long-acting beta-blockers (e.g. atenolol) in severe renal impairment • Dosage reduction generally not required for other beta-blockers
• CCBs (e.g. amlodipine, felodipine, verapamil)	• No dosage adjustment required
Anti-inflammatory agents and analgesics	
• Aspirin	• No dosage adjustment required
• NSAIDs (e.g. indomethacin, COX-2 inhibitors)	• Review clinical indications and consider other alternatives in patients with risk of renal impairment • Avoid use in eGFR < 30 mL/min/1.73 m^2
• Paracetamol	• No dosage adjustment required although accumulation of inactive glucuronide/sulfate conjugates with unknown clinical significance
Antimicrobial agents	
Antibacterial agents	
• Aminoglycosides	• Renal clearance is the main route of elimination • Use with caution and require significant dosage reduction in patients with renal impairment • Therapeutic drug monitoring is recommended
• Carbapenems	• Dosage reduction according to CrCl
• Cephalosporins	• Need renal dosage adjustment except for cefoperazone and ceftriaxone

182

Table 19.1 (continued)

Drugs	Adjustments and precautions in renal impairment
• Cloxacillin	• No dosage adjustment required
• Doxycycline	• No dosage adjustment required
• Penicillins	• Dose adjustment depends on CrCl, especially when large doses are used
• Linezolid	• No dosage adjustment required
• Macrolides	• Dosage reduction in clarithromycin depends on CrCl; no dosage adjustment for erythromycin and azithromycin • Beware of QTC prolongation in renal failure patients
• Metronidazole	• Metabolites may accumulate in severe renal impairment; monitor for adverse events
• Nitrofurantoin	• Avoid use in patients with renal impairment
• Quinolones	• Dosage reduction depends on CrCl except for moxifloxacin and gatifloxacin which require no adjustment
• Sulfamethoxazole-trimethoprim	• Dosage reduction depends on CrCl; avoid use in severe renal impairment
• Tetracycline	• Avoid use in renal impairment
• Vancomycin	• Requires significant dosage reduction in patients with renal impairment • Serum trough concentration should be monitored with parenteral use • Dialysis: High-flux membranes and CRRT increase clearance, require replacement dosing
Antifungal agents	
• Amphotericin B	• Monitor renal function, as well as K and Mg levels in patients receiving amphotericin B • Consider liposomal formulation (AmBisome) if no alternative
• Azoles (e.g. Fluconazole, 5-Flucytosine, ketoconazole, fluconazole, itraconazole, voriconazole, posaconazole)	• Dosage reduction required
• Echinocandin (e.g. caspofungin, micafungin, anidulafungin)	• Dosage reduction required
Antituberculous agents	
• Ethambutol • Pyrazinamide • Streptomycin	• Dosage reduction depends on CrCl
• Isoniazid	• Mild dosage adjustment generally required, although the main route of clearance is hepatic • Increase risk of neurotoxicity and high-dose supplemental pyridoxine required in patients with renal impairment
• Rifampicin	• Mild dosage adjustment generally required, although the main route of clearance is hepatic • Has multiple significant drug–drug interactions in renal patients (e.g. CNI or mTOR inhibitors)
Antiviral agents	
• Acyclovir	• Dosage reduction depends on CrCl • Monitor renal function closely and watch out for neurotoxicity
• Antihepadnavirals (e.g. lamivudine, telbivudine, entecavir, tenofovir)	• Dosage reduction depends on CrCl
• Ganciclovir, valganciclovir, foscarnet	• Dosage reduction depends on CrCl
• Oseltamivir	• Dosage reduction depends on CrCl
Diuretics	
• Hydrochlorothiazides	• Use with CrCl < 10 mL/min not recommended. Usually ineffective with CrCl < 30 mL/min unless used in combination with a loop diuretic
• Loop diuretics (e.g. furosemide)	• Doses up to 1 – 3 g daily may be necessary for desired diuretic response
• Potassium-sparing diuretics	• Avoid in advanced renal failure

Table 19.1 (continued)

Drugs	Adjustments and precautions in renal impairment
Drugs for asthma	
• Beta-2 receptor agonist	• No dosage adjustment required
• Phosphodiesterase inhibitor	• No dosage adjustment required
Gastric protective agents	
• H2 receptor antagonists	• Dosage reduction depends on CrCl
• PPI	• Generally require no dosage adjustment (esomeprazole not recommended in severe renal impairment)
Lipid lowering agents	
• Ezetimibe	• No dosage adjustment required
• Gemfibrozil and clofibrate	• Dosage reduction required
• Statins	• Atorvastatin and fluvastatin do not require dose adjustment in CKD and are the statins of choice in patients with severe renal impairment. Other statins usually require dosage reduction
Oral hypoglycemic agents	
• Acarbose	• Avoid use eGFR < 30 mL/min/1.73 m^2
• Biguanide: Metformin	• Contraindicated in eGFR < 30 mL/min/1.73 m^2 • Dosage adjustment in between eGFR < 30 – 45 mL/min/1.73 m^2 • May precipitate severe metabolic acidosis in patients with significant renal impairment
• DDP-4 inhibitors	• Dosage reduction generally required except for linagliptin
• GLP-1 receptor agonists	• Liraglutide and dulaglutide should be used with caution in renal impairment • Exenatide and lixisenatide contraindicated in eGFR < 30 mL/min/1.73 m^2 • No dosage adjustment required for semaglutide
• SGLT2 inhibitors	• Empagliflozin: contraindicated when eGFR < 30 mL/min/1.73 m^2 • Canagliflozin: no dosage adjustment if eGFR > 60 mL/min/1.73 m^2; contraindicated when eGFR < 30 mL/min/1.73 m^2 • Dapagliflozin: No dosage adjustment if eGFR > 45 mL/min/1.73 m^2. Contraindicated in eGFR < 30 mL/min/1.73 m^2
• Sulphonylurea	• Avoid long-acting sulphonylurea; dosage reduction generally required
Psychotropic agents, tranquilizers, and sedatives	
• Diazepam	• No adjustment required but should be used with caution
• Haloperidol	• No dosage adjustment required
• Lorazepam	• No dosage adjustment for oral form or parenteral acute doses; risk of propylene glycol toxicity with repeated dosing
• Morphine	• No specific dosage adjustment but active metabolite may accumulate, causing severe and prolonged respiratory depression
• Pethidine	• Avoid use in renal impairment
Xanthine-oxidase inhibitors	
• Allopurinol	• Dosage reduction depending on CrCl. Allopurinol and azathioprine should not be co-prescribed as this may result in fatal myelosuppression
• Febuxostat	• Dosage reduction depending on CrCl

ACEI, angiotensin-converting enzyme inhibitor; ARB, angiotensin receptor blocker; CCB, calcium channel blocker; CKD, chronic kidney disease; CNI, calcineurin inhibitor; COX-2, cyclooxygenase 2; CrCl, creatinine clearance; CRRT, continuous renal replacement therapy; DDP-4, dipeptidyl peptidase-4; eGFR, estimated glomerular filtration rate; GLP-1, glucagon-like peptide 1; LMWH, low molecular weight heparin; mTOR, mammalian target of rapamycin; NOAC, novel oral anticoagulant; NSAIDs, nonsteroidal anti-inflammatory drugs; PPI, proton-pump inhibitor; SGLT2, sodium-glucose co-transporter 2 molecular sizes and high protein-binding capacities may exhibit a slight advantage in clearance.

Effects of Drugs on the Kidney

Drug toxicity is an important cause of AKI, CKD, and renal tubular disorders. Most drugs that cause renal dysfunction have their distinct mechanisms of insult, although some medications may have multiple deleterious effects on the kidneys. The following overview will highlight the various nephrotoxic agents and their putative mechanisms to cause renal abnormalities.

Drugs that cause alterations in renal haemodynamics

Both nonsteroidal anti-inflammatory drugs (NSAIDs) and cyclo-oxygenase 2 (COX2) inhibitors inhibit the activity of cyclo-oxygenase enzymes involved in vasodilatory prostaglandins synthesis, thereby leading to intra-renal vasoconstriction and a decrease in GFR. Exposure to high concentrations of calcineurin inhibitors (CNIs) can lead to vasoconstriction and acute CNI toxicity.

Drugs that cause renal vascular endothelial injury

Antiplatelet agents (e.g. clopidogrel and ticlopidine), CNI, chemotherapeutic agents (e.g. mitomycin, gemcitabine), immunotherapy (e.g. alemtuzumab, apolizumab), anti-VEGF agents (e.g. bevacizumab), and tyrosine kinase inhibitors (e.g. imatinib) can cause direct endothelial injury, resulting in systemic or renal thrombotic microangiopathy (TMA).

Drugs that cause direct renal tubular toxicity

Aminoglycoside is the prototypic class of drugs that cause acute tubular necrosis (ATN). Aminoglycosides interfere with lysosomal protein synthesis and the mitochondrial function of proximal renal tubular cells, thereby inducing cell apoptosis. Vancomycin can cause ATN by mechanisms similar to aminoglycosides, but in addition can form casts with uromodulin to cause renal tubular obstruction. Colistin increases the permeability of renal tubular epithelial cells, leading to cellular swelling and apoptosis. Amphotericin B and ifosfamide can cause both direct renal tubular toxicity and distal renal tubular

acidosis (RTA). Cisplatin nephrotoxicity often manifests non-oliguric AKI and is related to direct injury to nuclear and mitochondrial DNA accompanied by activation of multiple apoptotic and inflammatory pathways in renal tubular epithelial cells. Isometric vacuolization of proximal renal tubules is observed with the administration of osmotic diuretics (e.g. mannitol) or IVIG with sorbitol.

Drugs that cause immune-mediated tubulointerstitial nephritis and glomerulopathies

Drugs are the leading cause of acute interstitial nephritis (AIN). Common offending agents include antibiotics (e.g. beta-lactams, sulphonamides, and rifampicin), NSAIDs, allopurinol, and proton-pump inhibitors (PPI) (Table 19.2). Chronic interstitial nephritis (CIN) can be caused by cyclosporine, lithium, Chinese herbs containing aristolochic acid (AA), and chronic analgesics consumption (e.g. paracetamol, NSAIDs, and phenacetin). CIN usually presents with insidious onset of renal impairment without overt signs of hypersensitivity.

A number of agents used to treat rheumatoid arthritis have been implicated in the development of membranous nephropathy, including NSAIDs, gold, penicillamine, and antitumour necrosis factor (anti-TNF) treatments. Exposure to bisphosphonates (specifically pamidronate and alendronate) is associated with collapsing focal segmental glomerulosclerosis (FSGS). ANCA-associated glomerulonephritis has been reported in patients receiving antithyroid medications (e.g. propylthiouracil and carbimazole) and anti-TNF therapy. There is growing application of immune checkpoint inhibitors (ICPIs) to treat malignancies, and these agents can induce AIN and various forms of glomerulonephritis (GN) (see below).

Drugs that cause intra-renal obstruction

Some antiviral medications (e.g. acyclovir, adefovir, tenofovir, indinavir, foscarnet) and antifungal agents can precipitate in the renal tubular lumen, leading to crystal nephropathy. Methotrexate, particularly in high doses, can precipitate within renal tubular lumens to cause AKI. In patients with high tumour loads, especially those with haematological malignancies, the administration of chemotherapy or CAR-T cell therapy may result in tumour lysis syndrome and AKI due to intra-tubular uric acid or

Table 19.2: Drugs that commonly cause acute interstitial nephritis

Antimicrobials	Analgesics	Anticonvulsants	Diuretics	Others
β-lactams	*NSAIDs*	*Phenytoin*	*Furosemide*	*Allopurinol*
Fluoroquinolones	*COX2-inhibitors*	Carbamazepine	Hydrochlorothiazide	*Proton pump inhibitors*
Sulphonamides	Aminopyrine	Phenobarbital	Indapamide	*H2 receptor antagonists*
Rifampicin		Valproate		Cyclosporine
Erythromycin		Diazepam		Captopril
Vancomycin				Interferon
Minocycline				Carbimazole
Nitrofurantoin				Propranolol
Colistin				Fenofibrate
Ethambutol				Warfarin
Abacavir				Aspirin
Indinavir				
Atazanavir				
Acyclovir				

COX-2, cyclo-oxygenase 2; NSAIDs, nonsteroidal anti-inflammatory drugs; H2, Histamine-2
#Drugs most commonly involved are shown in italics.

calcium phosphate crystal deposition. Both prescribed drugs (e.g. statins, colchicine, daptomycin, volatile anaesthetics) and substances of abuse (e.g. heroin, cocaine, amphetamines) can cause rhabdomyolysis and AKI.

Drugs that cause renal tubular disorders

Various drugs such as cisplatin, adefovir, valproate, and zolendronate can cause proximal renal tubular dysfunction, resulting in Fanconi syndrome. Lithium impairs aquaporin fusion in the collecting duct by inhibition of cyclic adenosine monophosphate (cAMP) formation, thereby leading to unresponsiveness to antidiuretic hormone and hence diabetes insipidus (DI) (Table 19.3).

Drugs that have multiple deleterious effects on kidneys

NSAIDs can cause renal dysfunction via intra-renal haemodynamic disturbances, glomerulonephritis (e.g. minimal change disease and membranous nephropathy), and AIN. Another example is CNI, which can cause both acute and chronic nephrotoxicity. Acute CNI toxicity is often related to exceedingly high CNI concentrations, leading to intra-renal

Table 19.3: Drugs that can cause renal tubular disorders

Proximal RTA	Distal RTA	Diabetes insipidus
Aminoglycosides	Amphotericin B	Lithium
Carbonic anhydrase inhibitors (acetazolamide, topiramate)	Lithium	Demeclocycline
	Ifosfamide	Foscarnet
	Ibuprofen	Cidofovir
Cisplatin/ oxaliplatin		Vasopressin receptor antagonists (tolvaptan, conivaptan)
Tenofovir		Amphotericin B
		Ifosfamide
		Ofloxacin
		Orlistat

RTA, renal tubular acidosis

vasoconstriction and a drop in renal function. Prolonged CNI exposure can affect different renal parenchymal and vascular components, with typical histologic findings of nephrotoxicity such as striped interstitial fibrosis, tubular atrophy, medial arteriolar hyalinosis, tubular microcalcifications, and glomerular capsular fibrosis.

Toxicology for Nephrologist and Extracorporeal Removal

Exposure to substances known to be 'toxic' does not necessarily incur adverse health effects. One may instead unexpectedly suffer from excessive exposures to substances that are commonly acknowledged as harmless. The median lethal dose (LD$_{50}$), defined as the dose needed to kill half of the tested population within a defined duration, is used as a measure of toxicity. Other parameters, such as no-observed-adverse-effect level (NOAEL), lowest-observed-adverse-effect level (LOAEL), therapeutic index, (TI) and margin of safety (MOS) may also indicate the toxicity of a drug/substance. A drug/substance is usually regarded as 'very toxic' if all these parameters are low. Furthermore, the toxic effects of a drug or substance are also significantly influenced by individual susceptibility. Kidneys have substantial exposure to toxic substances and the renal tubular cells are metabolically active, which renders them one of the most vulnerable organs in drug/substance intoxication. The toxic effects on kidneys can be dose-dependent or idiosyncratic, although the risk is generally increased with exposure to higher doses and longer duration, intravenous route of administration, and concurrent use of nephrotoxic drugs. Drug/substance intoxication can give rise to several common toxic renal syndromes which include: (1) AKI related to ATN, AIN, or obstructive uropathy; (2) chronic renal impairment (e.g. CIN by analgesics and AA-containing herbs); (3) nephrotic syndrome (e.g. inorganic mercury, NSAIDs, cocaine, heroin); (4) RTA (e.g. toluene); and (5) nephrogenic DI (e.g. lithium).

General approach to patients with suspected drug-induced kidney disease or intoxication

A detailed drug history, including any over-the-counter medications, herbal remedies, and use of recreational drugs, helps elucidate the culprit agent. Very often, a clear temporal relationship accompanied by compatible blood and urinary findings (e.g. blood or urine eosinophilia, or presence of urine crystals) may suffice to establish the clinical diagnosis. Renal biopsy is generally not required in mild cases or when there is prompt and satisfactory clinical improvement after discontinuation of inciting agents. Withdrawal of the offending medication is usually followed by renal recovery, which typically occurs within 2 – 4 weeks, although in some cases the damage can be irreversible and is associated with progressive renal failure. The use of corticosteroids and other immunosuppressants (e.g. mycophenolate mofetil, anti-CD20, cyclophosphamide) in drug-induced AIN remains controversial, but may be considered in selected patients, such as those with ICPI-associated AIN. Re-challenging with the offending agent should only be attempted in exceptional cases where there is a clear clinical indication and no other appropriate alternatives are available.

In patients with suspected drug or substance intoxication, additional investigations such as blood electrolytes, glucose, lactate, acid–base, and blood and urine toxicology screening as well as electrocardiogram are also indicated. Clinical specimens should be saved to analyse for potential culprits. It is also important to monitor the vital signs, urine output, serum and urine pH, electrolytes, and organ functions to detect early clinical deterioration. Depending on poison and patient factors, the general approach of management includes: (1) exposure termination and prevention; (2) supportive treatment; (3) decontamination; (4) use of antidote; and (5) enhanced elimination. After discontinuing exposure to the culprit agent, supportive measures such as stabilisation of airways, ventilation and circulation, close observation for progression of toxidrome, maintenance of acid–base and electrolytes balance, glycaemic control, and urinary bladder catheterisation should be instigated. Specific antidotes are not always available. Decontamination can be considered for early presenters before poisons are substantially absorbed. Depending on the route of exposure and site of poison retention, the methods can be surface decontamination, gastric lavage, activated charcoal, whole bowel irrigation, and surgical removal. Induced emesis is no longer recommended for toxic ingestions. The elimination can be enhanced for selected substances, using pharmacotherapies like multiple-dose activated charcoal (MDAC), urine alkalinisation, or extracorporeal removal techniques.

Most drugs exist partly as non-ionised molecules at physiological pH. Urine alkalinisation is based on the principles of pH partition theory and ion trapping. For example, salicylic acid is a weak acid (pKa = 2.98) that remains ionised in a more basic pH environment. Upon passing through the glomeruli, the salicylate anions in the ultrafiltrate are 'trapped' in the renal tubular lumen and excreted without tubular reabsorption. The administration of sodium bicarbonate serves the dual purpose of enhancing renal elimination of ionised salicylates (target urine pH is 7–8), and reducing the availability of non-ionised salicylates to pass the blood-brain barrier. However, such a strategy is only applicable for substances with renal excretion as the major route, and does not necessarily confer a more favourable clinical outcome. Also, potential drawbacks of sodium bicarbonate infusion include fluid overload, hypernatraemia, hypokalaemia, hypocalcaemia, and metabolic alkalosis. Forced alkaline diuresis is no longer recommended due to the lack of efficacy for poison removal and the risk of overexpansion of extracellular compartment. Similarly, urine acidification for alkaline drugs (e.g. amphetamines and phencyclidines) is also not recommended because of its low efficacy and risk of precipitating systemic metabolic acidosis.

Extracorporeal elimination is indicated in life-threatening clinical toxicity, massive ingestions, very high blood levels, impaired intrinsic elimination, and unresponsiveness to standard treatment. Extracorporeal elimination also has the benefit of fluid, electrolyte, and acid–base corrections. The mnemonic 'METAL' (Methanol/Metformin, Ethylene glycol/Ethanol, Theophylline, Aspirin, Lithium) includes some common 'dialysable' poisons. The clearance of toxins or drugs by extracorporeal means is influenced by the characteristics of the substance (e.g. molecular weight or volume of distribution) (Table 19.4). Intermittent HD is the most effective way to eliminate toxic substances, but patients who are haemodynamically unstable should be admitted to the intensive care unit for continuous renal replacement therapy (CRRT). Lipid soluble and protein-bound drugs (e.g. phenytoin, digoxin, paraquat, and theophylline) can be removed by haemoperfusion—a process in which blood passes through a device containing adsorbent particles such as activated charcoal or resins. Plasmapheresis or exchange transfusion can be considered for 'non-dialysable' substances. PD only has a limited role in the elimination of toxic substances due to its low efficiency. In case of doubt in clinical management, one should consult the in-house clinical toxicology team (if available), or the local poison information centre and toxicology reference laboratory (TRL) for medical advice and toxicology analysis.

Specific Nephrotoxic Agents and Herbal Medicine

Immune-checkpoint inhibitors

The use of immune-checkpoint inhibitors (ICPIs) has transformed the management paradigm of various malignancies. Commonly used ICPIs include monoclonal antibodies that target programmed cell death protein 1 (PD1) and PD-ligand 1 (PD-L1), or cytotoxic T lymphocyte-associated protein 4 (CTLA-4). One important side effect of ICPIs is immune-mediated injury to different organ systems including the kidneys. The overall incidence rate of ICPIs-related AKI is around 3% and the risks are heightened in patients with pre-existing CKD, or in those who receive combination ICPIs or concomitant PPI. ICPIs-related AKI typically occurs at around 4 to 12 weeks after treatment and is sometimes accompanied by subnephrotic-range proteinuria or sterile pyuria. The most common histologic finding in ICPIs-related AKI is AIN, although ICPIs may also cause various forms of GN. Discontinuation of therapy and corticosteroids are the mainstays of treatment for ICPIs-related AKI, and are usually associated with satisfactory renal recovery. The decision for rechallenge should take into consideration the severity of prior AKI, tumour status, and whether alternative therapeutic options are available.

Lithium

Lithium is a common treatment for bipolar affective disorder. Lithium is not protein-bound, and is excreted unchanged in urine. Its clearance depends

Table 19.4: Characteristics of substances that allow improved clearance with renal replacement therapy

For all 3 techniques	For haemodialysis	For charcoal haemoperfusion	For haemofiltration
Low Vd (< 1 L/kg)	MW < 500 Da	Adsorbable by activated charcoal	MW < 10,000 or < 40,000 Da depending on filter type
Single compartment kinetics	Water-soluble	Not precluded by plasma protein-binding	
Low intrinsic clearance (< 4 mL/min/kg)	Not plasma protein-bound		

MW, molecular weight; Vd, volume of distribution

on GFR and proximal tubular function. The therapeutic range in plasma is narrow (0.6 – 1.2 mmol/L), and severe toxicity is usually observed in acute overdoses by chronic lithium users ('acute-on-chronic'). Chronic accumulation of lithium is more common, and predisposing factors include prolonged excessive exposures, dehydration, drug interactions, congestive heart failure, and liver cirrhosis. Features of severe lithium toxicity include cerebellar signs, peripheral neuropathy, serotonin syndrome, cardiac arrhythmia, seizure, coma, and haemodynamic instability. Nephrogenic DI and hypercalcaemia secondary to lithium-induced hyperparathyroidism can also occur. Management includes discontinuation of lithium, supportive measures, and consideration of gastrointestinal decontamination other than activated charcoal. Extracorporeal removal is indicated in severe toxicities.

Inorganic mercury

In Hong Kong, the majority of mercury poisonings occur following chronic exposure to inorganic mercury salts, which may be present in skin-lightening cream, traditional Chinese medicine (TCM), or contaminated proprietary products. Nephrotic syndrome (due to membranous nephropathy or minimal change disease) can occur with subacute or chronic exposures to low concentrations of inorganic mercury salts, as opposed to ATN in acute mercury poisoning. Patients may show neurological manifestations such as tremor, neurasthenia, mixed sensorimotor neuropathy, ataxia, tunnel vision, and anosmia. Diagnosis is made with a history of substantial exposure, compatible clinical features, and elevated whole-blood mercury (acute) or 24-hour urine mercury (chronic) levels. Treatment involves termination of further exposure of the culprit product, supportive measures, and chelation treatment for high mercury levels. Mercury-induced nephrotic syndrome is usually reversible. Haemodialysis has a limited role in removing mercury because of its large volume of distribution and significant protein binding.

Zopiclone

Acute overdose of zopiclone is typically associated with respiratory and central nervous system depression, but haemolysis and ATN can occur with massive ingestion. Treatment is largely supportive, but activated charcoal can be given if the patient presents

early. Intravenous methylene blue is indicated for symptomatic or significant methaemoglobinaemia (> 20%). Renal impairment and haemolysis are usually self-limiting and improve with supportive treatment.

Ketamine

Ketamine is a phencyclidine derivative originally used for procedural sedation and general anaesthesia, but has emerged as a drug of abuse since the 1980s. Acute toxicity is characterised by reduced consciousness, psychosis, and abdominal pain. Chronic use is associated with neuropsychiatric sequelae, urological complications, and cholestasis with bile duct dilatation. Ketamine-induced urologic complications start to develop typically after 1 – 4 years of street ketamine use, which affect about one-third of chronic users. The proposed mechanisms are direct toxicity of ketamine and its metabolites, causing microvascular ischaemia and autoimmune reactions. Clinical features of ketamine-induced cystitis are dysuria, urinary frequency, urgency, urge incontinence, and painful haematuria. Ulcerative cystitis is the typical cystoscopic finding. Chronic obstructive uropathy, chronic renal failure, and urothelial carcinoma are some potential long-term complications.

Traditional Chinese medicine

Some TCMs may cause renal dysfunction via various mechanisms. These can be systemic toxins in multiple organ systems, such as poisonous metals (arsenic, inorganic mercury), 雷公藤 (Tripterygium wilfordii), 蒼耳子 (Fructus xanthii), 斑蝥 (Mylabris species), 蓖麻 (Ricinus communis). AA-containing herbs (e.g. 尋骨風 [A. mollissima], 關木通 [A. manshuriensis], 廣防己 [A. fangchi], 青木香 [A. debilis], 天仙藤 [A. debilis], 馬兜鈴 [A. contorta], 漢中防己 [A. heterophylla], and 細辛 [Asarum species]) are directly nephrotoxic. AA nephropathy was first reported in 1993 when a cluster of patients who took 廣防己 (Aristolochia fangchi) for slimming presented with renal interstitial fibrosis, rapid progression to end-stage kidney disease (ESKD), and urothelial malignancies. Circulatory albumin-bound AA is transported through the basolateral membrane of proximal tubular epithelial cells via receptors OAT1, OAT2, and OAT3. AA binds to DNA to form AA-DNA adducts. Fanconi syndrome can occur following proximal tubular dysfunction. AA nephropathy is dose-dependent, in which AKI occurs after exposure to high cumulative doses, while CIN occurs after chronic low-dose exposure. AA is a class 1 human carcinogen and can cause urothelial carcinoma even in the absence of pre-existing AA nephropathy. It is essential to collect herbal formulae and unused herbal remnant to identify AA-containing ingredients, or erroneous substitution of benign herbs with AA-containing herbs. Fibrosing interstitial nephritis is the typical histopathologic finding.

20

Critical Care Nephrology

Hoi Ping Shum, Desmond Yap, and Wing Wa Yan

Introduction

Critical care nephrology is a new discipline formally established in 1998 worldwide. It is a multidisciplinary branch of medicine that deals with issues of critical care medicine and nephrology. Acute kidney injury (AKI) is a centre of attention in the arena of critical care nephrology and internists, critical care physicians, surgeons, and nephrologists all participate in the management of this important and serious condition. Moreover, chronic dialysis patients who become critically ill may also require renal support in the intensive care unit (ICU). This chapter will highlight the spectrum of renal problems in critically ill patients and the application of renal replacement therapy (RRT) in these settings.

Disease Spectrum in Critical Care Nephrology

AKI is a common condition in the critical care setting, and the reported incidence ranges from 22% to 57% depending on the definition used. The development of AKI in critically ill patients is associated with substantial morbidities, mortality, and treatment costs. Furthermore, patients with prolonged or improperly managed AKI may also progress to chronic kidney disease (CKD) or even end-stage kidney disease (ESKD). Common conditions that are associated with AKI in critical care settings include severe infection and septic shock, cardiogenic shock, liver failure, intra-abdominal hypertension, malignancy, recovery from major operation (especially cardiac and vascular surgery), trauma, burns, and exposure to iodine-based contrast or other nephrotoxic agents.

The pathogenesis of AKI from the above-mentioned conditions are highly complex and contributed by macro- and micro-circulatory disturbance, the surge of inflammatory mediators and reactive oxygen species, activation of the coagulation cascade, glycocalyx degradation, and renal venous congestion. Once AKI occurs in a critically ill patient, the cause of AKI should be identified as quickly as possible to tailor a set of actions to prevent further progression of AKI and avoid irreversible kidney damage. Another commonly encountered clinical scenario in critical care nephrology is when patients on chronic haemodialysis (HD) or peritoneal dialysis (PD) become critically ill and require ICU care. In this context, their usual modality and regimen of dialysis may be significantly modified to suit their clinical conditions and metabolic demands.

Renal Replacement Therapy in the Critical Care Setting

About 10% of AKI patients require RRT to compensate for the loss of renal function, manage acid–base and electrolyte disturbances, remove excessive fluid gain, and allow time for renal recovery. RRT in critically ill patients can be provided continuously or intermittently depending on patients' needs. Continuous renal replacement therapy (CRRT) is a slow and continuous process that removes fluid and uremic toxins from the patients. CRRT is the predominant form of RRT in the critical care settings due to its accurate volume control, steady acid–base and electrolyte correction, and good maintenance of blood pressure during the treatment. It is frequently prescribed in critically ill patients with hemodynamic instability

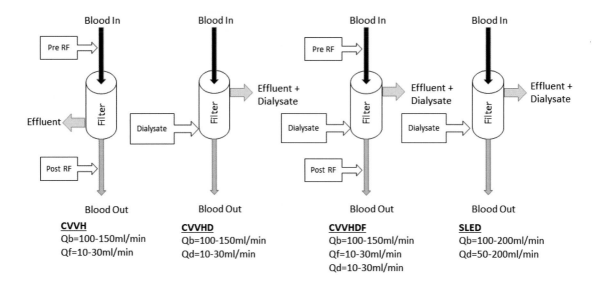

RF= replacement fluid

Figure 20.1: Typical set-up of different modalities of continuous renal replacement therapy in critically ill patients Qb, blood flow rate; Qf, replacement fluid flow rate; Qd, dialysate flow rate; RF, replacement fluid

and multi-organ failure who cannot tolerate the relatively fast removal of fluids and solutes by intermittent renal replacement therapies (IRRT) like HD. CRRT is based on four main physiologic processes: (a) diffusion, (b) convection, (c) ultrafiltration, and (d) adsorption to achieve treatment targets. Diffusion allows rapid removal of small molecules and can achieve good ionic stability, whereas convection confers more efficient elimination of medium to large molecules. Ultrafiltration allows steady water removal while adsorption captures cytokines, chemokines, or super-antigens through hydrophobic interaction, Van der Waal's forces, or ionic interactions to the surface of the semi-permeable membrane. Depending on the membrane structures of the haemofilter or dialyser, and the treatment modalities used, there is often more than one principle involved in achieving the goals of required treatment. Inflammatory mediators like cytokines play an important role in the pathogenesis of AKI. Most cytokines are relatively large molecules of more than 10 kDa and therefore it is unlikely that a significant amount will be removed by conventional HD, which is largely based on a diffusive mechanism. Therefore, in theory, haemofiltration based on a convective mechanism may show better elimination of inflammatory cytokines. The typical set-up of the different modalities of CRRT is illustrated in Figure 20.1.

Continuous venovenous hemodiafiltration (CVVHDF), continuous venovenous hemodialysis (CVVHD) and continuous venovenous hemofiltration (CVVH) are three of the most commonly prescribed modalities in the local critical care setting. In general, there is no significant difference in mortality among the various CRRT strategies in patients with septic AKI although CVVH may be associated with short filter lifespan compared with the other two modalities. CRRT is usually delivered by regular CRRT machines, though it can also be provided by a hemodiafiltration machine incorporated with the water treatment system. Synthetic, biocompatible, and high-flux membranes are routinely used to achieve good convective solute removal. Replacement or substitution solutions are prescribed in modalities that involve convective solute removal (e.g. CVVH and CVVHDF) and this can be infused before (i.e. predilution) or after (i.e. post-dilution) the dialyser, or both before and after the dialyser (i.e. pre- and post-dilution). Dialysate should be used in modalities that make use of diffusion for solute removal (e.g. CVVHD and CVVHDF). Both the replacement or substitution solution and the dialysate solution are sterile, bicarbonate-buffered, and balanced electrolyte solutions that resemble the composition of the ultrafiltrate.

Options of IRRT include intermittent haemodialysis (IHD), intermittent haemodiafiltration (IHDF)

Table 20.1: A comparison of the different modalities of renal replacement therapy in critically ill patients

Parameters	IHD	SLED	CRRT
Principle	Diffusion	Diffusion	CVVH: Convection CVVHD: Diffusion CVVHDF: Both
Blood flow (ml/min)	200–300	100–200	100–150
Dialysate flow (ml/min)	> = 500	50–200	CVVHD: 10–30 CVVHDF: 10–30
Treatment duration (hours)	3–5	6–12	>24
Hemodynamic stability	Unstable	Marginally stable	Stable
Fluid removal	Rapid	Intermediate	Very slow and gentle
Efficiency	High	Medium	Low
Anticoagulation	LMWH/UFH/ anticoagulation free	LMWH/UFH	RCA/LMWH/UFH/ pre-dilution
Nursing workload	Low	Intermediate	High
Nurse requirement	Renal nurse	Renal nurse	ICU nurse
Treatment cost	Low	Low	High

CRRT, continuous renal replacement therapy; CVVH, continuous venovenous haemofiltration; CVVHD, continuous venovenous haemodialysis; CVVHDF, continuous venovenous haemodiafiltration; ICU, Intensive care unit; IHD, intermittent haemodialysis; LMWH, low molecular weight heparin; RCA, regional citrate anticoagulation; SLED, sustained low-efficiency dialysis; UFH, unfractionated heparin

and sustained low-efficiency dialysis (SLED). In general, IRRT should be considered in situations requiring rapid correction of electrolytes or urgent fluid removal, or in acute poisoning. While there is no proven survival benefit of CRRT over IRRT, CRRT appears to confer advantages to hemodynamic stability, control of fluid balance, renal recovery, and dialysis dependence. Furthermore, CRRT is also associated with a smaller increase in intracranial pressure compared with IRRT and thus more preferable in patients with liver failure, acute brain injury, or conditions that create a predisposition to cerebral oedema. The current guidelines recommend that CRRT and IRRT be used as complementary therapies in critically ill patients with AKI, and the choice of modality should take into consideration the patient's condition (e.g. diagnosis, hemodynamic status etc), availability of nursing staff, equipment, and other relevant resources (Table 20.1). In this context, patients with haemodynamic instability generally receive CRRT and are often transferred to IRRT once they are free from vasopressor use.

Acute PD is often an overlooked dialysis modality for critically ill patients with AKI. It is technically easy to perform and is associated with low cost and good haemodynamic stability. PD is a safe and viable option for dialysis support in AKI patients, especially for neonates, children, and those with a PD catheter

in-situ. The current data suggest that acute PD is comparable to HD as regards the incidence of renal recovery and mortality in critically ill patients with AKI. The slow rate of solute removal in acute PD incurs a lower risk of disequilibrium syndrome but is also a drawback in patients with high physiological and metabolic stresses. Acute PD is contraindicated for those with recent abdominal or cardiothoracic surgery, severe respiratory failure, extreme volume overload, and very poor glycaemic control.

The right timing to commence RRT in critically ill patients with AKI remains debatable due to a lack of consensus on the parameters to define timing and threshold for initiation of RRT. Starting RRT before a patient develops absolute indications (e.g. fluid overload resistant to diuretics therapy, severe metabolic acidosis with pH < 7.15, hyperkalaemia > 6.5 mmol/L, or symptomatic uraemia) is a common practice in ICUs. However, commencing RRT too early may subject patients who could have naturally recovered kidney function to unnecessary risks of complications. Although current evidence suggests that early initiation of RRT in critically ill patients with AKI does not improve mortality when compared with standard or late initiation, early RRT is associated with a significant reduction of the length of hospitalization. The appropriate timing of initiating RRT should be individualized and take into consideration patients' comorbidities, current diagnoses, the severity of illness, extra-renal organ dysfunction, fluid burden, as well as laboratory and physiological parameters.

The adequacy of IHD is usually assessed by the removal of urea (a surrogate of low molecular weight products of metabolism) and is often reflected by the urea reduction ratio (URR) or the fractional clearance of urea (Kt/V_{urea}, where K is the instantaneous clearance, t is the treatment time, and V is the volume of distribution of urea). For CVVH, the clearance of small molecules like urea is equal to the ultrafiltration rate as the sieving coefficient should be 1, which indicates free passage with complete equilibration. During CVVHD, the dialysis flow rate is much slower (10–30 ml/min) than the blood flow rate (100–150 ml/min), and hence urea in the dialysate will equilibrate with that in the plasma and its clearance will be approximated by the dialysate flow rate. Thus, in the absence of infusion with predilutional replacement fluid, the treatment dose can be quantified based on effluent flow rates, which is equal to the sum of the ultrafiltrate and dialysate flow. The current evidence suggests performing CRRT at a minimum delivered dose of an effluent flow rate of 20–25 ml/kg/hr. Importantly, one should appreciate that the prescribed dose is not necessarily equal to the actual delivered dose due to circuit clotting, machine alarms, or other logistical issues like interruptions for investigative or surgical procedures.

Anticoagulation in CRRT

Activation of platelets and the coagulation cascade occurs with the exposure of blood to the haemofilter/dialyser membrane. Protein coating and clogging together with clot formation compromise the haemofilter performance, and therefore anticoagulation is necessary to prevent clotting of the extracorporeal circuit. The appropriate choice of anticoagulation in CRRT is key to maintaining circuit patency and minimizing bleeding complications in high-risk populations. Adequate anticoagulation can effectively prevent clot formation over the membrane surface, which translates into longer treatment duration and less discrepancy between the prescribed and delivered treatment doses. Moreover, less circuit clotting is associated with reduced blood transfusion requirement, less consumption of nursing manpower for circuit change, and lower treatment costs. An ideal anticoagulation strategy should be regional, inexpensive and easy to implement, simple to monitor

the anticoagulation effect, readily reversible, and with minimal side effects.

Unfractionated heparin (UFH) and low molecular weight heparin (LMWH) are commonly used systemic anticoagulants for CRRT and IRRT (Table 20.2). They are inexpensive, readily available, and have an extensive history of clinical usage. The CRRT circuit lifespan using UFH or LMWH as anticoagulant ranges from 26 to 52 hours. LMWH shows less protein binding than UFH, and so its anticoagulation effect is more predictable and may also confer better circuit patency. The bleeding risk and chance of heparin-induced thrombocytopenia of LMWH are also lower than that of UFH. Both UFH and LMWH may induce variable degrees of systemic anticoagulation, which limit their use in patients with bleeding tendency or postoperative conditions.

Regional citrate anticoagulation (RCA) represents an emerging way of anticoagulation in patients receiving CRRT. Citrate chelates ionized calcium, which is crucial for the activation of various clotting factors and thrombin formation. An ionized calcium concentration of 0.25–0.35 mmol/L is essential for achieving the anticoagulation effect in an extracorporeal circuit. The majority of citrate is removed by either filtration or dialysis during CRRT. Calcium is replaced intravenously before the blood is returned to the patient to compensate for the extracorporeal loss and to normalize the systemic calcium levels. Compared with heparin-based anticoagulation, RCA is associated with lower bleeding risk and longer haemofilter lifespan (27–72 hours), but with similar overall mortality. However, RCA is technically more demanding than a heparin-based regimen. Conditions associated with reduced metabolism of citrates, such as chronic liver disease, ischaemic hepatitis, hypoxemia, and impaired muscle perfusion, are not uncommon in the ICU setting. Excessive citrate accumulation leads to low ionized calcium levels and acidosis, thereby causing hypotension secondary to decreased myocardial contractility and vascular hypotonia. Other metabolic disturbances of citrate accumulation include hypomagnesaemia and hypernatremia.

Anticoagulation-free RRT can be considered for patients with high bleeding risk or those with contraindications for citrate use. In this context, higher blood flow rates and predilution with replacement fluids can be used to improve circuit lifespan. Despite these measures, the circuit lifespan is still often shorter compared with UFH or LMWH circuits.

Table 20.2: Different anticoagulation strategies for renal replacement therapy in critically ill patients

Methods	Pros	Cons
Anticoagulant-free/ saline flush	• Easy implementation • Safest in those with bleeding risks	• Short haemofilter lifespan and more blood loss due to circuit clotting • Labour intensive for repriming of circuit
Pre-dilution	• Easy implementation • Can be used in those with bleeding risk and minimal monitoring is needed	• Short haemofilter lifespan • Compromised treatment efficacy due to pre-dilution
UFH	• Effective anticoagulation • Anticoagulation effect is titratable • Extensive clinical experience	• Causes systemic anticoagulation and thus increased risk of bleeding • Less predictable PK than LWMH • Risk of HIT
LMWH	• Easy implementation • Effective anticoagulation • Extensive clinical experience • Lower risk of HIT than UFH	• Causes systemic anticoagulation and thus increased risk of bleeding • Anticoagulation effect is not readily reversible
RCA	• Longer haemofilter lifespan and lower risk of bleeding compared with UFH or LMWH	• Risk of citrate toxicity and metabolic/electrolyte disturbance • Complicated protocol and higher manpower demand
Direct thrombin inhibitors/ heparinoids	• Can be considered in patients who develop HIT	• Limited local experience • High cost

HIT, heparin-induced thrombocytopenia; LMWH, low molecular weight heparin; PK, pharmacokinetics; RCA, regional citrate anticoagulation; UFH, unfractionated heparin

21

Imaging in Nephrology and Interventional Nephrology

Ferdinand Chu, Victor Lee, and Kelvin Choi

Introduction

Imaging and interventional procedures in nephrology can be quite sophisticated and costly. Each modality has its own edge, while their scopes may overlap. The choice of modality should take into consideration the local availability, expertise, and cost, as well as clinical indications.

Imaging and Intervention of Common Renal Problems

Radiological examinations are clinically important investigations for identifying potential causes of acute and chronic renal impairment. Renal imaging is useful in various clinical situations including acute and/or chronic renal impairment, gross haematuria, polycystic kidney disease, renovascular disease, and suspected urological malignancy. Commonly used imaging modalities include ultrasonography (US), Doppler US, magnetic resonance imaging (MRI), and renal arteriography. The growing application of MRI in renovasculature assessment avoids the use of computed tomography (CT) and conventional renal arteriography, thus reducing the overall incidence of contrast-induced nephropathy.

US is often the initial choice of investigation as it is non-invasive, readily available in most centres and does not involve ionizing radiation. US of the urinary system gives a real-time overview of the kidneys with regard to their size and echotexture, and is useful for excluding obstruction, structural anomalies, and mass lesions in the kidney (Figure 21.1). While alterations in corticomedullary differentiation and parenchymal echogenicity could signify chronic kidney disease (CKD), these ultrasonographic abnormalities can be nonspecific and do not provide histopathological differentiation. Also, renal ultrasound findings can sometimes be unremarkable in affected individuals.

Hypertension and diabetes mellitus are two common causes of CKD, accounting for up to two-thirds of cases. While 95% of hypertensive cases are related to essential hypertension, identifying secondary causes such as renovascular and glomerular abnormalities will facilitate early initiation of appropriate management and retard the progression of CKD. In this context, patients with renal artery stenosis (RAS) may show renal size discrepancies, with the affected side being significantly smaller (size difference of 1.5 cm). In patients with suspected RAS, the renovascular status can be further assessed by Doppler US to quantify motion; processed information is displayed graphically, which provides

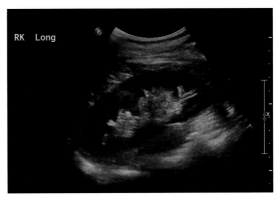

Figure 21.1: Ultrasound image of the right kidney with normal cortical thickness and clear corticomedullary differentiation

information such as velocity and spectral waveform to determine vessel patency and degree of stenosis (Figures 21.2 and 21.3). US, however, is highly operator-dependent and image quality is limited by body habitus and bowel gas. MR angiography (MRA) with contrast offers three-dimensional evaluation of the main/proximal renal arteries with high sensitivity and specificity (> 90%) (Figure 21.4). Not only is it more tolerable for patients with renal impairment, but it also provides more accurate information for planning of renal revascularization strategy. Wider application of MRA in renovascular disease is still restricted by its availability and long acquisition time when compared to ultrasonography. In addition, MRI

is an increasingly popular imaging modality used for the assessment of total kidney volume in patients with adult polycystic kidney disease (APKD). Such MRI findings can help risk stratification and guide treatment decisions in APKD patients.

Invasive investigations such as renal biopsies are often required to resolve the diagnostic uncertainty. USs offers real-time guidance for kidney biopsies and are readily available in most centres. For non-targeted renal biopsies, diagnostic accuracy could be affected by glomerular yield, and therefore samples should be obtained from the peripheral portion of the kidney targeting the lower pole cortex to minimize the risk of bleeding (Figure 21.5). CT

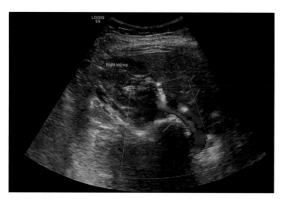

Figure 21.2: Colour Doppler image of the right kidney shows patency of the main renal artery (red arrow) and renal vein (blue arrow)

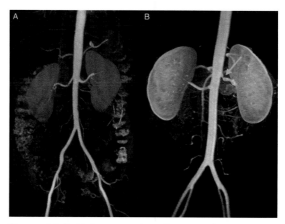

Figure 21.4: Volume-rendered magnetic resonance angiography (MRA). (A) Normal renal arteries with no evidence of renal artery stenosis; (B) in a different patient, MRA demonstrates high-grade stenosis in the left renal artery, with post-stenotic dilatation (arrow).

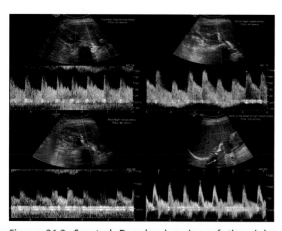

Figure 21.3: Spectral Doppler imaging of the right kidney assessing the velocity and spectral waveform of the renovascular structure. Measurements should be made at the proximal/mid/distal renal artery and the aorta (arrow). In normal individuals, a waveform obtained from the renal artery should demonstrate a rapid upstroke in systole and a low resistance waveform with continuous forward flow, peak systolic velocity (PSV) < 180 cm/s, and Renal (PSV)/Aorta (PSV) < 3.5.

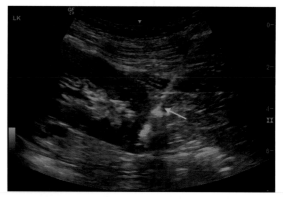

Figure 21.5: Ultrasound-guided left renal biopsy with 16G biopsy needle (arrow), aiming at the peripheral portion of the lower pole

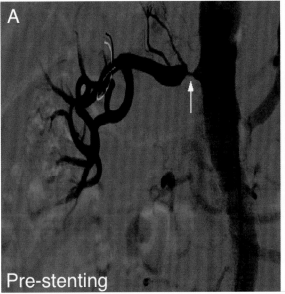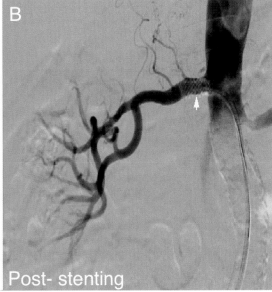

Figure 21.6: Patient presented with stage 4 chronic kidney disease found to have severe right renal artery stenosis. (A) Pre-stent right renal angiogram confirmed high-grade stenosis in proximal right renal artery; (B) satisfactory luminal gain achieved following stent insertion.

guidance is often reserved for difficult cases, such as patients with large body habitus or inconspicuous lesions.

Renal arteriography, the 'gold standard method of renal artery imaging, is largely reserved for therapeutic purposes in managing patients with significant RAS (Figure 21.6) or traumatic events. Renal artery stenting is indicated in patients with symptomatic RAS and the following comorbidities:

- cardiac disturbance syndromes (e.g. flash pulmonary oedema)
- uncontrolled hypertension, despite being on at least three antihypertensive agents in patients with bilateral or solitary severe RAS
- Severe CKD without an explanation, provided the kidney is not significantly atrophic (bipolar length must be > 7 cm)

Renal arteriography is also increasingly being used to achieve haemostasis in traumatic or iatrogenic renal injury (e.g. after renal biopsy or lithotripsy) (Figures 21.7 and 21.8). By identifying the feeding vessels on a renal angiogram, the bleeding culprit can be selectively embolized by various haemostatic materials (e.g. glue, particles or mechanical plugs). Such strategy has significantly improved patient outcomes by avoiding nephrectomy and minimizing the sacrifice of renal parenchymal tissue. Furthermore, oncological therapies can also

be delivered by the renal arteriographical approach to achieve tumour devascularization and size reduction.

Imaging and Intervention of Dialysis-Related Complications

Dialysis is a life-saving treatment to replace the loss of kidney function in patients with ESRD. Up to 80% of ESRD patients in Hong Kong receive peritoneal dialysis (PD). Ultrafiltration (UF) failure is a commonly encountered clinical problem in PD patients, and is frequently caused by a malpositioned catheter or PD fluid leakage into spaces outside the peritoneum. In this context, radiological examinations can help identify the various causes of UF failure. Simple investigations like abdominal X-ray/KUB can reveal malpositioning of PD catheters, whereas chest X rays can often give a clue to the presence of pleuroperitoneal communication. CT peritoneogram is a crucial imaging modality for suspected leakage into the retroperitoneal (Figure 21.9) or scrotal area. Radiological investigations can also help the assessment and management of infective complications in PD patients. Tunnel tract infections and abscesses adjacent to the PD catheter can be assessed by ultrasonography. CT of the abdomen or pelvis is also useful for recognizing intra-abdominal pathologies in PD patients suffering from severe peritonitis.

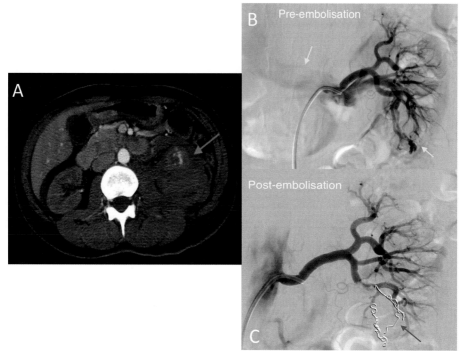

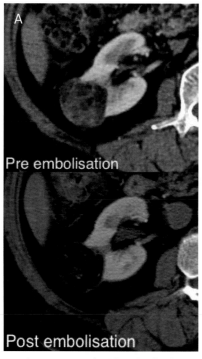

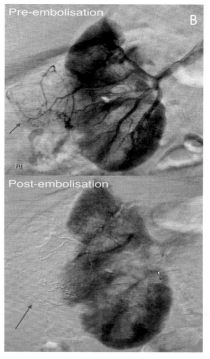

Figure 21.7: Patient underwent a renal biopsy and presented with hypotension and drop in haemoglobin. (A) computed tomography (CT) showed left perinephric haematoma with left lower pole pseudoaneurysm; (B) selective left renal angiogram confirmed left lower pole pseudoaneurysm, note of spontaneous drainage via left renal vein, suggestive of concurrent arteriovenous fistula (AVF); (C) following coil embolization, both pseudoaneurysm and AVF are no longer evident.

Figure 21.8: Patient presented with right flank pain and found to have a 4.8 cm right renal angiomyelipoma; subsequently underwent embolization with alcohol/ lipiodol mixture. (A) computed tomographic (CT); and (B) fluoroscopic images demonstrate significant devascularization following embolization.

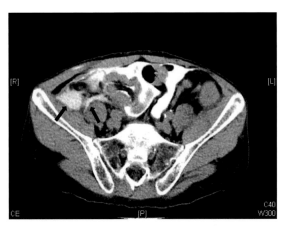

Figure 21.9: Computed tomography (CT) peritoneogram showing evidence of retroperitoneal leakage on the right side (black arrow)

US- or CT-guided drainage is indicated in patients who developed intra-abdominal abscesses or collection after peritonitis.

Haemodialysis (HD) is the predominant modality of renal replacement therapy in many countries. In Hong Kong, only approximately 20% of patients receive chronic HD, often because of contraindications to PD or peritoneal failure secondary to severe peritonitis. Vascular access is the prerequisite to the successful delivery of HD. Common vascular accesses include catheters (temporary or tunnelled cuffed catheters) and more permanent accesses such as arteriovenous fistula (AVF) or arteriovenous grafts (AVGs). Interventional radiology plays an important role in managing vascular access problem in HD patients. Nowadays, HD catheters are usually inserted into large veins under ultrasonographic guidance using Seldinger's technique. Common sites of insertion in the order of desirability are the right jugular vein, left jugular vein, femoral veins, and subclavian veins. For jugular and subclavian catheter insertion, it is preferable to avoid the side where an AVF is to be created in the future. Tunnelled cuffed catheters have a tissue cuff buried in the subcutaneous skin tunnel, which helps block direct communication between the external milieu and the bloodstream and also secure the catheter's position by inducing fibrosis around the cuff. During tunnelled cuffed catheter insertion, the jugular or femoral veins are first cannulated under US guidance. The guidewire and vascular sheath are then inserted and their positions confirmed with real-time fluoroscopy. After the creation of a subcutaneous skin tunnel, and the cuffed catheter is inserted along the guideline and

vascular sheath and its final position confirmed again by fluoroscopy. Long-dwelling HD catheters can develop complications such as superior vena cava (SVC) stenosis or fibrin sheath, which are both amenable to radiological interventions. In this context, SVC stenosis can be managed by balloon angioplasty +/- stenting of the affected vascular segments. The fibrin sheath is a flimsy fibrous tissue membrane formed at the opening of the catheter, and is characterized by smooth inflow but unsatisfactory outflow. The fibrous sheath can be mechanically removed by an interventional radiological procedure called catheter stripping.

AVFs or AVGs are the vascular accesses of choice in HD patients due to better blood flow and lower infection risks compared to catheters. Venous mapping by Doppler US can provide detailed assessments of the patency and calibres of the venous anatomy, and thus aid surgical planning of the AVF or AVG creation. AVFs or AVGs can develop complications such as stenosis or pseudoaneurysms after prolonged use or repeated needling. AVF or AVG stenosis is suspected when there is poor blood flow, high venous pressure during HD, prolonged bleeding after an HD session, or vascular recirculation. Stenosis of the arterial or venous limb of the AVF or AVG can be confirmed by a fistulogram and managed by balloon angioplasty (Figure 21.10). Permanent metallic stents can be deployed in recurrent AVF or AVG stenosis. Acute thrombosis of AVFs or AVGs can be dissolved by direct infusion of urokinase or recombinant tissue plasminogen activator into the vascular access. Mechanical methods can be attempted to dismantle and remove older and more organized clots. While most AVFs or AVGs are created surgically at the time of writing, various minimally invasive gadgets have emerged to facilitate the creation of AVFs by endovascular means alone without open surgery.

Imaging and Intervention of Kidney Transplantation

Pretransplant imaging for live kidney donors

Live donor kidney transplantation, is the preferred treatment for ESRD patients due to the significantly superior clinical outcomes compared with deceased donor kidney transplantation and dialysis. Nowadays, donor kidneys are often harvested using the laparoscopic approach. Renal imaging is part of the standard workup for live kidney donors, and allows accurate anatomic delineation for surgical

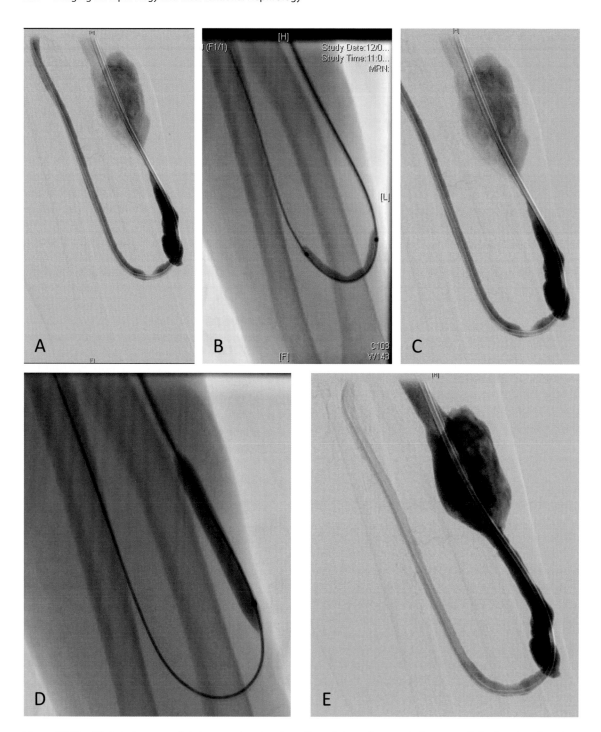

Figure 21.10: (A) Arteriovenous fistulogram showing two sites of stenosis, one at the apex of the looping denoting the arteriovenous anastomosis, and the second one on the venous side of the arteriovenous fistula just distal to the puncture site denoted by the aneurysmal dilatation. (B) A dilated angioplasty balloon covering the site of the stenosis at anastomosis. (C) Arteriovenous fistulogram after first balloon dilatation, showing persistent residual stenosis at both sites. (D) Second angioplasty performed over both sites; only the inflated angioplasty balloon over the stenosis on venous side of the fistula is shown. (E) Completion arteriovenous fistulogram showing reopening of both stenotic sites.

planning and exclusion of contraindications for kidney donation. Contrast-enhanced CT is the imaging modality of choice for pre-operative assessment of live kidney donors. A typical CT protocol includes the unenhanced, arterial, nephrographic, and delayed excretory phases. The arterial phase is used to delineate vascular anatomy and variants, which have important surgical implications. In general, the kidney with less complex vascular anatomy will be harvested. In most individuals, each kidney is supplied by a single renal artery arising from the abdominal aorta. Accessory renal arteries, seen in up to one-third of individuals, usually arise from the aorta or iliac arteries between T11 and L4 levels (Figure 21.11). If the main and accessory renal arteries are wide apart, the surgeon needs to carry out a double arterial anastomosis in the recipient, increasing the complexity of the operation. Detection of venous anomalies is also essential before donor nephrectomy to minimize haemorrhagic complications. The unenhanced phase is highly sensitive in detecting nephrolithiasis. Kidneys with a renal stone larger than 5 mm or multiple stones are excluded from donation unless the stones are removed and metabolic analysis is performed. The nephrographic phase allows the detection of renal masses such as renal cell carcinoma. The delayed excretory phase is helpful in the depiction of pelvicalyceal and ureteric anatomy and also in the detection of small transitional cell carcinomas.

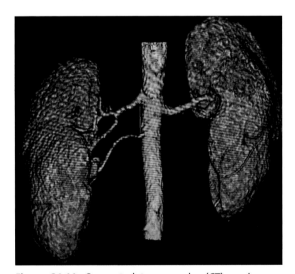

Figure 21.11: Computed tomography (CT) angiogram with volume rendering showing double right renal artery in a potential live kidney donor

Imaging and intervention in renal transplant recipients

US is the principal imaging modality to evaluate vascular and non-vascular complications in kidney allografts. B-mode US depicts pathology through acquisitions of two-dimensional grey-scale images. Duplex US permits assessment of arterial and venous complications, while spectral US allows the graphical display of renal artery waveform (i.e. blood flow velocities over time). The renal arterial resistive index (RI), demonstrated by spectral US and calculated as (peak systolic velocity – end-diastolic velocity) ÷ peak systolic velocity, is a potential sonographic marker to indicate abnormalities in the kidney allograft.

Evaluation of vascular complications in kidney transplant recipients

Graft RAS and graft renal artery or vein thrombosis are important vascular complications that can occur after kidney transplantation. In this context, graft RAS represents the most common post-transplant vascular complication and frequently manifests as resistant hypertension requiring multiple antihypertensive agents for control. Direct sonographic signs of graft RAS include elevated peak systolic velocity (PSV) (> 250 cm/sec), presence of aliasing on Duplex US at the site of narrowing (Figure 21.12) and an elevated ratio of PSVs between the main renal artery and the upstream iliac artery (> 1.8). The first-line treatment for graft RAS is percutaneous transluminal angioplasty +/– stent placement. Renal artery thrombosis is rare and usually develops in the early postoperative period. On US, there are absent Doppler signals throughout the graft kidney and the presence of intra-renal hypoechoic 'mass-like' lesions is suggestive of a renal infarct. Graft renal vein thrombosis usually occurs within five days after kidney transplantation. Sonographic features include oedematous renal allograft with loss of corticomedullary differentiation and reversed diastolic flow in the graft renal artery on spectral US.

Evaluation of non-vascular complications in kidney transplant recipients

Perinephric fluid collections after renal transplantation, such as haematoma, lymphocele, urinoma, and abscess, can be characterized by US (Figure 21.13). Haematoma appears as a complex hyperechoic collection with central hypoechoic areas, while both urinoma and lymphocele occur as simple hypoechoic fluid collections. Perinephric abscess

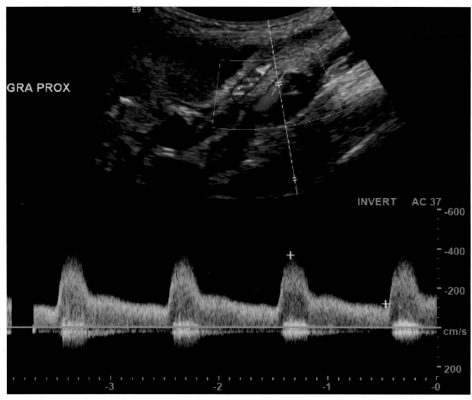

Figure 21.12: Spectral ultrasonography at the proximal graft renal artery demonstrating elevated peak systolic velocity up to ~400 cm/sec

usually presents as a triad of fluid collection, fever, and leucocytosis. Sonographic features include complex hypoechoic collection with internal debris and increased peripheral Doppler signals due to hyperaemia. These different types of perinephric collections after kidney transplantation can be further differentiated by biochemical and microbiological analysis of the drained fluid. While small non-infected fluid collection may resolve spontaneously, percutaneous catheter drainage can be considered if a perinephric collection exerts a significant mass effect. Percutaneous drainage, if technically feasible, should be performed on top of systemic antibiotic treatment for perinephric abscesses in kidney transplant recipients. US also enables the recognition of graft hydronephrosis or other obstructive lesions in patients who present with deterioration of renal allograft function. US can also pick up nonspecific changes in other renal allograft diseases such as acute tubular necrosis, allograft rejection (hyperacute, acute, or chronic), drug-related nephrotoxicity, and infection. This can be accompanied by elevation of intra-renal RI (> 0.7), although such an increase

may often be quite nonspecific. The confirmation or exclusion of these kidney allograft complications often requires a US-guided allograft biopsy.

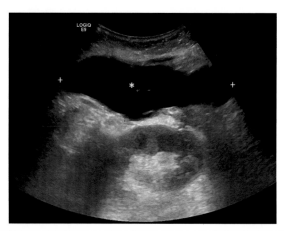

Figure 21.13: B-mode ultrasonography (US) demonstrating a large hypoechoic perinephric fluid collection (asterisk) superficial to the graft kidney, confirmed to be a lymphocele on US-guided aspiration

22

Geriatrics and Palliative Nephrology, and Renal Rehabilitation

Yat Fung Shea, Kwok Ying Chan, Terence Yip, and Maggie Ming Yee Mok

Introduction

Geriatrics nephrology, renal palliative care, and renal rehabilitation are emerging fields in nephrology and have growing service demands. This chapter provides an overview of managing elderly patients with renal failure, palliative nephrology, and renal rehabilitation.

Management of Renal Failure in Geriatric Patients and Related Psychosocial Aspects

Management of elderly patients with chronic kidney disease (CKD) can be challenging. The severity of renal impairment may be under-estimated if serum creatinine (Cr) level or Cr-based equations were used to assess kidney functions in frail elderly with reduced muscle mass. Geriatric patients with polypharmacy are also more susceptible to the side effects of medications when they have renal insufficiency. Elderly patients may also develop other sinister medical conditions along the clinical course that adds to the difficulty of the decision to start or terminate renal replacement therapy (RRT) when they reach end-stage kidney disease (ESKD). When formulating a management plan for geriatric patients, it is important to take into consideration the comorbidities, frailty, and functional status of the patient in order to predict the need for dialysis and survival after the commencement of dialysis. Attending clinicians should fully inform these elderly patients regarding their illness and prognosis, and explore their fears and worries (e.g. symptoms) as well as the perspectives of functional status that are important to them (e.g. the ability to eat or go to the toilet independently). Together with the primary caregivers, the goals of care—including health-related goals (e.g. maintaining function or independence) and personal goals (e.g. travel hopes, spending time with loved ones)—should be discussed with patients and their caregivers. The involvement of geriatricians facilitates the referral of suitable patients to community care services that provide escort services, meal delivery, dietary or fluid advice, home-based physiotherapy, and occupational therapy. Geriatric patients with ESKD should be considered for RRT when they are in stable medical condition and have a reasonable expected quality of life. However, the decision to initiate RRT can be difficult especially during the acute setting in patients with multiple pre-existing comorbidities or in those with poor family support. Kidney transplant recipients in the geriatric age group are increasingly common due to improved survival of existing renal transplant patients and the use of expanded criteria donors. Careful pre-operative assessment, appropriate modification of immunosuppressive regimens, vigilant surveillance of malignancy, and cardiovascular complications are all important measures to optimize the outcomes of geriatric kidney transplant recipients.

Both geriatric patients with CKD and their carers often experience high levels of stress. These stresses can emanate from symptoms of CKD such as anorexia, generalized pruritus, recurrent fluid overload with dyspnoea, reduced exercise tolerance, and cognitive impairment. Complications arising from RRT and the time spent in performing dialysis can also induce significant stress in patients and their caregivers. Advanced care planning should be discussed and regularly reviewed to explore the patient's expected goals of care. Termination of RRT may need to be considered if new debilitating comorbidities develop (e.g. major stroke, incurable, and terminal malignancies), especially if the original goals of care cannot be attained. Under these circumstances, it would be appropriate to also discuss the Do-Not-Attempt Cardiopulmonary Resuscitation (DNACPR) order (including when the patient is out of hospital) and initiate early referral to renal palliative care (RPC) services.

Renal Palliative Care

While dialysis and renal transplantation are important options of RRT for patients with ESKD, those with advanced age or multiple comorbidities often opt not to undergo dialysis or kidney transplantation. Some ESRD patients who choose conservative management may survive up to 6–9 months, but in general, the lifespan of these patients remains limited and varies from individual to individual. Furthermore, ESKD patients who develop other severe medical comorbidities (e.g. metastatic cancers, massive strokes) may also be considered for withdrawal from dialysis and these patients usually have very short lifespans (often a few days or 1–2 weeks). Owing to the substantial symptom burdens and shortened life expectancies, patients with ESKD who choose conservative management can benefit from good RPC programmes. In this context, RPC achieves symptom control, psychosocial support to the patients and their caregivers, and end-of-life (EOL) care through a multidisciplinary approach and coordination of community care services.

Symptom management in renal palliative care

Owing to the high symptom burden in ESKD patients who opt not to undergo RRT, symptom management constitutes a pivotal component of the RPC programme. These symptoms may be related to the primary kidney disease (e.g. polycystic kidney disease), complications arising from severe renal impairment (e.g. anaemia, fluid overload, pruritus, and renal osteodystrophy), or concomitant medical conditions (e.g. cancer, congestive heart failure).

Fluid overload and dyspnea

Development of oligo-anuria in ESKD patients who opt for RPC will invariably lead to fluid overload and dyspnea. Fluid overload can be managed with high-dose furosemide diuretics in patients who still have a reasonable amount of residual urine. Thiazide diuretics (e.g. metolazone) can sometimes be used as add-on therapy to augment urine output. Opioids can be used to alleviate severe dyspneic symptoms in ESKD patients on conservative management. Psychoeducation can also help optimize fluid management in ESRD patients who opt for RPC.

Pain

About half of the ESKD patients on conservative management experience various forms of pain, with prevalence increasing to 60–70% when approaching EOL and up to 80% being graded as moderate to severe. Degenerative joint diseases and gouty arthritis are common causes of pain in elderly ESRD patients. The World Health Organization (WHO) analgesic ladder is also applicable in ESRD patients who opt for RPC, starting from acetaminophen and nonsteroidal anti-inflammatory drugs (NSAIDs) for mild to moderate pain, then weak opioids (e.g. tramadol), and strong opioids (e.g. fentanyl or methadone). Analgesics should be used with caution in ESKD patients who opt for RPC. For instance, the prescription of NSAIDs can precipitate complete anuria in patients with advanced kidney disease. Dosage modification is required for tramadol in patients with renal impairment. Opioids which are primarily metabolized by the liver (e.g. oxycodone, fentanyl, or methadone) are preferred in patients with advanced renal failure. Adjuvant agents such as pregabalin or gabapentin can be added for control of neuropathic pain, but generally require dosage adjustment in ESRD.

Fatigue

Factors contributing to fatigue in these patients include anaemia, depression, insomnia, malnutrition, and side effects of medications. Correction of anaemia with erythropoietin-stimulating agents and iron therapy can improve fatigue and quality of life in ESKD patients who opt for RPC. Treatment with antidepressants may significantly improve fatigue symptoms related to depression. Moderate exercise may also alleviate fatigue in some patients.

Sleep disturbance

Sleep disturbances have been reported in 40% of ESKD patients who opt for conservative management. Sleep problems may be related to symptoms such as pain but may also be attributed to primary sleep disorders. A thorough history and physical examination should be performed to screen for primary sleep disorders (e.g. obstructive sleep apnoea, restless leg syndrome, and periodic leg movement disorder) and patients should be referred for sleep studies for confirmation. The practice of sleep hygiene is a useful and safe way to manage sleep problems in ESKD patients who opt for RPC. Non-benzodiazepine hypnotics can also be considered in these patients.

Pruritus

Pruritus is one of the most frustrating symptoms in patients with ESKD on conservative management. The pathophysiology of pruritus in ESKD is not well understood although putative mechanisms include hyperparathyroidism, calcium/phosphate disturbances, excessive histamine release from mast cells, chronic skin inflammation, and altered peripheral nerve perceptions. Simple measures such as adequate skin hydration and avoidance of scratching may help alleviate itchiness in ESKD patients. Control of calcium and phosphate can improve pruritus but can be challenging in patients receiving RPC. Topical therapies (e.g. emollients or capsaicin cream) and antihistamines are common treatments for pruritus in ESKD patients, and sertraline or pregabalin can be considered in those who experience persistent itchiness despite antihistamines. Non-pharmacologic options (e.g. UVB therapy) can also be attempted as adjunctive therapies.

Anorexia

Anorexia is another common symptom in ESKD patients who opt for RPC, and can be related to uraemia per se, side effects of concomitant medications, alteration in taste and gastroparesis due to underlying diabetes, and mechanical causes. Antiemetics such as haloperidol can be prescribed in patients whom nausea is a major complaint while promotility agents such as metoclopramide can be used with caution in those with gastroparesis. Appetite stimulants such as megestrol, dronabinol, or prednisone may also be attempted in patients with uraemic anorexia.

Psychosocial aspects and healthcare utilization in renal palliative care

The EOL care in ESKD patients should be individualized with a focus on comfort care and minimization of unnecessary interventions. Evidence from randomized controlled trials has shown that enhanced

psychosocial support in patients who received RPC services can result in an early and significant reduction in caregiver burden and anxiety. Emerging data shows that good RPC service can decrease acute hospital admissions and attendance to the emergency department.

Renal Rehabilitation

Patients with CKD are often physically inactive. This can be due to anaemia, sarcopenia, frailty, malnutrition-wasting, fluid overload, depression, concomitant heart failure, fractures, or cognitive impairment with apathy. Physical inactivity has been shown to increase the morbidity and mortality of ESKD patients requiring dialysis. Renal rehabilitation, which focuses on physical exercises in CKD patients with or without RRT or after renal transplantation has long been studied to combat physical inactivity. However, the importance of renal rehabilitation remained under-recognized among healthcare professionals who provide care to patients with CKD.

Most exercise therapies include treadmill or cycling exercises, but some programmes also focus on the provision of mobilization (e.g. sitting, standing, transfer, and locomotion) and training on activities of daily living (e.g. eating, dressing, grooming, and cognitive training). These exercises often last between 45 to 60 minutes and are provided around twice per week for three months. These programmes are generally well tolerated in CKD patients and have been shown to improve physical and functional capacity, self-reported levels of fitness, anxiety, and depressive symptoms. Renal rehabilitation should adopt a multidisciplinary approach that involves nephrologists, renal nurses, physiotherapists, occupational therapists, and dieticians. Renal physicians should identify reversible factors contributing to inactivity (e.g. depression, anaemia, and fluid overload). The presence of physical inactivity can be detected by simple assessment tools for sarcopenia or frailty (Table 22.1). A brief assessment of cognitive function (e.g. by the Hong Kong version of Montreal Cognitive Assessment) is important to gauge the ability of patients to follow instructions in a renal rehabilitation programme. Patient safety is of utmost importance in renal rehabilitation programmes. Nephrologists should be alerted to contraindications to exercise programmes such as unstable cardiovascular conditions or brittle diabetes. Inputs from cardiologists are warranted in patients with concomitant ischaemic heart disease. Resuscitation facilities should be available and the initial exercise intensity should aim at 60–65% of the predicted maximal heart rate. Blood pressure and pulse should be monitored before and after (e.g. 5–10 minutes) the cessation of exercise. Blood glucose measurement by finger-prick tests should be performed before and after exercise in diabetic patients.

Cognitive impairment is common among patients with CKD. It is believed to be a form of vascular cognitive impairment and executive functions can also be impaired. A recent meta-analysis demonstrated that the pooled prevalence of cognitive impairment in patients receiving peritoneal dialysis (PD) was up to 28.7%. Cognitive impairment is recognized to be a risk factor for PD-related peritonitis, and it remains unclear whether retraining of PD techniques in patients who are cognitively impaired may reduce the risk of peritonitis. In summary, renal rehabilitation in the form of physical activity has been shown to improve the physical performance of patients with CKD. The incorporation of cognitive training in renal rehabilitation program may benefit PD patients with cognitive impairment.

Table 22.1: Simple tools to assess frailty and sarcopenia among patients with chronic kidney disease

The simple 'FRAIL' Questionnaire Screening Tool

Fatigue: Are you fatigued?

Resistance: Are you able to walk up 1 flight of stairs?

Aerobic: Are you able to walk 1 block?

Illnesses: Do you have more than 5 illnesses?

Loss of weight: Have you lost more than 5% of your weight in the past 6 months?

0 = Normal; 1–2: prefrail; 3 or greater: frailty

SARC-F screen for sarcopenia

Strength: How much difficulty do you have in lifting and carrying 10 pounds?

(None = 0; some = 1; a lot or unable = 2)

Assistance in walking: How much difficulty do you have walking across a room?

(None = 0; some = 1; a lot, use aids or unable = 2)

Rise from a chair: How much difficulty do you have transferring from a chair or bed?

(None = 0; some = 1; a lot or unable without help = 2)

Climb stairs: How much difficulty do you have climbing a flight of 10 stairs?

(None = 0; some = 1; a lot or unable = 2)

Falls: How many times have you fallen in the past year?

(None = 0; 1–3 falls = 1; 4 or more falls = 2)

0–3: no sarcopenia; 4–10: sarcopenia

Index